Good Housekeeping

FAMILY GUIDE TO MEDICATIONS

And Dictionary of Prescription Drugs

Good Housekeeping

FAMILY GUIDE
TO
MEDICATIONS

And Dictionary of Prescription Drugs
(Revised edition of <u>Good Housekeeping Guide to Medicines and Drugs</u>)

Judith K. Jones, M.D., Ph.D.

HEARST BOOKS
NEW YORK, NEW YORK

Library of Congress Cataloging in Publication Data

Main entry under title:

Good housekeeping family guide to medications and
   dictionary of prescription drugs.

   Includes index.
   1. Drugs—Popular works. 2. Pharmacology—
Popular works. 3. Medicine, Popular. I. Jones,
Judith K. II. Good housekeeping. III. Title:
Family guide to medications and dictionary of
prescription drugs. IV. Title: Dictionary of pre-
scription drugs.
RM301.15.G66 1980   615.1   80-36867
ISBN 0-87851-041-9

About the Author

Judith K. Jones formerly practiced internal medicine and clinical pharmacology in San Francisco where she was Chief of the Division of Clinical Pharmacology at Presbyterian Hospital, Pacific Medical Center, and Assistant Clinical Professor of Medicine at the University of California in San Francisco. She also served as Adjunct Professor of Physiology and Pharmacology at the University of the Pacific School of Pharmacy, a post she continues to hold in addition to her present duties as Director of the Division of Drug Experience of the Food and Drug Administration in Rockville, Maryland.

The views expressed by the author are her own and should not be interpreted as those of the Food and Drug Administration.

SPECIAL EDITORIAL ADVISERS

Joseph E. Snyder, M.D., Director of Medical Affairs, Columbia-Presbyterian Medical Center, New York City.

Peter Rheinstein, M.D., J.D., M.S., doctor of internal medicine, consultant in legal medicine, and Director, Division of Drug Advertising, Food and Drug Administration.

Acknowledgments

The author wishes to express her continuing gratitude to those who originally helped her with the first edition, including Dr. Donald Shirachi, John Peck, Ed Elzarian, Kenneth Low, Sharon Mauldin, and Martha Lowery. In addition, special gratitude is due to Martin Self for helping the fledgling author prepare the first edition; to Bonnie Mettee for her gracious help on the revisions; to Stephen Jones for assistance in preparing the revised manuscript; and to Wendy Rieder and Diana Childress for their editing.

Contents

Foreword
to the Revised Edition

Since writing the first edition of this book in 1977 (published as the *Good Housekeeping Guide to Medicines and Drugs*), there has been increasing recognition of the need for public understanding of medications, how they should be used and what dangers they may present. The purpose of this revised edition is to make available, in the clearest form possible, the latest information about specific medical problems and the drugs and therapies used to treat them. With this knowledge a patient will be able to develop a useful dialogue with the physician. In almost all cases, however, the actual setting in which a drug is prescribed and taken is highly individual and is influenced by each patient's disease and sensitivities as well as by many other factors, so that only the physician and the patient together can develop the best possible therapeutic regimen.

Preface

As a physician and pharmacologist with a long-time interest in educating other physicians, medical and pharmacy students, paramedical health workers, and my own patients about how medicines act and work, I found the preparation of an everyday guide for the public a welcome, if difficult, task.

Pharmacology, or the study of how drugs affect animals and man has usually been restricted to schools of medical sciences. In the past, few courses on pharmacology could be found at the college level and public interest in the subject was very low. But now several factors appear to have changed all that. Among these have been several highly publicized tragedies resulting from the use of certain drugs: the thalidomide infants, blood clots caused by oral contraceptives (the pill), and, more recently, vaginal tumors in teenage women whose mothers had been given the hormone diethylstilbestrol (DES) to prevent miscarriage during pregnancy.

Another event that brought the word drug into the public consciousness was the association of the hippie movement with psychedelic drugs. Then came the sudden growth in hard street drugs and the abuse of amphetamines, heroin, and "downers," which include barbiturates and other tranquilizers.

In the past decade or so there has also been a rise in the number of prescriptions per capita in the United States of about the same magnitude as the rise in health-care costs. The drugs Valium and Librium, probably the two best-known medicines, appeared in the early 1960s, and within a decade they were in occasional use in an estimated seven to ten percent of U.S. and European homes.

On the heels of these events came the rise of the U.S. consumer movement, which has lately turned its attention to medical care. As a result, a mostly well-intentioned, wide array of books, pamphlets, and manuals has been produced on how to obtain and maintain good health within and without the traditional medical system. Demand has also increased for the inclusion of information leaflets in the packages of all medicines. These package inserts will soon be available for some drugs, and, with the growing interest of drug consumers, it is probable that all patients will one day be provided with the same information received by their physicians. In the long run, this may allow for joint decisions to be made on the proper medication between patients and doctors.

That day is still in the future, but, for now, it is hoped this guide will provide a full, independent reference of drug information that should suit most needs. It is based on the concept that an informed patient can obtain the best medical care in the traditional medical system. By this means the author hopes to encourage a better relationship between patient and physician and thus speed the growth of their dialogue, which will improve the patient's overall medical care and reduce the risk of problems. Such knowledge can be particularly helpful when medication must be taken for long periods or for several illnesses simultaneously and risk/benefit considerations become complex.

The book has been structured to provide general information on drugs: how, why, and when they are used both in general and for treating specific ailments. Also, it very clearly spells out informative details about the most commonly prescribed drugs, including their therapeutic actions, possible adverse effects, and interactions.

The introduction, Part 1, defines drugs and describes where they come from, how they work in the body, and why they cause changes, lead to side effects, and interact with other medication(s), food, and drink. This section explains many words and ideas mentioned later on in the text so it is worth skimming through quickly to familiarize yourself with the subject before getting down to specifics.

Part 2 considers the causes and treatments of various health problems such as high blood pressure, diabetes, and asthma. It explains why certain drugs are used and how they cure or relieve the symptoms of a disease, and why a doctor will often change one specific drug for a different but probably related one. This section will help you to understand the broader view of treatment and provide an insight into how your doctor is thinking about the medication he is prescribing for you.

Part 3 is an alphabetical listing of the 200 most frequently prescribed drugs, some other commonly used medications, and several newly introduced drugs. Medicines are listed in alphabetical order, by either their trade (brand) name or generic name, whichever is most common. Each drug description includes other brand names for the drug, as well as its actions, side effects, interactions, and any precautions to be taken when using it. Each drug is also cross-referenced to the section in Part 2 that discusses the general class of medication to which it belongs. For example, if you want to look up *digoxin,* the drug will be found under its generic name in Part 3; below the main heading are listed its trade names (Lanoxin and SK-Digoxin) and following is a discussion of the drug's action, dosage, adverse effects, and interactions, as well as a reference to the section on *Heart failure,* for which the drug is prescribed.

Other valuable information for the consumer is provided in two handy tables at the back of the book. The first is a summary of drugs by use, drug group, and generic and trade names. In a graphic way it points out a number of important factors about drugs. First, it shows that many similar drugs are used to treat the same condition. Not only may several products be sold under the same generic name, but drugs grouped in the same category generally have similar effects. By checking this list, a patient taking more than one medication can make sure none is a duplication. Too often physicians consulted for unrelated problems will prescribe similar medications with different names. This could lead to adverse effects that could be prevented if a patient knows enough to ask his physician the right questions.

In addition, the table provides a quick way of finding generic and trade names for the major drugs, and it indicates those medications that are combination drugs, so the reader can then turn back to the alphabetical listing in Part 3 to find out what the constituents of such drugs are. It is also interesting to note from this list that certain drugs with multiple effects may be used as treatment for more than one kind of medical problem.

The second table represents a careful selection of the most common and critical drug interactions that may cause serious health problems, those that really deserve public attention. It presents the major drugs, such as tranquilizers and blood thinners, that are known to interact with other drugs, food, or drink; those things with which they interact; and the effects on the body of such interactions.

Concluding the book is an index that lists all the drugs mentioned by both their generic and trade names and also refers to them under the common symptoms or disorders for which they are prescribed. Entries for trade-name drugs are followed by the generic name (if it is a single drug) in parentheses. Page references in heavy type indicate where the subject is discussed most thoroughly.

Since there are thousands of medicines available in the United States, it was impossible to describe every prescription drug in detail within the confines of this volume, but many drugs are mentioned in Part 2 that are not listed in Part 3. It has already been noted that a medication usually behaves similarly to other drugs with which it is grouped, so the same general description often applies for all. However, you should consult a recognized reference book (available at most libraries) for more specific information on any drug that is not fully discussed here.

It is hoped that this guide will prove to be as valuable a source of information about specific drugs as it is about the general diseases they are meant to treat, and that it will promote better health by encouraging informed dialogue between patient and physician.

JUDITH K. JONES, M.D., Ph.D.
Rockville, Maryland

Basic Information about Drugs

Definition, Origins and Regulations

The world of drugs and medicines today is considerably different from what it was 50 or 100 years ago. In the past, medicines were usually mixtures of many plant and mineral substances, prescribed in Latin by physicians and then deciphered and made up by pharmacists into elixirs, powders, or ointments that were often strange-smelling and tasting. Some of these unusual concoctions contained ingredients still used in drugs today but many of the old medicines appear to have been effective as much through patients' expectations of good results as from anything else. We now call this phenomenon a *placebo effect,* from the proven capacity of patients to benefit even from a harmless unmedicated preparation—a placebo—provided they believe it is a medicine that will do them good.

Modern drugs and their regulation Today we are in an entirely different era of drugs and medicines. Rarely are prescriptions written in Latin and rarely does the pharmacist himself prepare the mixtures, except for some elixirs. Instead, most medicines are manufactured in large quantities in the form of tablets, capsules, creams, suppositories, and liquids (such as cough syrups or insulin) whose exact contents are carefully measured and standardized. Production, distribution, and availability of each type of drug are now controlled by legislation that chiefly dates from the first half of this century, although new laws have been passed as recently as 1962.

Before a drug can be introduced onto the market, it has to meet stringent standards of safety and effectiveness. To determine whether it meets these requirements, it is first tested in many animals, and later in human volunteers and in persons with specific diseases.

These requirements for safety and effectiveness (laid down by the Food and Drug Administration) have long been the subject of controversy. On the one hand, there is the real fear that another tragedy like the one produced by thalidomide (the sedative/sleeping pill that produced crippling birth defects in many children abroad) will occur if every drug is not carefully tested. On the other hand, such testing takes much time and delays the introduction of many promising drugs. This has led to a frequently expressed fear that the American public is being deprived of good, useful drugs that are available in many other countries, because the Food and Drug Administration's requirements are too strict. There is no simple solution to this controversy.

Under a "grandfather clause" in the regulations, aspirin and other drugs which were in use before the stricter laws governing the testing of drugs were passed, were not required to be tested as stringently owing to their presumed safety as demonstrated by many years of use.

Definitions of drugs and medicines Drugs and medicines can be defined in terms of several characteristics—their use, their origins, and their actions, both helpful and harmful. In very general terms, a drug or medicine is any substance or mixture of substances that is taken into the body to improve one's physical or mental condition.

Sources of drugs Drugs and medicines come from many different sources. In ancient times, medicinal preparations were made from extracts of plants, from certain animal materials, and occasionally from mineral sources. In fact, many of our modern drugs are still derived from plants. For example, quinine, used for muscle cramps, and quinidine, used to control heart rhythm, both come from the bark of the cinchona tree. Likewise, animal materials are still the major sources of certain drugs. Thyroid hormone, for instance, is obtained from animal thyroid glands, and insulin from animal pancreases. Minerals such as calcium and iron supplements still come from natural mineral sources. And, since it was discovered that the simple bread mold produced the invaluable antibiotic penicillin, living fungi have been important sources of drugs—especially of antibiotics and the drugs used in cancer therapy. Finally, some drugs such as Valium and Librium are synthesized from organic chemicals—a major source of modern medicines.

Drugs versus poisons By definition, drugs are substances which are used to produce benefit, and poisons are substances which can, either intentionally or accidentally, cause harm. But any substance can, in fact, be either beneficial or poisonous depending on the dose taken, the intent of the individual taking it, and sometimes the presence or absence of disease in the person taking it.

For example, any drug taken in excessive amounts may be likely to cause adverse effects or poisoning. Conversely, some traditional poisons, such as curare, the poison used by South American Indians on their arrows, is a very useful muscle-relaxant drug in the controlled setting of a surgical operation. From another viewpoint, antibiotics often act as a "poison" to bacteria, but do not affect the patient. Similarly, many cancer drugs act as "poisons" to the tumor, and may also be somewhat toxic or "poisonous" to other organs, but are used because their overall benefit to a cancer patient is greater than the risk they entail.

Drug Actions and Side Effects

Drugs can also be frequently defined or classified according to their actions. For example, a chemical that relieves pain, such as aspirin, is often classified as a pain reliever (analgesic), even though it may be equally effective as an anti-in-

Figure 1.

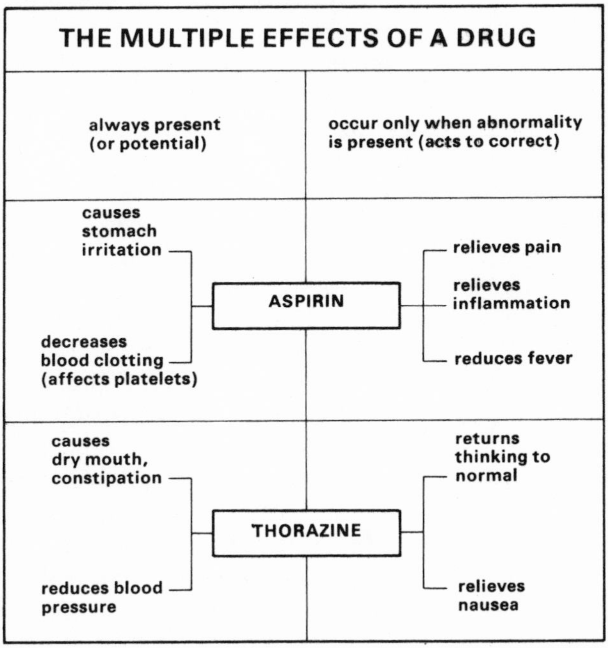

THE MULTIPLE EFFECTS OF A DRUG

always present (or potential)	occur only when abnormality is present (acts to correct)
causes stomach irritation —	— relieves pain
ASPIRIN	— relieves inflammation
decreases blood clotting — (affects platelets)	— reduces fever
causes dry mouth, constipation —	— returns thinking to normal
THORAZINE	
reduces blood — pressure	— relieves nausea

flammatory drug (to relieve inflammation) and as an anticoagulant (to prevent clotting). These actions may be seen as desirable effects in some cases (the relief of pain) and as "side effects" in other instances, as when aspirin's anticoagulant effect is not desired. We have to consider drugs and medicines both from the point of view of their intended actions and uses and from the point of view of their other, sometimes undesirable, actions or adverse effects.

How drugs act and interact Drugs, if taken internally, can act on many organs, sometimes altering their function. For example, certain drugs can adversely effect the functions of the kidney. Equally important, if two or more drugs are taken, there is sometimes a possibility of the two drugs interacting with each other. This can result in a *drug interaction*—an increased, a decreased, or sometimes a wholly new effect from either or both of the drugs. For example, when the anticoagulant drug Coumadin interacts with vitamin K in the liver, the two drugs cancel each other out. An interaction of this kind can be very significant for the health of the patient, and important drug interactions are noted at the end of each drug entry in Part 3.

The journey of a drug in the body When a drug is swallowed, where does it go? It is useful to consider the journey of a drug through the body since this journey often determines how long and how strongly the drug acts. Once the drug is swallowed, it goes to the stomach, which often contains food, and almost always contains strong hydrochloric acid. Many drugs will begin to dissolve here, even before they pass along into the intestines and bowel. As they dissolve, they pass through the walls of the stomach, intestine, and bowel into the blood vessels supplying those organs. They are then transported in the bloodstream directly to the liver. Sometimes the presence of food or diarrhea can interfere temporarily with their absorption into the blood.

The liver acts as a type of processing "roundhouse" for all foods and chemicals, altering them in such a way that they can be either used or eliminated from the body. Through the long history of evolution, men and animals have developed very sophisticated livers that can process the many complex chemicals present in plants and other foodstuffs. Some of the chemicals in the things we eat are toxic, and these the liver converts, by a process called *metabolism,* to less toxic sub-

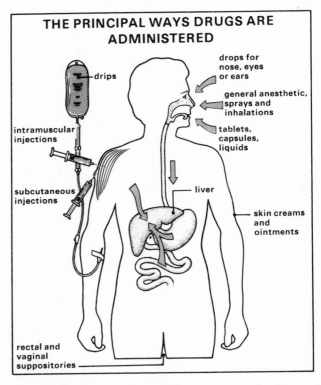

THE PRINCIPAL WAYS DRUGS ARE ADMINISTERED

drips

intramuscular injections

subcutaneous injections

rectal and vaginal suppositories

drops for nose, eyes or ears

general anesthetic, sprays and inhalations

tablets, capsules, liquids

liver

skin creams and ointments

Figure 2. *The liver is a great chemical factory equipped with special enzymes capable of transforming the chemical structure of almost any substance they encounter. Most drugs active in the body dissolve in fat, but not in water or urine. The liver changes such drugs into water-soluble substances by combining them with another chemical so they can be excreted by the kidneys. Apart from metabolizing drugs, the liver also manufactures "carrier" proteins that bind to drug molecules and circulate them around the body.*

stances which can be eliminated or used. Most drugs arriving at the liver are partly metabolized at this "first stop." Sometimes the metabolized drug is more, sometimes less, active than the original drug. Obviously, if the patient has a liver disease, for example, hepatitis, the liver's metabolic function may be affected. This is why people with liver disease sometimes require lower doses of the drugs they take.

In the liver the drug can "hop onto" a carrier protein which will carry it around the bloodstream to the various organs, although some drugs will travel freely in the bloodstream to all organs of the body. Once it reaches an organ it can attach to a protein molecule called a *receptor,* and at this point the action of the drug is seen. At the end of its journey,

19

the drug is eliminated, usually via the bloodstream to the kidney, where it is excreted in the urine. A good example of this journey can be seen if a person takes a multi-vitamin pill containing riboflavin. The vitamin will soon appear in the urine, turning it a yellowish-green.

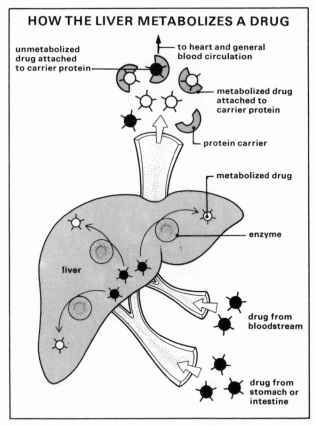

Figure 3. *Drug action occurs where drug molecules bind to receptors on a cell membrane (upper illustration). Many drugs are transported around the body bound to carrier proteins, but it is only the free or unbound drug molecules that are active at the cell receptors. The lower drawing depicts the two main routes by which drugs are excreted from the body after a period in the circulation. Most drugs are extracted from the blood by the kidneys and excreted in the urine, but the liver secretes some drugs into the bile for excretion in the feces.*

Occasionally drugs are also eliminated into the bile and therefore pass into the bowel. Obviously, if there is kidney failure, the drug cannot leave the body; patients with this problem are therefore given smaller doses or told to wait for

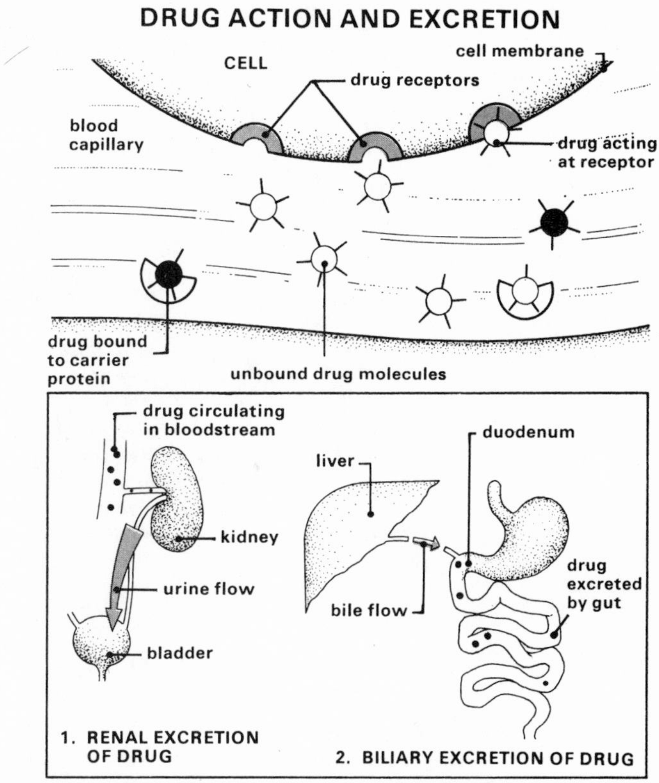

DRUG ACTION AND EXCRETION

Figure 4. *Most drugs are excreted from the body in urine, but a patient who has kidney failure produces very little urine and needs much more time than a normal person to excrete a dose of drug from his bloodstream, as shown above.*

longer intervals between doses of drugs to prevent large amounts of the drug accumulating in the body.

When drugs are given by other methods—for example, intravenously, by injection, or in the form of suppositories—they enter the bloodstream directly and can go to the liver and from there to the rest of the body. Some drugs, like creams and ointments, are for direct use on the skin or in the eye. These drugs do not usually enter the bloodstream, but they may if used in large amounts.

Proper Dosages and How They Vary

What determines how often a drug must be taken? In earlier years it was generally felt that any drug was usually best taken in divided doses, usually three or four times a day—a

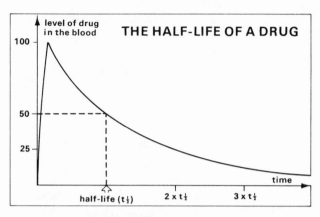

Figure 5. *Drugs can be taken orally, injected directly into the bloodstream, breathed into the lungs, introduced as suppositories, or applied locally as drops, sprays, ointments, or creams. Those that enter the bloodstream (either directly by injection or indirectly by absorption) are transported to the liver where they are metabolized (see Figure 2).*

view based, in many cases, on the fact that the effect of the drug appeared to wear off in six to eight hours. More recently, however, two factors have changed this approach.

First, a great deal of work has been directed to measuring the amount of the drug in the blood at various times after its administration. This has resulted in much closer scrutiny of drug effects and their length of action. It has also allowed a calculation of the drug's *half-life*. The half-life of a drug is the length of time it takes for the body to eliminate half the amount of the drug present in the body. If a drug is given at intervals corresponding with its half-life, relatively constant amounts of the drug will remain in the body. The major discovery of these studies was that many drugs that had been frequently prescribed in three or four times daily doses, such as Dilantin, allopurinol, and Elavil, have half-lives of longer than 24 hours and therefore could be taken only once daily and have a similar effect.

This development has contributed greatly to a general trend, that of trying to make it easier for patients to follow the drug regimen prescribed by their physicians. It was found that patients who were required to take many pills a day tended either to forget or simply to refuse. This difficulty, defined as a problem in *compliance* (adherence to a prescribed regimen), can clearly have serious implications for the health of patients. Such patients would obviously benefit from drug

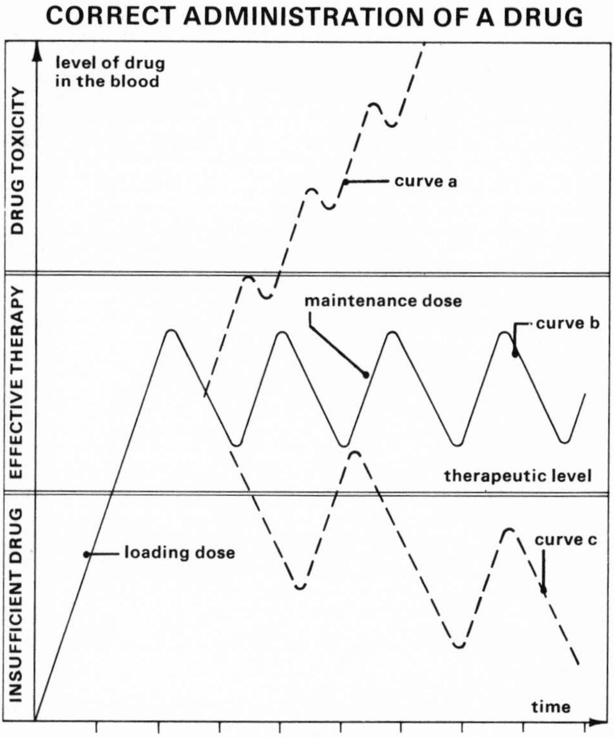

CORRECT ADMINISTRATION OF A DRUG

Figure 6. *The half-life (t½) is the time taken to clear one-half the quantity of a drug from the body; this determines how frequently the drug should be administered. The half-life is not always the same for a particular drug but varies from person to person. However, most drugs have half-lives of between 8 and 24 hours.*

regimens that required less frequent doses of the medicines they need. As interest in the problem of patients' compliance has increased, so has the search for drugs and drug dose forms which have longer actions and half-lives. This quest has already begun and is helping to improve therapy.

What determines dose? The dose of a particular drug is usually standardized, although in fact there are often variable responses to the same amount of a drug. Doses of different drugs vary greatly—from grams, as in many antibiotics, to millionths of a gram, as in the synthetic thyroid preparations. The best dose of any drug is usually established by extensive testing—first on animals and then on humans.

It is important to note that the dose of any two drugs, even those with similar actions, should not necessarily be

23

compared as to size or magnitude of effect. For example, 5 mg (5 milligrams, or thousandths of a gram) of Valium is often just as strong and effective a sedative as 100 mg of phenobarbital. The dose of any particular drug is the amount of that particular drug found to be effective.

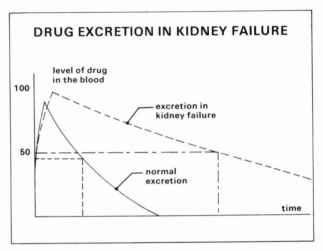

Figure 7. *The effect of most drugs depends on their concentration in the bloodstream. In order to establish the correct level of a drug in the blood—the therapeutic level—one large loading dose is given initially followed by smaller maintenance doses. Curve (a) demonstrates that if maintenance doses are given too frequently, an excess of the drug builds up, leading to toxic effects. Curve (b) shows the ideal result where the amount of drug in the bloodstream remains at the therapeutic level because the maintenance doses are properly spaced. Curve (c) shows that if the maintenance doses are not given often enough, the amount of the drug in the bloodstream soon falls, thereby ceasing to be effective.*

Drugs in children The prescribing of medicine for children, and especially for infants, presents certain problems because their reactions to drugs tend to differ from those of adults. For example, the liver, which metabolizes drugs in an adult body, may not be completely developed in an infant, and so cannot process drugs properly. In some cases this can lead to poisoning. Drugs can also have an opposite effect on children from the effect they have on adults. A classic example is the drug Ritalin, which is used to calm hyperactive children, while in adults it produces hyperactivity. These factors, plus the fact that the amount of drug needed to produce an effect in a child is much smaller, make the use of medicines in children a specialized subject. *Although some of the drugs pre-scribed in this book are also used to treat children, the doses for children are generally much lower than described here and are not specifically noted.*

Drugs in pregnant women Since the thalidomide tragedy, there has been a much greater and more widespread aware-ness of the potential danger of drugs taken during preg-nancy, especially during the first eight to twelve weeks of pregnancy, when the development of vital fetal structures is taking place and can easily be adversely affected. Thalido-mide, which was often prescribed as a sedative/sleeping pill during this critical period, produced deformities in the de-velopment of the arms and legs of unborn infants.

Unfortunately, partly because of the time-lag between the critical developmental period early in the pregnancy—of-ten before pregnancy is discovered or even strongly sus-pected—and the birth of the infant, it has been difficult to identify the factors or drugs which cause developmental problems in the fetus. Collecting exact information on the re-lationship between drugs and malformations also presents problems of various kinds. Animal studies, for example, do not necessarily provide results which correspond exactly with what occurs in humans. Certain drugs can affect fetal devel-opment at only one critical time during pregnancy, but are otherwise not harmful. Other drugs are thought to be harm-ful throughout the pregnancy or for longer periods of time. For example, the antibiotic tetracycline can affect bone and tooth development and thus cannot be used in pregnancy at all and is contraindicated during most of childhood for the same reason. (Interestingly enough, tetracycline appears to cause ill-effects in the mother as well as in her unborn child.)

Excessive consumption of alcohol and cigarettes by the pregnant woman may also affect the developmental process in the fetus at several stages. But the adverse effects pro-duced by alcohol and cigarettes do not occur in every case! In fact, even a drug which is known to cause specific effects may cause those effects only in five to twenty percent of cases, or even less. This may be because of the dose, the timing, or other unknown factors, and it makes the precise relationship between cause and effect very difficult to establish.

Still another problem is that the harmful effect of a drug taken during pregnancy may not be easily discovered for some period of time. This would be the case, for example,

25

with adverse effects on the intelligence or neurological development of the baby. A classic example of this type is the DES or diethylstilbestrol problem. For a period of time, beginning in the mid-1940s, women who were in danger of miscarrying were given the hormone diethylstilbestrol to prevent the loss of the baby. Some 13 to 16 years later a small percentage of the female children born to these mothers had developed cancer of the vagina—a form of cancer that previously was very rare. Only very careful detective work on the part of pathologists who became suspicious about the increased rate of this rare cancer revealed the connection with DES. Not surprisingly, their discovery has increased the concern about drugs in pregnancy to an even greater extent. The state of knowledge about this subject will continue to be limited since in many cases adequate testing cannot be carried out. However, the general rule of obstetricians is that pregnant women should avoid most drugs during pregnancy, except vitamins, iron, and a few other drugs which may be essential to the mother's health, such as thyroid hormone or insulin. However, the use of *any* drug during pregnancy is usually carefully supervised because of concern about the dangers.

The major problem still lies, not with women who are aware of their pregnancy and are therefore more cautious, but with potentially pregnant women who are taking drugs such as tetracycline, Valium, or Librium, which are now suspected of causing some birth defects in a small number of cases. Clearly, any woman of childbearing age who is having sexual relations and is liable to become pregnant must exercise great caution where drugs and medicines of all kinds are concerned.

Drugs in the elderly The third group of people who may have special responses to drugs is the elderly. Just who belongs in this classification is a moot point, since physiological aging does not necessarily correspond to age in years. Nonetheless, when physiological aging becomes apparent, it is often associated with changes in response to some drugs. One factor that contributes to this change is the gradual decline in the efficiency of the kidney in eliminating wastes (and therefore drugs). This is one of the reasons for the need for elderly people to use lower doses of some drugs. Since the decline in kidney function does not take place at the same rate in everyone, individual dosage adjustment may often be called for.

The use by elderly people of various sedative and tranquilizing drugs, such as chloral hydrate, Seconal, Valium, Librium, and Dalmane, can be problematic for two reasons. First, as noted above, smaller doses may be needed, especially if regular use is planned, since the drug may accumulate and cause drowsiness. Second, some elderly people may experience excitation rather than sedation in response to some of these drugs, as is also often the case with children. The reason for this is not known, but it can cause confusion since often the response is to give more sedative!

Genetic factors Genetic differences between people can also influence a drug's effect. For example, some individuals are more sensitive than others to small doses of the tricyclic antidepressant drugs, such as Elavil, Tofranil, and Sinequan. Studies of those drugs have shown that equal doses given to several people would result in different levels of drug in their blood. However, identical twins would have very similar blood levels. This suggests that at least some of the differences in blood levels are due to genetic factors affecting the body's ability to deal with the drug. The genetic causes of variable drug effects are only just beginning to be studied and defined at present, but in the future they may play an important part in determining the exact drug dose administered to each individual. Some individuals have genetic traits which can make common drugs harmful, though fortunately this is a relatively rare phenomenon. People with the rare metabolic disease porphyria, for example, cannot take phenobarbital and certain related drugs because of the severe adverse reactions these drugs produce in them. Likewise, approximately 13% of the black population and a certain percentage of persons of Mediterranean origin have a deficiency of a certain enzyme in their red blood cells which makes them particularly susceptible to drugs used to treat malaria (primaquine), some sulfa drugs, and the drugs Furadantin and Macrodantin used to treat bladder and kidney infections. When any of these drugs are taken by persons with this enzyme deficiency, their blood cells begin to break down and they may develop fever and generalized discomfort. Fortunately, this enzyme deficiency can be detected by a simple blood test and the problematic drugs avoided. In many other cases, the genetic differences which cause these special effects cannot be anticipated. Further research may increase the chances of doing so in the near future.

Placebo effects Another factor that strongly influences the way in which a drug will affect someone is the so-called *placebo effect*. In Latin, the word placebo means "I will please." In medical terminology, the word refers to a pill or other treatment that by itself has no chemical activity or drug-like effects on the body. Frequently it is simply a pill made of sugar or lactose. However, when a placebo is given, it may, in fact, bring about certain changes in a patient's condition simply because the patient, or the doctor, or both, expect it to cause a change. These changes are called placebo effects. Placebos are most often used in studies of drugs to ascertain the effects of a real drug. This is very important since many people have marked responses to placebos. For example, most mild, pain-relieving drugs are tested against a placebo. Two groups of patients are tested in a double-blind test where neither the patients nor the doctor knows which is the real drug, one group receiving the drug under review and the other a placebo. Frequently 20–40% of people receiving the placebo will experience pain relief! Further, if the study is geared to checking for side effects, it is frequently found that people may experience nausea, vomiting, itching of the skin, or even rashes and other effects after taking the placebo. This is why the placebo effects of taking a drug must be set against the final result of a drug test to determine the actual pharmacologic effect of the drug.

Why do people experience effects from a placebo? The answer must lie in the *expectations* both of the patient *and* of the therapist. For example, if a person has a headache and takes a pill which he expects will relieve his headache, he frequently will experience relief, even if the pill is completely inactive (a placebo). It appears that if this expectation of relief is enhanced by the enthusiastic expectations of the prescribing doctor, the pill is even more likely to produce relief.

The placebo effect tends to be particularly noticeable in connection with drugs used for pain, sedation, tranquilization, or other consciously experienced sensations. It is very much less noticeable when the anticipated effect is not directly perceived, as in the case of antibiotics or heart medication.

Sometimes placebo drugs are administered when the physican feels that relief, often of mild anxiety, may be obtained as readily by the placebo effect as by an active, possibly harmful, drug. This is often done to protect the patient against chronic use of sedatives or pain relievers, and not just to fool him.

Effects of disease on drug actions The effect of any given drug also varies in the presence of disease. For example, if a person has a fever, either aspirin or Tylenol will tend to bring the temperature back down to normal, but these drugs will not significantly lower body temperature that is already normal. In a person suffering from a disordered perception of reality, as in schizophrenia, the use of phenothiazine drugs such as Thorazine will tend to normalize the thinking process, but the same drug will not markedly affect the thinking of a person in touch with reality. Other diseases simply change the way a drug is absorbed, metabolized, or excreted. Thus, a person with severe diarrhea might not absorb much of a drug taken orally. A person with kidney failure may be unable to eliminate certain drugs, so they must be used in lower doses or less frequently lest they build up in his system.

Drug Reactions

There is considerable public and medical concern over side effects and adverse reactions to drugs. It is contended by some that drug reactions are a significant cause of hospitalization and of problems during hospitalization. Various frightening statistics have been cited in the popular press. However, some of these figures represent general conclusions drawn from small studies; whether these are really accurate is questionable. One recent large study of drug reactions in eight hospitals over a period of several years indicated that the rate of adverse reactions was not as high as previously thought. The controversy nevertheless continues.

Several points about drug reactions should be borne in mind when considering the problem:

1. Any drug is likely to have effects on many parts of the body. Some of these effects are desired, some are of little consequence, and some are not desired and are usually termed side or adverse effects. A side effect in one setting, such as the tendency of aspirin to inhibit blood clotting when it is used for arthritis, may be the desired effect when it is used in another setting, for example, to prevent stroke.

2. Unwanted reactions to drugs fall into two main categories:

   a) First are the known side effects of the drug, which can be anticipated and either accepted, prevented, or treated. For example, the potassium loss that is a side effect of taking a strong diuretic ("water pill") such as Lasix, can be prevented by adding potassium to the diet.

   b) Side effects of the second type are not so predictable, since they occur in only a small percentage of people receiving the drug. They can be true allergic reactions, such as the rashes some people develop in response to penicillin, or they can be the so-called "idiosyncratic" reactions, which are probably not allergic in nature but are rather related to the distinct genetic makeup of individuals and the way their particular bodies handle the drug. This latter type of reaction is much more difficult to anticipate or predict, since it may occur in only one out of 10,000 or 100,000 persons and may not be discovered before the drug is released for use. In contrast to the first category of reactions, these unwanted reactions cannot necessarily be prevented, but their possible occurrence is usually noted and considered in the risk/benefit analysis which accompanies the prescribing of any drug.

3. Very few drugs are free of unwanted side effects. Fewer still are free of the possibility of unpredictable allergic or idiosyncratic reactions. Some drugs have a greater potential for producing side effects than others. Thus, the prescribing of the drug by a physician is usually the result of a careful calculation of the benefits to the patient (i.e., relief of symptoms or cure of the disease) versus the risks and cost to the patient. The seriousness of the disease and the seriousness and frequency of the side effects are very important factors in this consideration; it is never a simple calculation. For example, in the treatment of arthritis, the benefits of higher-dose aspirin (effective relief of pain and inflammation at a relatively low cost) must be weighed against its disadvantages and risks (frequent dosing, possible hearing disturbances, gastric upset, bleeding or ulceration). A more difficult calculation is

called for with the anti-cancer drugs: in this case, the possibility of prolonging life must be weighed against their often very serious side effects, the need they entail for frequent and costly medical supervision, and, sometimes, their very high cost.

Clearly, the decision as to whether the benefits of taking a drug outweigh the risks involved can be very difficult, and the problem is often complicated by a lack of sufficient information about the likelihood of side effects.

4. Certain conditions seem to increase the likelihood of drug reactions. The longer a drug is taken, for example, the more likely it is to cause side effects. Likewise, a higher dose of the drug may cause more side effects than a lower dose. A person who has already had allergic reactions (rashes, swelling of various areas of the body, or anaphylactic shock and wheezing) to one or more drugs is more likely to have an allergic reaction to another drug, particularly if it is chemically related to the drugs that have produced allergic reactions in the past. It is important to note, however, that in most cases nausea or vomiting after taking a drug (as for example, after taking codeine, Demerol, or morphine) seldom represents a true allergic reaction, but rather an increased sensitivity to one of the known and expected effects of the drug. Further, alcohol can interact with many drugs to produce toxic effects.

5. The greater number of drugs a person takes, the more likely he is to experience side effects, not only because the individual effects of multiple drugs add up, but also because with several drugs there is a greatly increased possibility of drug interactions.

Pinning down what is, and what is not, a genuine reaction to any one drug is not always easy. Just because a symptom occurs after taking a drug does not necessarily mean the drug caused that symptom. It may, for example, represent a placebo side effect or a totally separate problem. On the other hand, it sometimes happens that a side effect, such as headache or nausea, is ascribed to the underlying disease, while the drug as a cause is missed. In such cases, a simple discussion with a physician about whether a particular sign or symptom could be caused by a drug might clarify the situation early on and save valuable time and discomfort for the patient.

Indeed, when a side effect is suspected, the doctor should always be consulted. In some cases the drug will be stopped, not only to prevent further reaction, but also as a test to see if the effect goes away. In other cases, the side effect may be treated directly, as when antacids are given during treatment with aspirin or cortisone or prednisone to prevent the gastric irritation that is so often a side effect of these drugs.

Avoiding drug reactions In general, it is a good rule for each individual not only to know what drugs he or she is taking, and to know as much about them as possible, but also to carry a list of those drugs being taken currently and any that have caused reactions in the past. In our highly mobile society, visits to unfamiliar clinics, doctors, or emergency rooms are a frequent occurrence, and specific information about a patient's drug history before treatment is given is often very helpful. A simple drug information card can be made from a three by five card and carried in a prominent place in your wallet. An alternative plan is to use a metal bracelet or necklace that carries this information. Your physician can often help in providing the relevant information.

Generic versus Brand-name Prescriptions

Many drugs today are fairly expensive. Some people, in fact, have to pay a dollar or more a day for their drugs, and when these drugs must be taken over a period of months or years, the daily expense can add up to a heavy financial burden.

What determines the cost of a drug? In general, the cost of a drug to the patient is based on the costs of research and development, manufacture, advertising, packaging, shipping, and pharmacy handling. But the price of an individual drug may not be related to any of these elements. An additional factor is whether the drug is a *generic* product or a *brand-name* preparation.

Most drugs begin life as a basic chemical substance which is produced by several manufacturers. These drugs, in tablets, capsules, ointments, and other forms, are sold directly to pharmacists or hospitals under generally accepted chemical names—the generic names. Alternatively, the manufacturers may apply trade or brand names to their products to differentiate them from the same products manufactured by other companies. Thus tetracycline may be sold by its generic name, tetracycline hydrochloride, or by one of its trade names, such as Achromycin. Some manufacturers sell only generic products, both to pharmacists and to other companies, which apply their own brand names. Other drug manufacturers sell their products only under trade names, although the same drugs may be available by generic names from another manufacturer.

Frequently, drugs are developed by one company and then produced and manufactured by that company under a drug patent giving it exclusive rights to make and market the drug for 17 years. Once the 17 years have elapsed, the particular company holding the patent no longer has exclusive rights to the drug, so it may be produced and manufactured under its generic name as well as under new trade names. For example, because the patent of Librium has expired it is now available under its generic name, chlordiazepoxide. In some cases, drugs sold under their generic names are also sold by three or more companies under different trade names. Thus, tetracycline hydrochloride is available under that generic name *or* as Achromycin, Robitet, SK-Tetracycline, and Retet. Ampicillin (generic name) is available under that name as well as under the brand names Supen, Amcill, Omnipen, Polycillin, Pensyn, Pen A, Penbritin, and Principen. This multiplicity of brand names for one generic drug creates confusion both for the prescribing doctor and for his patient, but the drug industry argues that it allows for healthy competition on the drug market. It is doubtful, therefore, that the situation will change, although the trend seems to be toward prescribing more by generic name than by brand name.

A company will usually spend some money promoting its brand-name product and this cost is usually added on to the basic cost of the drug. This means that, in general, a trade-name drug is more expensive—sometimes by several times—than its generic equivalent. For this reason, many consumer groups have advocated that generic drugs be used in preference to brand-name drugs. Several factors, however, complicate this straightforward approach. First, many companies with brand-name products argue that their drugs are more carefully tested and regulated than generic equivalents produced by other companies. Indeed, it has been found that several products containing the same generic drug may be absorbed by the body at very different rates, so that one may produce definite effects and another none at all. This has raised the issue of *bio-availability*—how much of the drug can be absorbed by the body and thus produce an effect—and has led to stricter requirements by the Food and Drug Administration for each manufacturer to prove that its drug is as bio-available as equivalent drugs.

In the long run, the drug companies' argument that their brand-name products represent better quality-control may tend to counteract the trend toward generic prescribing. Many drug companies have also implied that their long-standing reputation as manufacturers of quality drugs is good reason for continuing to choose their products. Unfortunately, this generalization about quality may not apply, as almost every drug company has been subject to drug recalls and manufacturing problems at some point in its history.

Adding to the confusion, many states have passed "generic substitution" laws. These regulations allow a pharmacist to substitute one brand of a generic drug for another if he deems this necessary for reason of better quality, lower price, or stock supply. Thus, a prescription for erythromycin tablets in 250 mg strength might be filled with large, red, round tablets (Ilotycin), large, blue-green tablets (Robimycin), or large, peach-colored tablets (E-Mycin), or a variety of other products. Any would contain the prescribed amount of erythromycin and the effect would in all probability be the same. If the physician simply wrote the brand name on the prescription, any equivalent erythromycin could be substituted for it at the pharmacist's discretion. If, however, the physician also wrote "no substitution" on the prescription, the pharmacist would be required to fill the prescription with the particular brand of erythromycin specified by the physician, even if it cost considerably more. Sometimes a physician has a very definite reason for prescribing a brand-name product (as, for example, to avoid confusion in the case of a patient taking several drugs) and sometimes not. It is often worth discussing the matter with your physician, because when there is no special reason for prescribing a brand-name drug, a switch to a generic prescription may save money.

The cost of a drug, whether it is a generic or a brand-name product, can vary considerably depending on several factors. Prescriptions for large numbers of pills or capsules are usually relatively less expensive, partly because medicines packaged in larger lots can be dispensed more easily and partly because each prescription includes a handling fee for the pharmacist, so that the more prescriptions needed by an individual patient, the more handling fees he must pay. Although smaller, private pharmacies tend to have somewhat higher prescription prices than larger chain store operations, this is by no means always the case. Private pharmacies may also offer certain convenient extra services such as home delivery, drug profiles, counseling on the effects of the drugs, and so forth. Many states require pharmacies to post their drug prices so that people who take drugs over long periods of time (as do people with high blood pressure) may check prices at various sources and even report their findings back to their physician if they wish.

Another factor influencing the cost of prescriptions affects only those people on health plans such as Medicaid and Medi-Cal that grant allowances for prescriptions, provided they are on an approved drug list. If they are not on this list, the patients must either pay for the prescriptions themselves or justify the use of those particular drugs before qualifying for their allowance. Since a limited number of allowances is available, the size of individual precriptions is usually larger, creating problems where drug abuse is a possibility.

How, then, does one get the best-quality drug at the most reasonable cost? First, it is helpful to indicate to the doctor a preference for a generic-named drug in maximum quantity (100 to 200 pills is customary) if it must be used for long periods. This recommendation is based on the generally valid assumption that in most cases generic drugs *are* equivalent and *are* less expensive than their brand-name counterparts. The doctor may have objections—both to prescribing a generic equivalent and to prescribing in quantity—but these questions should generate a useful dialogue. There are, of course, good reasons for small prescriptions of sedatives and narcotics, for example.

Second, in addition to comparing prices at various pharmacies, it is wise to consider the quality of the service those pharmacies provide. A good pharmacist, whose thorough training equips him to provide useful information about differences between drugs and advice about over-the-counter products, may well be worth some extra charge.

This book does not give the price of any drug, but each listing includes both the generic name and one or more trade names. In Part 3. "An Alphabetical Guide to Over 200 of the Most Frequently Prescribed Drugs," drugs that are most frequently prescribed by their generic name (such as ampicillin) are listed under that name with the trade names following. Other drugs are listed by their trade names, but the generic name is also given. For identification, the trade names are always capitalized; the generic names are not, except in the individual listings in Part 3.

Part 2

Medications for Specific Disorders

Pain and/or Inflammation

Pain is often our first indication that something is wrong, but sometimes treating the pain is all the therapy that is needed—and in some types of disease this is still the only therapy possible. In general, there are three types of pain and three corresponding categories of drugs to treat them, though the categories overlap somewhat:

1. Moderate to severe pain, for which narcotic drugs are usually prescribed
2. Mild pain, such as headache
3. Pain combined with inflammation, usually of the joints, as in arthritis

Before considering the three basic drug groups, it will be helpful to review the whole subject of pain and the principles behind the methods used to relieve it.

Definition Pain can be defined as the perception of discomfort due to irritation, chemical stimulation, or stretching of a pain nerve ending. Pain nerves are located throughout the body, except inside the brain; when stimulated, they send signals indicating pain to the brain, where they are registered and perceived. The brain may then send return signals back to the body, usually to the muscles, initiating withdrawal from the pain.

Prevention Prevention or relief of pain can be accomplished in several ways. We all know, for example, that the perception of pain in major surgery can be totally eliminated by general anesthesia, which simply puts the perceptive organ (the brain) to sleep. Perception of very localized pain as in dental treatment can be avoided through the use of a local anesthetic such as procaine (Novocaine) that prevents the pain nerves in the region from sending signals to the brain. In rare cases of severe chronic pain, the pain nerves themselves can be cut, usually near the spinal cord. These methods of preventing or relieving special kinds of pain do not involve the drugs and

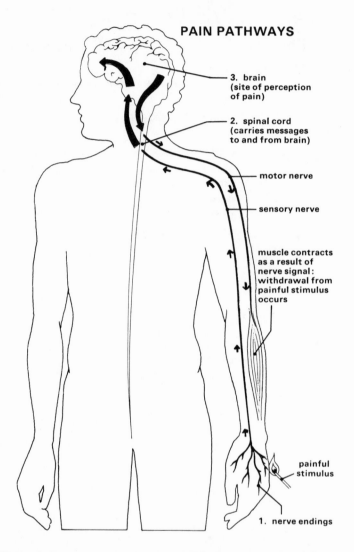

PAIN PATHWAYS

3. brain
(site of perception
of pain)

2. spinal cord
(carries messages
to and from brain)

motor nerve

sensory nerve

muscle contracts
as a result of
nerve signal:
withdrawal from
painful stimulus
occurs

painful
stimulus

1. nerve endings

Figure 8. *Pain is a vital mechanism that causes us to withdraw from potentially dangerous stimuli. This illustration shows in diagram form an everyday withdrawal reflex from a painful stimulus—in this case fire. Pain may also result from internal disease, in which case simple withdrawal is not possible. However, the pain pathway can be interrupted at the following points to produce relief:*
1. *At the site of the pain, for example, by anti-inflammatory drugs such as aspirin or by an injection of local anesthetic.*
2. *In the spinal cord, by surgically cutting the pain fibers. This is done only in cases of continual severe pain.*
3. *In the brain, by general anesthesia or narcotics such as morphine.*

medicines we normally use, and so are not discussed further in this book.

For most types of pain the means of relief is usually to remove or eliminate its cause, or, alternatively, to decrease the sufferer's perception of the pain. The pain of red, swollen, inflamed joints can be relieved in part by drugs such as aspirin that decrease the inflammation. The perception of pain from an uninflamed joint, however, can only be relieved by a drug that changes a person's perception of what he describes as pain.

The subject of pain and its relief is a very complex matter because of the considerable variation in pain perception between individuals and the difficulty of objective measurement. For example, ask a few people to describe the pain of an ordinary headache and the responses are likely to vary from "a dull ache," to "a sharp, shooting pain," to a "band around the head" or other descriptions. Why the variation? One reason is that the cause of headache pain varies: it can be muscle spasm, injury, hangover, sinusitis, eye fatigue, or a true migraine headache. In turn, differing causes may affect the *quality* of the pain—sharp or dull, for example. Another reason has to do with the duration of the pain. What begins as a relatively sharp headache pain (and is newly perceived) may take on a dull, throbbing character as the headache persists.

Psychological factors Psychological factors may also have an important effect on the perception of pain. These include learned (or cultural) influences and perhaps even genetic or inherited ones. They also include the emotional impact of the pain. (If the pain arouses a suspicion of cancer or a heart attack it will always be very noticeable until the suspicion is disproved.) The presence or absence of other distracting factors can also make a difference. For example, a headache may suddenly be dismissed at the beginning of a long-awaited party. Just as the perception of pain is influenced by all these factors, so are the effects of any drug designed to change that perception. And, of course, the effectiveness of any drug is partly dependent upon the *expectations* of the person taking it and of the doctor prescribing it.

Placebos A tablet or capsule that someone strongly believes in will be effective more frequently—even if it is really only a sugar pill (a *placebo,* with no chemical effect)—than a pill believed to be useless in the first place. This placebo effect, the result of expectation rather than of the true chemical or pharmacologic effect of the drug on the body, often leads doctors to prescribe sugar pills to "cure" non-existent diseases. It is a very powerful phenomenon, as demonstrated by tests showing that 30–40% of people with mild pain will get relief from a sugar pill if they believe it is a pain killer. This factor makes the evaluation of pain medicines, and in fact of all medicines, fairly difficult, especially when the pain or symptoms involved are only mild.

Analgesics Most drugs for relief of pain primarily alter preception and are called, as a group, *analgesics.* They can be divided into drugs for severe pain and drugs for mild pain. Some of the latter drugs that also help to relieve inflammation are considered separately later.

Acute (temporary) and chronic (continuous and recurring) pain are often perceived in different ways. Pain-relieving drugs also act in more than one way, with the possible exception of local anesthetics that temporarily "deaden" the nerve carrying pain signals to the brain. While most pain medications act primarily to decrease perception of the pain, some, especially aspirin and related anti-inflammatory drugs, also act locally at the site of the pain.

Narcotic pain relievers (see next section) primarily decrease perception of pain, often by producing a transient feeling of well-being or euphoria. Non-narcotic pain relievers (see page 42) also decrease perception of pain, acting both near the site of pain and on the brain. They are less potent than narcotics and are not generally addictive, at least physically.

Side effects
Those pain relievers that also have anti-inflammatory properties (see *Pain with inflammation,* page 43) usually have more side effects, particularly gastrointestinal upset. Frequently these drugs are formulated as combinations of aspirin, phenacetin, and caffeine, with or without other analgesics such as codeine (a narcotic) and Darvon (propoxyphene). The relative usefulness of these combinations is discussed under the individual products. In general the actual function of caffeine in these drugs is unknown and the use of phenacetin, which may cause kidney damage with long-term use, has been challenged and even discontinued in some countries.

Pain perception
Two recent research breakthroughs hold out the hope of even more effective and better-controlled methods of treating

pain. One is the notion of a central biasing mechanism—a sort of "gate-control" in the brain that can affect the perception of pain. Researchers believe that stimulating the mechanism that controls pain "feeling" can effectively shut the gate to pain sensations. In part, this helps explain the usefulness of electrical stimulation therapy and acupuncture, as well as age-old "natural" remedies for pain such as hot cups, ice packs, and even mudpacks.

The other research discovery is that the human body itself produces its own natural potent pain relievers, called enkephalins (meaning "in the head"). When these substances were identified, it was hoped that by synthesizing them chemically useful non-narcotic, non-addictive pain relievers could be produced. So far this has not been successful but intensive research continues. Taken together, these two ideas have given scientists new paths to follow in their search for better medications for the treatment of all types of pain.

Narcotic pain relievers Most of the drugs used for severe pain are considered narcotics and are related to morphine. All of these drugs act to decrease perception of pain and tend to produce a temporary sense of well-being or euphoria. This in part accounts for the abuse of these drugs, even those taken under the supervision of a physician.

When a narcotic drug is used repeatedly and regularly for many days or weeks, the dose needed to effectively relieve pain or cause a feeling of well-being must be increased because the body develops a tolerance to the drug. If the narcotic is suddenly discontinued, withdrawal symptoms (e.g., marked nervousness or stomach cramps) may occur, indicating physical dependence upon the drug. These symptoms are relieved rapidly when the drug is taken again, and thus a cycle can develop in which it is difficult to permanently discontinue the drug. The presence of tolerance and physical dependence are indications of addiction to the narcotic.

Side effects The potent narcotic analgesics remain highly valuable drugs; however, they must be used with caution and only when needed for the relief of severe pain. Because of the hazard of addiction, this class of medication is restricted in its use and distribution in hospitals and pharmacies by regulations established by the U.S. Drug Enforcement Agency.

Listed below are some of the commonly prescribed narcotic pain relievers. Those with an asterisk are individually described in Part 3.

A.S.A. Compound codeine*
Demerol*
Dilaudid
Empirin Compound with codeine*

Fiorinal with codeine*
morphine*
Percodan*
Phenaphen with codeine*

Synalgos-DC*
Tylenol with codeine*

Non-narcotic pain relievers Although a very large number of products for relief of mild-to-moderate pain are available both over the counter and by prescription, it is important to point out that they are generally composed of one or more of three basic components, all of which can relieve mild pain: aspirin; acetaminophen, or phenacetin, which the body converts to acetaminophen; and the Darvon (proxyphene) group of drugs. These are often combined with each other or with small amounts of the mild stimulant caffeine and sometimes with smaller amounts of codeine or tranquilizers. Frequently the drugs are essentially equivalent except for their cost and packaging, although it can be reasonably argued that both these factors increase the expectation of greater effect!

Muscle relaxants There is an additional group of drugs called muscle relaxants, which includes Parafon-Forte, Robaxin and Soma Compound. These are believed to act on special nerve cells in the spinal cord with the effect of allowing relaxation of nerves at a local level. It has been proposed that Valium acts in this way as well. It has been very difficult to prove the effectiveness of these drugs, but they are often used for this effect nevertheless.

Listed below are some of the commonly prescribed non-narcotic pain relievers and muscle relaxants. Those with an asterisk are individually described in Part 3.

Non-narcotic pain relievers:
acetaminophen*
aspirin*
Darvocet-N*
Darvon*
Darvon Compound-65*
Equagesic*
Fiorinal*
Norgesic*
Talwin*

Tylenol*
Muscle relaxants:
Parafon-Forte*
Robaxin-750*
Soma Compound

Pain with inflammation The word inflammation is a general term which is applied to the occurrence of swelling, along with pain and often external redness. Inflammation is a very complex response of the body to various noxious stimuli, including insect stings; local infections or abscesses; injuries, such as a broken bone or burn; and chronic diseases like rheumatoid or gouty arthritis. In all of these, the area affected becomes red, swollen, and painful.

Anti-inflammatory drugs and arthritis The treatment of inflammation often involves eliminating the cause through means other than medication, for example, by draining an abscess or treating an infection. However, some types of inflammation, particularly arthritis, are fairly consistently relieved by a group of drugs called anti-inflammatory drugs. The term arthritis applies to a group of diseases that affects the joints of the body causing chronic pain and often swelling, and eventual destruction of joints. Some types of arthritis are associated with acute inflammation (that is, swelling, redness, and pain) of several joints. The most common of these "inflammatory" arthritis disorders are rheumatoid arthritis and gouty arthritis. Both these diseases have varying courses of acute "flare-ups" alternating with periods of normality where there are no symptoms. Several drugs that slow the inflammatory process and relieve pain are effective in treating the acute phases and sometimes even prevent them altogether. Drugs effective in one disease, such as colchicine in acute gout, are not necessarily effective in the other, and sometimes their application is actually used by doctors as a kind of diagnostic aid. For example, if colchicine doesn't work, then the problem is probably not gout.

A very common type of arthritis, called *osteoarthritis,* does not usually cause much inflammation, but can cause tenderness of many joints, especially the larger ones. Pain of a chronic nature is a greater problem here than inflammation. This type of arthritis can often be treated with pain relievers with no anti-inflammatory effect, such as acetaminophen.

Side effects The drugs used for arthritic pain generally have the property of causing a slow-down of the inflammatory process, although they do this in diverse ways. Unfortunately, most of the drugs that have this anti-inflammatory effect also share the tendency to promote ulceration or irritation of the stomach. M ost of these drugs tend to relieve pain more by helping to relieve the inflammation causing the pain than by changing perception of the pain (aspirin is an exception in that it acts in both ways). Several new anti-inflammatory drugs, usually known as non-steroidal anti-inflammatory drugs, have recently been put on the market and the most widely used, Motrin, is discussed in Part 3. Although these drugs have been shown in short-term studies to be equal in effectiveness to aspirin in relief of chronic arthritic pain, they are far more costly and share many of the side effects of aspirin and the other anti-inflammatory drugs.

Listed below are some of the commonly prescribed anti-inflammatory drugs. Those with an asterisk are individually described in Part 3.

aspirin*	Indocin*	Naprosyn*
Butazolidin	Nalfon*	Tandearil*
Butazolidin Alka*	Motrin*	Tolectin*
Clinoril		

Sleep Disorders and Problems with Anxiety, Mood, or Thought

The most commonly prescribed group of drugs are those used for treating anxiety and mood, sleep, or thought disorders. Although sedative and tranquilizing substances (not the least of which is alcohol) have been used for centuries, it is only in the last 20 years that such a range of drugs for treating nervous disorders has become available. Development of more sophisticated drugs in this area has increased the number of problems treatable with medication, although the origins of many of these disorders and the mode of action of the drugs themselves remain mysterious.

Drugs in this category fall into two major classes:

1. Those used for mild, self-limited problems that are part of the ordinary stresses of life, such as sedatives or tranquilizers for anxiety, and sleeping pills for the occasional disturbance of normal sleep patterns

2. Those used for more disrupting disturbances that seriously interfere with day-to-day behavior, such as the major tranquilizers for thought disorders and the antidepressants and lithium for disabling problems of mood

Stimulants, another group of drugs, are usually used in problems with weight control and are therefore discussed in the chapter on that subject (see *Weight Loss,* page 106).

Minor tranquilizers Minor tranquilizers, also called anti-anxiety agents, are in the most frequently prescribed drug group, along with sleeping pills. In fact the leading minor tranquilizer, Valium, is the most prescribed medicine in the United States. Since the introduction of Librium and Valium the percentage of the population taking minor tranquilizers has sharply increased, reflecting intensive promotional efforts directed at physicians by drug companies, increased access to health care, and, possibly, heightened environmental stress.

Minor tranquilizers, sleeping pills, and sedatives have very similar effects—their differences are more related to dosage and use than to pharmacological activity. For example, Dalmane, which is used most often for sleep, is not significantly different from Valium or Librium, which are usually prescribed as anti-anxiety agents.

Benzodiazepines By far the most commonly taken group of anti-anxiety agents is known as the *benzodiazepines* and includes the related drugs Librium, Valium, Serax, Ativan, and Tranxene. The major difference between these and the other tranquilizers lies in the fact that the benzodiazepines appear to have a lower potential for (1) abuse, (2) death, when taken in overdose, and (3) drug interactions.

Barbiturates Conversely, the *barbiturate* group, including phenobarbital and Seconal, as well as Quaalude and Doriden (which are more commonly used as sleeping pills) have high potentials for all of these and require very judicious use. Another minor tranquilizer, very similar in effect to the barbiturates, is meprobamate (Equanil).

Antihistamines The antihistamines, which include Vistaril and Atarax, have significant sedative effects in certain individuals, although their actions differ from other drugs in this group (see *Antihistamines,* page 121). Since they are relatively safe, antihistamines are often used as both tranquilizers and sleeping pills; they have long been major components of over-the-

45

counter sleep preparations, although one, methapyrilamine, has been withdrawn because of fears that it may cause cancer.

Dosages All of these drugs lower anxiety and often allow a calmer, though altered, perception of life at "tranquilizing" doses. In tranquilizers as in most other medications, the effect of any dose appears to vary among individuals. For example, 5 mg of Valium (the usual anti-anxiety dose) may calm one person, put another to sleep, make a third feel dizzy, and have no effect on a fourth. Occasionally, these drugs can actually *excite*—especially children or the elderly—but most people are tranquilized at this dose. At higher doses, especially when taken at night, these drugs can help induce sleep, though the sleep is different from unassisted sleep and with habitual use, real sleeping and dreaming time may decrease, an effect discussed in detail in the following section on sleeping pills.

Side effects The most significant side effect of minor tranquilizers is drowsiness, which is often a function of dose. Of course this can be a useful effect if the drug is used at night. A very small percentage of people taking these drugs also experiences confusion, disorientation, or even vertigo.

All these drugs share characteristics which can make them hazardous in certain situations:

1. They can depress breathing in persons with significant lung disease or when taken in excessive doses.
2. They are "additive" to one another and to alcohol in producing sedation or sleep and in depressing breathing (this explains some accidental deaths due to intake of slightly excessive amounts of sedatives with alcohol).
3. They can be habit-forming. Once a habit is established, not only is it difficult to stop, but withdrawal symptoms can follow sudden drug stoppage. In mild cases this may only mean nightmares or some anxiety for several days. In more severe cases, seizures can result.

Mild tranquilizers are often prescribed for use two to four times a day, but in many cases this may be excessive or unnecessary. First, anxiety is often transient and may require only occasional doses rather than continuous use. Second, drugs like Valium, Librium, and phenobarbital stay in the body for long periods, so often they can be taken just once a day.

Listed below are some of the commonly prescribed minor tranquilizers. Those with an asterisk are individually described in Part 3.

Atarax*	meprobamate*	Tranxene*
Ativan*	phenobarbital*	Valium*
Equanil*	Serax*	Vistaril*
Librium*		

Sleeping pills Most tranquilizers can be used as sleeping pills, and vice versa, as noted in the previous section. However, drugs such as chloral hydrate, Dalmane, Seconal, and Nembutal are more commonly prescribed as sleeping pills, though in lower doses they have essentially the same effects as daytime tranquilizers.

The nature of sleep Before some recent studies of sleep characteristics, sleeping pills were routinely administered in hospitals and nursing homes and frequently prescribed for use at home for treating common insomnia. But greater understanding of the phenomenon we call sleep has cast doubt on the wisdom of using sleeping pills routinely. Studies of brain waves show that normal sleep consists of several stages numbered from 0 to 4. After going to sleep, there is a gradual progression through each of these stages beginning at zero, then the cycle is repeated three or more times. Dreaming usually occurs after return to stage 1, and since it is accompanied by eye movements, this stage is known as rapid eye movement sleep, or *REM sleep.*

Side effects REM sleep appears to be important, because anyone deprived of it for long periods tends to become irritable, anxious, or even begins to hallucinate. It has also been discovered that the majority of sleeping pills tend to change the normal sleep cycle. For example, barbiturates such as Seconal, Nembutal, or Tiunal, or the drug Doriden, tend to suppress REM sleep. Drugs such as Dalmane, or chloral hydrate in low doses, do not affect REM sleep, but they can eliminate stage 4 sleep. Studies on long-term users of sleeping pills indicate that not only do they skip REM sleep, but they tend to wake up several times during the night. The full meaning of these and other studies still needs to be clarified, but they do

THE EFFECT OF BARBITURATES ON SLEEP PATTERNS

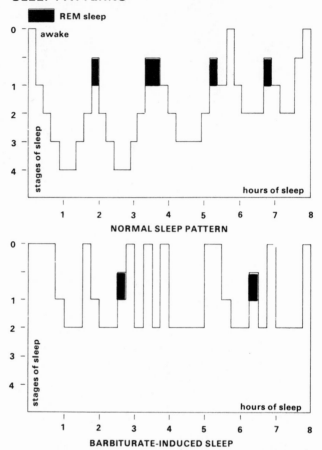

Figure 9. *EEG recordings of brain waves have shown that depth of sleep normally fluctuates throughout the night. A typical pattern, illustrated in the upper diagram, varies from Stage 0 (awake) to stage 4 (deeply asleep). At about 90-minute intervals, the sleeper has periods where his eyes move quickly from side to side (Rapid Eye Movement sleep) and these probably coincide with dreaming. If a person is repeatedly awakened whenever he is starting REM sleep he becomes anxious and irritable. The lower diagram demonstrates how barbiturate drugs alter the sleep pattern and reduce REM sleep in particular. However, they do not produce the adverse psychological effects that would be expected from sleep deprivation.*

indicate that *sleeping pills do not produce normal sleep.* Because of this, most doctors have become more selective in prescribing sleeping pills, and caution should be exercised in using any non-prescription products to aid sleep.

Overuse and overdosing
Another significant problem in the use of sleeping pills is abuse of such drugs as Seconal, Nembutal, and Quaalude. As a result, the prescribing of many of these drugs has been restricted in a manner similar to that for narcotics. The use of sleeping pills in suicide attempts, especially in certain age groups, must also be considered in prescribing them. Furthermore, insomnia, like pain, is often a symptom of other physical or mental problems. Sometimes it reflects depression, and when that is resolved, sleep improves. At other times, insomnia may be a transient reaction to specific life stresses and will disappear in its own good time. For all these reasons, the therapeutic approach to insomnia is changing. Although sleeping pills are still helpful in some situations for short-term assistance, their use should become much more selective in the future.

Listed below are some of the commonly prescribed sleeping pills. Those with an asterisk are individually described in Part 3.

Butisol*	Nembutal*	Seconal
chloral hydrate*	Noludar	Tiunal
Dalmane*	Quaalude	
Doriden*	Placidyl*	

Major tranquilizers   The group of drugs called major tranquilizers, or anti-psychotic drugs, must not be confused with the more commonly used minor tranquilizers or anti-anxiety agents such as Librium or Valium, discussed under *Minor tranquilizers,* page 45. Major tranquilizers, although they have the ability to cause sedation, have a broader range of physiological effects and strong adverse reactions, so they are used only in special controlled situations for treating disorders of thinking.

Phenothiazines and thinking disorders
True major tranquilizers came into being in the early 1950s, revolutionizing the care of severely disturbed patients. These drugs, called *phenothiazines,* enabled many persons previously confined to mental hospitals to return to a relatively normal life because one of the drugs' major actions is to normalize thought processes. In people with severe thought dis-

49

orders who experience hallucinations or loss of contact with reality, as in schizophrenia and certain types of neurological diseases, the effects can frequently be dramatic. Although the major tranquilizers do not always eliminate the need for other types of therapy, they have very wide usage. Often the most effective treatment for thought disorders involves a major tranquilizer in combination with psychiatric and/or social therapy.

Anxiety and nausea problems
Major tranquilizers are also promoted and sometimes used for treating anxiety problems that do not involve disorders of thinking. Although the sedative effect provided by many of the major tranquilizers can help in these cases, it is very questionable whether such potent drugs are needed. Other actions of these drugs permit their use in different clinical settings. For example, one drug, Compazine, is primarily used to treat nausea.

Dosages
Sometimes called "neuroleptics," major tranquilizers work by acting on nerve endings in the brain and elsewhere in the body. Individual response to these drugs varies greatly, and there is a correspondingly large variation in the effective dose. Major tranquilizers stay in the body for a long time, so when prescribed over extended periods, they are usually taken once daily and sometimes skipped on weekends to prevent accumulation in the body. These drugs must be used selectively because they have a wide variety of side effects, some of which are predictable, others not.

Side effects
Almost all major tranquilizers can produce neurological effects, the most common being symptoms resembling those of Parkinson's disease, which is characterized by hand tremors, some rigidity of the arms and legs, and a "mask-like" facial appearance. These symptoms can be overcome with a standard anti-Parkinsonian drug such as Cogentin (see *Parkinson's disease,* page 131) without interrupting treatment, or by changing to a different major tranquilizer.

Other neurological effects, such as grimacing of the face and twitching in the extremities, are less predictable. A marked withdrawal symptom that occurs after major tranquilizers are stopped is characterized by uncontrolled trembling and circular movement of the tongue and lips. This unpredictable effect, called tardive dyskinesia may be aggravated by anti-Parkinsonian drugs, although sometimes it lessens with increased doses of the major tranquilizer. For such reasons, these drugs must be used quite selectively and with frequent medical checkups.

Mild sedation can also be produced by many of these drugs, particularly Thorazine and Mellaril. This effect is sometimes put to use by giving the daily dose at bedtime to avoid interference with daytime activities.

Low blood pressure is another effect of some of these drugs, again especially Thorazine and Mellaril. This effect tends to decrease with time, but when present, may produce dizziness when the patient moves from a reclining to a sitting position. Changing position slowly, or switching to a related drug with less of this effect, such as Prolixin, Stelazine, or Haldol, will prevent dizziness.

Like the antispasmodic drugs, such as Pro-Banthine, and the tricyclic antidepressant drugs (such as Elavil), major tranquilizers block the substance acetylcholine that is produced by the nervous system. This substance controls many body functions and blockage of it may cause a dry mouth; difficulty with bladder function (especially in older people); constipation; and changes in the eye, which can predispose to glaucoma. These effects may decrease with time, but can worsen if an anti-Parkinsonian drug, such as Cogentin, is used in conjunction with the tranquilizer.

Other side effects   Certain other adverse effects of the major tranquilizers are relatively rare. These include jaundice—yellow discoloration of the skin, eyes, and urine—due to liver damage; a marked decrease in the white blood cell count, predisposing to severe infection; and various allergic reactions such as skin rash. These serious effects usually appear within the first few months of treatment and should be reported immediately. If allergy develops to one of the phenothiazine-type major tranquilizers, an agent with a different chemical structure, such as Haldol, is usually substituted.

One major tranquilizer has now been combined with a tricyclic antidepressant (see the following section) in two identical products under different trade names, Triavil and Etrafon, which are frequently used in various types of depression with anxiety. For several reasons there is considerable question whether this drug combination has any appropriate use. The response to both a major tranquilizer and a tricyclic antidepressant is highly variable and seldom can a fixed combination provide the proper dose of each. Furthermore, the anticholinergic effects of each drug are additive, so, in most

51

cases, either one drug or the other is preferable.

Listed below are some of the commonly prescribed major tranquilizers and drugs that combine a major tranquilizer with an antidepressant. Those with an asterisk are individually described in Part 3.

major tranquilizers:
Compazine*
Haldol*
Mellaril*
Navane
Prolixin
Sparine
Stelazine*
Taractan
Thorazine*
Trilafon
major tranquilizer
with a tricyclic
antidepressant:
Etrafon
Triavil*

Antidepressants and lithium Variations in mood from elation to depression occur normally in almost everyone, but in some people the degree to which moods are felt may be exaggerated. When a person sees himself and his life in a wholly negative way the mood can lead to an inability to work and, occasionally, to suicide. However, such a state is almost always temporary, and after a time the mood lightens. In certain people the mood may lighten to the point of elation, which can be so excessive that the individual thinks he can achieve things well beyond his means or capacity. Whereas most of us experience all of these moods occasionally, when a person has long-standing, repeated, excessive mood changes, they interfere with day-to-day activities and relationships, and therefore require treatment. Recurrent depression is called *unipolar endogenous depression,* while fluctuations from depression to marked elation is called *manic-depression,* a bipolar state.

Normal mood changes Though serious, long-standing problems of mood are treatable with specific medications, such drugs are sometimes used inappropriately to treat minor mood problems, especially depression. Many life changes, such as the death of someone close or even moving to an unfamiliar place, can cause depression. But unless there is a history of recurrent, serious depression, drug treatment is usually unnecessary; these passing episodes will normally improve by themselves or with supportive therapy—often before drugs used in recurrent mood disorders could take effect, which may be more than three weeks. Thus, problems that will truly be helped by antidepressant drugs are fairly specific.

Treatments Until the 1960s, the treatment of serious depression included the use of stimulant drugs, such as amphetamines (which cause even worse depression when withdrawn); electroshock therapy; and another class of drugs still in occasional use called MAO inhibitors, after their effect on the enzyme monoamine oxidase.

MAO inhibitors MAO inhibitors include the drugs Parnate and Nardil, which are also used on rare occasions to treat high blood pressure. The MAO inhibitors are relatively effective in reversing depression, but are seldom used today due to drug interaction that can result in severe hypertension and sometimes stroke when they are taken with certain types of cheese, red wine, and brewers' yeast.

Tricyclics Fortunately, a group of drugs related to the drugs used for thought disorders (e.g., Thorazine) was introduced shortly after the MAO inhibitors. Called *tricyclic antidepressants* because of their chemical structure, they are the most useful drugs for serious depression and include: amitriptyline (Endep, Elavil), imipramine (Tofranil, Imavate, Janimine, Presamine, SK-Pramine), doxepin (Adapin, Sinequan), nortriptyline (Aventyl), and desipramine (Norpramine, Pertofrane).

Side effects A major difficulty with tricyclics is that they may require up to three weeks to take full effect. This problem is compounded by the fact that when first given, they have anticholinergic effects that can result in a very dry mouth, difficulty in urinating (especially if prostate trouble is present), sleepiness and blurred vision, or constipation. In short, a person starting these drugs may actually feel worse and must be strongly supported until they take effect. Luckily, at about the time the antidepressant effect takes hold, the side effects tend to become less bothersome.

The sedative effect of tricyclic antidepressants is often put to good use. As these drugs tend to stay in the body for more than a day or two, they are often taken at night when they can also promote sleep.

In addition to the temporary side effects noted above, tricyclics occasionally affect heart rhythm, so their use in persons with heart disease requires careful observation.

Drug interactions Tricyclic antidepressants also tend to have serious drug interactions with two types of drugs: the antihypertensive drug guanethidine (Ismelin), which it renders less effective, and other anticholinergic drugs such as those for stomach spasm and gastrointestinal disorders and those for Parkinsonian symptoms where additive effects can cause marked constipation or bladder problem.

Two products, Triavil and Etrafon, combine the antidepressant amitriptyline (in Elavil and Endep) with the phenothiazine major tranquilizer perphenazine (Trilafon). Since the two disorders that these combinations are used to treat usually require individualized doses, the likelihood that a fixed combination can be effective is very low.

When mood swings tend more toward marked elation, alternating with mild or severe depression, a mineral salt called lithium carbonate (Eskalith and Lithane) is extremely useful in allowing people to function normally. When using this preparation, however, dosage and blood level must be carefully monitored since excessive doses can be very dangerous.

Other drugs, such as the major tranquilizers or antidepressants, are sometimes used in treating this euphoric condition, but response is highly individual.

Listed below are some of the commonly prescribed antidepressants and drugs that combine an antidepressant and a major tranquilizer. Those with an asterisk are individually described in Part 3.

antidepressants:
Aventyl
Elavil*
Norpramine
Sinequan*
Tofranil*
Vivactil
antidepressant with a major tranquilizer:
Etrafon
Triavil*

Heart and Vascular Disorders

Cardiovascular disease is a major cause of death and hospitalization and a principal contributor to the need for long-term medical care in the United States. Thus, it is not surprising that many of the most frequently prescribed drugs come into the general classification of cardiovascular drugs, nor that these fall into a large number of categories.

Before examining these important categories of drugs and what they do individually (they are discussed in separate sections on the following pages) it is necessary to consider briefly what the "cardiovascular system" is, how it works, and how drugs can affect it.

Cardiovascular system The term *cardiovascular* refers to the heart (cardiac), plus the associated blood vessels (vasculature) that include the arteries, veins, tiny vessels, or capillaries, connecting the arteries, veins, and tiny vessels, or capillaries, connecting the arteries and veins. Under normal conditions, the cardiovascular sels) with a pump (the heart) that moves the blood through the tubes. The main purpose of the system is to deliver oxygen (picked up when the blood passes through the lungs) and other nutrients by way of the arteries to the capillaries, where they are passed across the capillary walls to the tissues. Further along, the capillaries become veins and the blood is returned to the heart, pumped back to the lungs to pick up more oxygen and on to the heart to begin another cycle. This system is not unlike a mechanical pump system, and its ability to achieve efficient blood flow to the tissues is related to the efficiency of the pump, the size and openness of the blood vessels or tubes, and the pressure in the system, which is a function both of the strength of the heart contraction (heartbeat) and of the stiffness of the artery walls.

The cardiovascular system is very finely tuned, but flexible, so it is able to adapt quickly to many different demands placed on it in different situations, such as exercise and stress. But if damage occurs to the system, either from disease or injury, several problems can arise, and different types of drugs must then be used to try to return the system to normal.

Heart failure If the heart is not getting enough oxygen due to clogging of the coronary arteries that serve the heart muscles, the heart may not function as efficiently as it should or contract as well as it has in the past. This turn of events may result in a signal

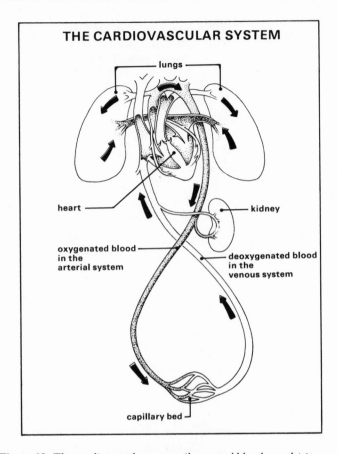

Figure 10. *The cardiovascular system (heart and blood vessels) is responsible for circulating the blood around our bodies. Actually, the heart is a double pump that feeds two circulations. One is the pulmonary circulation to the lungs where blood is oxygenated and then returned to the heart. The other is the systemic system that pumps oxygenated blood into the arteries, which eventually branch into tiny capillaries. Blood flows slowly through the capillaries giving up oxygen to the tissues and carrying away their waste products. This deoxygenated blood is returned to the heart through the veins.*

to the kidneys to retain salt and water in order to keep the maximum amount of volume and pressure in the system. On a short-term basis, this maneuver helps to maintain blood flow and volume, but the additional fluid to pump through the system can also increase stress on the heart. Because blood flow is less efficient, some of the retained salt and water goes out into the tissues causing edema (swelling of the tissues), especially in the lungs and the feet. This can result in a sensation of shortness of breath. This whole group of symptoms is called *heart failure.*

Diuretics and cardiac glycosides

One type of medication frequently given when the heart is not functioning at its peak is a diuretic (see *Diuretics,* page 63). A diuretic promotes loss of water and salt from the kidneys, thus decreasing the volume of liquid in the cardiovascular system and easing the load on the heart. The other medication usually prescribed for heart failure is a drug to stimulate the heart, usually one of the digitalis drugs, such as digoxin (see *Heart failure,* page 65). These drugs, called *cardiac glycosides,* increase the strength of the heart's contraction, improve the efficiency of its action (including the heart rate), and actually bolster the heart's ability to react normally to stimulation for additional output.

Abnormal heart rhythm

Heart failure can also result if the heart beats irregularly or too rapidly, failing to evacuate all the blood it holds with each beat. Abnormal rhythm can decrease blood flow to the capillaries and delivery of oxygen to the tissues. Many drugs are availble that act on the electrical conduction system of the heart (the mechanism by which the heart rate is controlled). These drugs can be used to slow heart rhythm and make it more regular (see *Abnormal heart rhythms,* page 67). These drugs include digoxin or Lanoxin (which affects the heart rhythm as well as the strength of contraction), quinidine, Pronestyl, Norpace, and Xylocaine.

Hypertension and angina pectoris

When the heart beats it is actually contracting in order to squeeze blood out of its chambers into the circulation. This is called *systole.* To beat, the heart must pump against both the pressure of the artery walls and the volume of blood in the closed tube system. If the arteries are constricted, as is often true in a condition of increased blood pressure (hypertension), the heart must pump harder than normal to generate sufficient pressure to get blood to the tissues and other organs. If the heart is already weakened, the need to generate further pressure puts it under even greater strain. Some drugs are now being used to decrease this pressure (called "afterload") by causing the arteries to open up or relax, thereby decreasing the work and strain on the heart. A secondary effect of these drugs is that they also improve blood flow to the heart muscle itself, which can bring a decrease in angina pectoris (intermittent pain in the heart). The drugs used in this way include nitroglycerin, Isordil, and a new class of medications called beta-blockers (see *Angina pectoris,* page 71).

Anticoagulants When the heart is functioning less efficiently, frequently the blood flow in the closed cardiovascular system may be less efficient. The tendency toward sluggish flow is greatest in the return system (the veins) with an increased likelihood of blood clotting within the blood vessels *(thrombosis)*. There are also many other causes of thrombosis that do not directly relate to failure of the cardiovascular system. If clots are formed that travel to the lung through the veins, they can cause a blockage in the lung *(pulmonary embolus)* affecting the heart and the exchange of oxygen in the lungs. To prevent further formation of clots, drugs called *anticoagulants* are used (see *Anticoagulants,* page 73). These include heparin, which is usually used in a hospital setting, as well as the oral drug Coumadin (warfarin) and its derivatives.

Arteriosclerosis Finally, one of the major causes of cardiovascular problems results from the formation of arteriosclerotic plaques in the arteries. These plaques, made of fatty materials including cholesterol, can block the flow of blood to various organs and tissues, such as the heart (where the result may be angina pectoris and coronary occlusion) or the brain (where blockage can cause a stroke). The actual mechanism by which the plaques of arteriosclerosis are formed and the ways in which it can be prevented are not known. However, it is thought that a lower dietary intake of saturated fats and cholesterol may help prevent further plaque formation. Some drugs are currently being used which are possibly effective in preventing arteriosclerosis in different ways and in different types of people. These drugs include Atromid and nicotinic acid (see *Circulaton problems,* page 68). Another group of drugs, prescribed to increase circulation in areas already affected by arteriosclerosis, includes Hydergine, Pavabid, and Vasodilan.

High blood pressure High blood pressure is one of the most common health problems in modern society, and many drugs are used to treat it. High blood pressure, also known as hypertension, occurs when pressure in the arterial blood vessels increases. The heart and blood vessels together make up a closed tubing system with a pump. The pressure in the system relates to how forcefully the pump works and to the size and strength of the tubes, especially the arteries.

Normal blood pressure in human arteries is expressed as

a ratio, usually less than 140 over 90 millimeters of mercury. (Mercury pressure is an arbitrary scale.) The higher figure, 140, is called the *systolic* pressure and measures the force of the heartbeat, as well as indirectly the openness and strength of the arteries. The lower figure, 90, is called the *diastolic* pressure and represents the pressure exerted by and the stiffness of the walls and the size of the arteries when the heart relaxes (diastole) between beats. A person with a normal heartbeat of 72 times a minute and a blood pressure of 140/90 has a pressure of 140 mm of mercury in the system each time the heart beats and a pressure of 90 mm between each beat.

VARIATIONS IN BLOOD PRESSURE

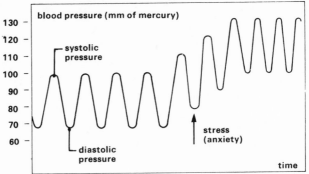

Figure 11. *With each heartbeat, blood pressure within the arteries rises from a diastolic level (maintained by the elastic artery walls) to a systolic level as the heart pumps blood into the arteries. In a state of anxiety, the blood pressure rises because the heart beats more quickly.*

Hypertension   Hypertension occurs when the heart contracts with unusual force or when the arteries become smaller in diameter, usually due to constriction of the muscular walls of the arteries, or both. It can also occur when there is more fluid (or blood volume) in the system. When taken on more than one occasion, a pressure of more than 140/90 in people below the age of 60 and 160/90–95 in older people is usually considered evidence of hypertension. The higher the pressure, the greater the problem.

   Over periods of months to years, high blood pressure is harmful because its constant pounding eventually damages small arteries and the organs that they supply, especially the brain and kidney. Also, of course, it affects the heart, since pumping against a higher pressure requires more work. Like any mechanical system that must work hard, it will eventually wear out. People with hypertension also have a higher incidence of other diseases, so its control can be seen as a form of preventive medicine.

One of the major determinants of blood pressure is the degree of contraction in the arterial blood vessels. This is controlled by many regulating substances in the body, as well as by the nervous system. For example, blood pressure can rise because of increased activity in the sympathetic nervous system. This releases a substance called norepinephrine or noradrenaline (similar to epinephrine, or adrenaline) that causes the arteries to constrict more tightly and increases the necessary force of heart contraction. In addition, the sympathetic nervous system (also called the "fight or flight" nervous system because it prepares the body for these activities) is sometimes activated under stress, which may, in turn, relate to periods of increased blood pressure. When this occurs, many people are aware of the heart "pounding," though normally they cannot feel the increased blood pressure. Many types of medicine, especially those used as general stimulants or appetite suppressants (such as amphetamines), decongestants (such as Neosynephrine nasal sprays), or drugs used to treat asthma or allergies (such as epinephrine) have very similar effects on the arteries and can cause or aggravate high blood pressure. They can also interact with drugs used to treat high blood pressure.

All of the drugs used to treat high blood pressure act to block one or more of the causes of the increased blood pressure. Thus, they can: 1) decrease the volume in the closed system and/or; 2) block the sympathetic nervous system or one of the substances causing blood vessel constriction and/ or; 3) dilate the arteries.

Diuretics The majority of antihypertensive drugs can be classified in three general categories. The first comprises the *diuretics,* which are usually the first drugs to be prescribed and also represent the mainstay of therapy in many cases because they actually enhance the effect and benefit of other drugs. Examples of diuretics include HydroDIURIL (hydrochlorothiazide) and Lasix (furosemide). Diuretics act to decrease the volume in the system by causing loss of excess water (often manifested as swelling of the feet, or edema) and salt.

They also dilate, or enlarge, the blood vessels to some extent. By virtue of these two effects they are widely used alone for mild cases of raised blood pressure and in combination with other drugs to treat more severe cases. They are discussed in detail in the section on diuretics, page 63.

Sympathetic blocking drugs The second general category of drugs for treating high blood pressure comprises the *sympathetic blocking drugs.* Their function, as the name suggests, is to block the activity of the sympathetic nervous system. Reserpine, Aldomet, and Ismelin are included in this category. Since the sympathetic nervous system can raise blood pressure by increasing the forcefulness of the heart's contractions and by causing constriction of blood vessels, these drugs usually act on both to decrease slightly the heart's contracting force and rate and to dilate blood vessels. The sympathetic nervous system originates in the brain and affects many other functions, such as bowel and bladder function and sexual response. This fact explains many of the side effects that sometimes accompany the sympathetic blocking drugs, such as drowsiness, depression, change in sleep or dreaming patterns, diarrhea, and change in sexual appetite. Since there is considerable variability in this system from person to person, dosage and side effects also vary widely.

Vasodilators The third category of drugs, the *vasodilators* (or "blood vessel relaxing agents"), acts primarily to relax the walls of blood vessels thus decreasing pressure in the system. Apresoline (hydralazine) and prazosin (Minipress) are the only drugs in this category for oral prescription available in the U.S. at this time, although other vasodilators are used in emergency treatment of high blood pressure. These drugs represent a very effective way to lower blood pressure, but their effectiveness is dependent on one's physical position, and they are associated with some severe side effects after long-term use. Thus if a person stands suddenly, much blood will go into the lower part of the body, cutting the supply of blood to the head and causing dizziness or a sense of faintness. This is called *postural hypotension,* or low blood pressure due to change in position. After a few moments, the heart and the blood vessels in the legs help readjust the circulation to bring the blood pressure back to normal. To readjust and increase the blood pressure, the heart sometimes beats rapidly and harder, which can be a bothersome side effect. This can be prevented by sympathetic blocking drugs, which are often given in conjunction with vasodilators. In addition, patients taking these drugs are usually instructed to move more slowly. The effect of vasodilators explains why a person with high blood pressure may get headaches when lying flat and why many doctors use positional changes in blood pressure to assess the effect of certain drugs.

Combination drugs Frequently, high blood pressure is treated by the combination of a diuretic, a sympathetic blocker, and a vasodilator. In fact, one of the major problems in drug therapy for hypertension is the need for a number of drugs, each of which must be taken several times a day; furthermore, the patient, who may have had no symptoms before treatment began, may suffer from so many bothersome side effects that he feels worse than before taking medication. Accordingly, many people fail to take their medicine regularly and continue to have hypertension, which eventually may lead to stroke, kidney failure, or heart failure.

One approach to this problem of multiple drugs has been the production of certain combinations for hypertension, tablets that contain drugs from two or all three categories mentioned above. Two examples are Aldoril and Aldactazide. Unfortunately, the establishment of an effective antihypertensive regimen for any particular individual often involves considerable adjustment to an individual drug, so the use of combinations in initiating or changing therapy makes the process more complicated. Once a regimen is established, however, the combination preparations may be useful, as their convenience may outweigh their higher cost.

Another approach is to find drugs that act for a long time and need to be taken only once or twice daily. In some cases this is possible, especially in the treatment of mild hypertension. Unfortunately, in many cases those drugs which are most effective and have the fewest side effects must be taken more frequently.

Listed below are some of the drugs commonly prescribed for high blood pressure. Those with an asterisk are individually described in Part 3.

Aldactazide*	Catapres*	Enduron*
Aldactone*	Diupres*	Esidrex*
Aldomet*	Diuril*	hydrochlorothiazide*
Aldoril*	Dyazide*	HydroDIURIL*
Apresoline*	Dyrenium	Hydropres*

DIURETICS ("WATER PILLS")

Hygroton*	Regroton*	Ser-Ap-Es*
Inderal*	Renese-R	Serpasil
Ismelin*	reserpine	Zaroxolyn
Lasix*	Salutensin*	

Diuretics ("water pills") Diuretic drugs are often referred to as "water pills" because they promote the loss of water, as well as salt, through the kidney into the urine. Common diuretic drugs include HydroDIURIL, hydrochlorothiazide, Lasix, Hygroton, Dyazide, and Aldactazide. Diuretics are the mainstay for treating two very common disorders: high blood pressure and heart failure. They are also used to treat edema (swelling due to the retention of water, usually in the feet and legs, but sometimes also in the hands, face, or abdomen), kidney disease (nephrosis), and liver disease (cirrhosis).

Effects of diuretics Diuretics have two related effects. The primary therapeutic effect—loss of water—can prevent overloading of the heart and blood vessels in cases of high blood pressure and heart failure. The second effect is the loss of salt (sodium chloride, or table salt). In many illnesses the kidney tends to retain excessive amounts of salt and water in the body; diuretics act on the kidney to block this effect.

Certain diuretics (Lasix, hydrochlorothiazide, HydroDIURIL) also cause loss of the essential salt (or mineral) potassium chloride, which must be replaced either through the diet or by medicine supplement. Other diuretics, such as Dyazide, Aldactazide, Aldactone, and Dyrenium, do not cause loss of potassium and are called *potassium-retaining diuretics*. Although potassium supplements are not required with the latter, these diuretics are not always considered drugs of choice due to other effects on the body's salt balance.

Thiazide-type diuretics Diuretics are commonly classified as *thiazide type, potent diuretics,* or *potassium-retaining diuretics.* Thiazide-type diuretics are so called after their chemical class, which relates them to the sulfa drugs and the oral antidiabetic drugs. They are the most commonly used diuretics, and hydrochlorothiazide (HydroDIURIL, Esidrix) and the longer acting Hygroton are the most frequently prescribed. Hydrochlorothiazide is also included in many combination diuretics such as Dyazide and Aldactazide and in combination antihypertensive drugs (see *High blood pressure,* page 58). Other thiazide-type diuretics are almost identical in their effects and side effects to hydrochlorothiazide, although some are longer acting. They include: Diuril, Enduron, Naturetin, Naqua, Oretic, Zaroxolyn, and Renese.

Side effects Major side effects of thiazide-type diuretics include a tendency to increase the level of sugar in the blood in people predisposed to diabetes and to increase the uric acid content in the blood, which can produce gout. A similar diuretic, Selacryn (tricrynafen) decreased the uric acid levels, but because of its toxic effects on the liver, it is no longer marketed. All the above drugs can cause, in some people, an excessive loss of water, potassium chloride, or sodium chloride. Thus, long-term therapy with any of these drugs usually requires occasional checks of blood values for sugar, uric acid, and potassium. Occasionally, they can cause rashes or muscle cramps. If a true allergic reaction occurs against one member of this group, it may also occur with others as well as with sulfa drugs.

Potent diuretics The potent diuretics include Lasix (furosemide) and Edecrin (ethacrynic acid). Although Lasix is sometimes used in routine treatment of high blood pressure or heart failure, the potent diuretics are usually reserved for treatment of severe edema, since they can cause the loss of considerably more water and salt than the thiazide-type diuretics. The potent diuretics show many of the same side effects as the thiazides, but in rare instances they may also lead to hearing problems, particularly if used with other drugs affecting the hearing nerves, for example, streptomycin or gentamycin.

Potassium-retaining diuretics The potassium-retaining diuretics, Dyrenium and Aldactone, are similar to thiazides but weaker. Because they don't cause potassium loss—eliminating the need to take extra potassium—they are often combined with a stronger thiazide diuretic, as in Aldactazide (Aldactone plus hydrochlorothiazide) and Dyazide (Dyrenium plus hydrochlorothiazide). Although sometimes useful, they can be associated with some loss of kidney function and retention of too much potassium. Aldactazide has been found to have one of the highest incidences of side effects of all drugs used in hospitals. Such combination drugs are also usually more costly than hydrochlorothiazide.

Diuretics for glaucoma A fourth kind of diuretic, Diamox, is essentially reserved for use in the treatment of glaucoma, partly because resistance to its effect develops rapidly and partly because it isn't particularly strong. It is useful in glaucoma therapy, where it can reduce the water pressure in the eye, but it should only be taken intermittently.

Listed below are some of the commonly prescribed diuretics and diuretic-containing combinations. Those with an asterisk are individually described in Part 3.

Aldactazide*
Aldactone*
Diamox Oral*
Diuril*
Dyazide*
Dyrenium
Enduron*
Esidrix*
Hydrochlorothiazide*
HydroDIURIL*
Hygroton*
Lasix*

diuretic-containing combinations:
Aldoril*
Diupres*
Hydropres*
Regroton*
Salutensin*
Ser-Ap-Es*
Renese-R

Heart failure Undoubtedly one of the most emotive descriptions of any disease is the term "heart failure." In fact, heart failure simply means that the heart is failing to do its job efficiently, not that it has stopped completely. Heart failure occurs in association with most other heart diseases since any failure of the circulatory pump can cause many changes. Except when the pump fails suddenly in an acute coronary occlusion (or heart attack), the changes are small. Often inefficiency results when the heart muscle doesn't receive enough oxygen because of obstruction or clogging of one of the coronary arteries that carries blood and oxygen to the heart itself. At other times, there is too much arterial pressure for the heart to pump against. The heart can also pump ineffectively if it beats too rapidly or irregularly, as in an *arrhythmia*. The most common arrhythmia is *atrial fibrillation,* which often oc-

65

curs in conjunction with heart failure.

When the heart pumps inefficiently, a signal goes to the kidneys to retain water in order to keep up the pressure in the circulatory system. This is a valuable protective mechanism in some acute situations such as shock (which can result from severe loss of blood or plasma), but otherwise it has a bad effect, creating extra work for the already overloaded heart. The heart cannot pump all of the extra fluid that, as a result, tends to accumulate in the legs (peripheral edema) or in the lungs (pulmonary edema). Meanwhile, the heart beats more rapidly. In very severe cases, the heart simply cannot get enough blood or oxygen to certain tissues, causing them to look purple or blue.

Reduced blood circulation helps to explain some of the other symptoms of heart failure, especially shortness of breath, which accompanies even light exercise since the heart cannot supply the body with enough oxygen. Even at night, or while the sufferer is at rest, the lungs can become congested with edematous fluid, causing breathlessness. Swelling of the feet and legs occurs, as does the sensation of rapid heartbeat. All of these symptoms can indicate a failing heart. However, they can also occur in other conditions, and diagnosis must be confirmed by such tests as electrocardiograms and chest x rays.

Treatments Since one acute problem of heart failure is the presence of excess fluid in the lungs and elsewhere in the body, initial treatment often involves the administration of diuretics such as hydrochlorothiazide (HydroDIURIL, Esidrix) and Lasix (furosemide) to reduce the load on the heart (see *Diuretics,* page 63). Often this alone will relieve many of the symptoms, but the specific causes of heart failure must also be treated. If the heart has been pumping ineffectively owing to a rapid irregular rhythm, then slowing it to a normal rate will ease the problem. Similarly, if the heart has been forced to pump against very high pressure in the arteries, as in severe high blood pressure, then reducing pressure will cut the load. Occasionally, in severe heart failure, blood pressure and work for the heart is decreased by dilating (widening) the blood vessels. A defective heart valve obviously affects the heart's ability to pump, so repair or replacement of the valve can sometimes improve functioning remarkably.

Digitalis drugs Sometimes, however, treatment of the specific causes of heart failure is not sufficient, and the heart must be directly treated to improve its performance. In 1775, an English physician, William Withering, found that a local countrywoman was very successful at treating a condition called dropsy, which was characterized by severe edema and was probably due to severe heart failure. Her treatment consisted of an herbal tea from the foxglove plant. Dr. Withering made good use of a chance observation and was instrumental in introducing the foxglove component, the digitalis leaf, to modern therapy as the primary drug for heart failure. Today, digitalis (or its purified derivatives) continues to be the mainstay of heart failure therapy. Digitalis drugs can overcome heart failure by actually increasing the strength of the heart's contraction. In addition, they improve the heart rate if it is rapid and irregular, which occurs in the very common abnormal rhythm, atrial fibrillation. Many people rely on these dual effects of the digitalis drugs (Lanoxin, digoxin, and digitoxin) to prevent recurring heart failure.

Listed below are some of the drugs commonly prescribed for heart failure. Those marked with an asterisk are individually described in Part 3.

digitalis   digoxin*   Lanoxin*

Abnormal heart rhythms The heart's muscle fibers are connected to an elaborate "wiring" or conduction system, which transmits electrical signals instructing the muscle fibers to contract. These impulses are normally sent about 72 times every minute. The conductive system starts at the top of the heart, runs through the middle (septum) and spreads out through the heart walls. If the heart is damaged, as after a heart attack, or stretched, as in heart failure, conduction of the signals can be affected and their rhythm may change. If the conduction system is blocked or damaged, the heart rate may slow down, or a type of short-circuiting may take place whereby the signals bypass the organized conduction system and fire more rapidly—sometimes irregularly, sometimes not. When normal conduction becomes disrupted, the resulting abnormal heart rate and/or rhythm is called an *arrhythmia*. The drugs used to treat this condition are called anti-arrhythmic drugs, and they come from a wide variety of unrelated classes.

Slow heartbeat   Arrhythmias can be a problem for several reasons, and they usually require treatment. If the heart beats too slowly, as in

67

certain blocks of the conducting system, the supply of blood to the brain and other organs is not sufficient and the person may have fainting spells. Although this kind of arrhythmia is occasionally treated with drugs, if it persists it often requires the surgical placement of an artificial pacemaker.

Fast heartbeat On the other hand, several problems can occur if the heart beats too rapidly and/or irregularly. If the heart beats rapidly for a few minutes, it's no cause for concern, although it may cause dizziness. However, when fast beating persists, the heart is working less efficiently, resulting in heart failure (see *Heart failure,* page 65). Certain rapid rhythms can progress to very dangerous conditions, even to cardiac arrest (heart stoppage). Other arrhythmias may not be as rapid, but can also be extremely dangerous—especially just after a heart attack when the heart muscle and conduction system may be damaged.

The drugs most commonly used in treating arrhythmias include quinidine, Pronestyl, lidocaine (Xylocaine) and Inderal (propranolol) and, more recently, Norpace (disopyramide). These drugs act in different ways on the electrical system of the heart, but they all make it less likely to "short-circuit" or to conduct extra beats causing irregular rhythm.

Listed below are some of the drugs commonly prescribed for abnormal heart rhythms. Those with an asterisk are individually described in Part 3.

Inderal*	quinidine*	Dilantin*
Pronestyl*	Xylocaine	

Circulation problems *Arteriosclerosis* describes a condition in which deposits of fat, cholesterol, and calcium build-up in the walls of arterial blood vessels. This causes narrowing of those blood vessels and may eventually progress so far as to obstruct the flow of blood, cutting off the vital supply of oxygen to the tissues. If the arteries serving the heart are affected, partial obstruction and a decreased blood supply can lead to the chest pain called angina pectoris. If total obstruction occurs, the person has a heart attack. Similar obstruction of arteries to the head can cause strokes, while obstruction of arteries to the leg can cause eventual gangrene and loss of a leg if not treated.

The build-up of these fatty deposits (plaques) is believed to occur gradually over many years, and some evidence suggests that the process starts in the early twenties. The build-up of the deposits generally proceeds unnoticed until a catastrophic event such as a heart attack or stroke signals the presence of this ailment.

Risk factors There is much controversy about the factors that cause the insidious build-up in arteries. Studies have identified several factors seemingly associated with arteriosclerotic disease, especially with its appearance early in life. Almost everyone has a fair amount of arteriosclerosis by the age of eighty. These factors, called *risk factors,* include elevated levels of such fatty substances in the blood as cholesterol and triglycerides; the presence of diabetes; a history of heavy smoking; a history of high intake of animal fats in meat and milk products; a history of high blood pressure; and, perhaps the most controversial factors at present, a history of high sugar intake and certain types of personality characteristics. Furthermore, a family history of early death (before the age of fifty-five) from heart attack or stroke or a history of elevated cholesterol or fat levels increases the likelihood of earlier problems with arteriosclerosis.

Prevention The medical approach to arteriosclerosis has been both preventive and therapeutic. There are some indications that preventive approaches may be having an impact in certain groups of people, among whom there is a decreasing incidence of arteriosclerotic disease. This reduction has been attributed to various factors, the most prominent being the lower animal-fat and cholesterol intake advocated for years by many heart associations and cardiologists. In fact, the true reasons are not known.

Preventive drug therapy Preventive drug therapy has been aimed at decreasing the amount of certain substances (such as cholesterol) available to make up the plaques. These efforts have been rather unsuccessful, although a number of drugs do reduce some types of blood fats (lipids). One of the most commonly used is Atromid-S (clofibrate). Other drugs that have been tried include nicotinic acid, a substance similar to thyroid hormone, Choloxin, Lorelco (probucol), estrogens, and drugs which prevent the absorption of fat and cholesterol from the bowel, e.g., Questran (cholestyramine). Cholesterol and other blood fats are key cellular building blocks, and many drugs that act to alter them do so while affecting other basic processes; they are not able specifically to reduce lipid levels to any great extent. However, these and other drugs continue to be studied for their usefulness early in life, or on particular groups of people that seem especially at risk. In the meantime, evidence continues to suggest that careful dietary regulation from an early age may play a key role in prevention.

A second approach to arteriosclerosis has been the attempt to prevent plaque formation and further obstruction that comes from the formation of clot-like material on the plaques. Common components of such clots are the *platelets* (a type of blood cell). Platelets have a tendency to adhere to a plaque, and, when several of them do so, they can increase the obstruction. Special drugs being extensively tested for prevention of recurrent strokes and heart attacks are the "antiplatelet" drugs, such as aspirin, Persantine, and Anturane, which decrease the stickiness of platelets. The usefulness of these drugs remains to be proven, but the small doses that seem necessary suggest they may be a relatively safe approach to some arteriosclerotic problems. Some physicians also use the blood-thinner Coumadin although, because of its many problems, it is usually reserved for situations where clotting is actively taking place rather than used as a preventive measure.

Surgery The other major approach to arteriosclerosis is surgical, and may be resorted to once there has been angina pectoris, a heart attack, a warning stroke, or poor circulation in the legs. If the arteriosclerotic plaques are in large blood vessels, they can often be surgically removed or bypassed with artificial arteries or veins made of dacron (although arteriosclerotic plaques tend to form on these as well).

Medications Drug therapy, on the other hand, is directed at opening up the arteries to improve circulation. Nitroglycerin has long been used to dilate arteries in the heart and elsewhere. Other drugs prescribed for opening up arteries elsewhere (and the use of these is somewhat more controversial) include Pavabid, Cerespan, Persantin, Cyclospasmol, Vasodilan, and Hydergine. All of these have some ability to dilate some blood vessels when they are tested in experimental animals, although a number appear to be active only when injected. Few studies, however, demonstrate that the drugs, taken orally, can have much effect in arteriosclerosis. Nonetheless, they are widely used, and fortunately most have relatively few side effects, although they are often expensive.

Listed below are some of the drugs commonly prescribed for preventing or treating circulation problems. Those with an asterisk are individually described in Part 3.

Atromid-S*	Hydergine*	Pavabid*
Cyclospasmol*	nicotinic acid*	Vasodilan*

Angina pectoris Angina pectoris is an ailment in which a person suffers chest pains below the breastbone that are due to temporary lack of blood supply, and therefore of oxygen, to the heart muscle. The usual cause of this lack is partial obstruction of the blood vessels going to the heart muscle (the coronary arteries). The obstruction is often due to fat-containing deposits (plaques) on the inner walls of the arteries, but also results from spasm of the arteries. Attacks of angina pectoris occur more often with exercise, when the heart needs more oxygen in order to pump harder. It can also occur at rest, in which case it is usually associated with stress. Angina attacks may persist for months or years before obstruction or heart attack occurs. However, these can never be predicted and a person with angina pectoris should therefore be under the direct care of a physician.

Drugs traditionally used to treat angina pectoris help to prevent the attacks in two ways:

1. By dilating (opening up) the coronary arteries to the heart, as nitroglycerin is thought to do, in part
2. By decreasing the work the heart must do, especially during exercise

Medications The drugs most commonly used to treat angina pectoris belong to a family of medications related to nitroglycerin and include Isordil and Peritrate. Nitroglycerin is taken in tablet form under the tongue or in a paste on the skin, while the other drugs are taken orally and have a longer action. They are believed to act both by opening up the arteries to the heart, allowing a larger blood supply, and by opening up other blood vessels in the body, easing the load on the heart.

Another type of drug used to treat angina pectoris is characterized by Inderal (propranolol), which decreases the work the heart must do and thus decreases the angina pectoris. It is usually taken on a regular basis, but once started, it can only be discontinued gradually. Inderal belongs to a group of drugs called *beta blockers* that block the effects of certain stimulations aimed at increasing the heart's rate and

71

the strength of its contractions. The use of beta blockers for many heart conditions, and for hypertension as well, is gaining acceptance.

Frequently a person with angina pectoris will be on a general program for heart disease, which includes changes in diet, smoking and drinking habits, and exercise, as well as medication. Often one drug, e.g., Inderal or Isordil, is taken on a regular basis, with nitroglycerin carried for use in the event of an acute attack. Each program should be highly individualized and supervised and regularly reviewed with the physician. It is difficult to judge if success in treatment is due to medication or to the change in physical habits, especially when the primary cause of the attacks is stress.

Listed below are some of the drugs commonly prescribed for angina pectoris. Those with an asterisk are individually described in Part 3.

Inderal*	Nitrobid*	Sorbitrate*
Isordil*	nitroglycerin*	

Anticoagulants ("blood thinners") There are three major types of drugs used to alter the blood's clotting mechanism: heparin, which is given only by injection; Coumadin-type drugs; and a third group called antiplatelet drugs, which include aspirin. These drugs all act to prolong the time it takes blood to coagulate or clot. Thus they prevent clot formation and are called *anticoagulants*. None of these drugs, however, actually dissolves clots which are already formed.

Thrombosis
Prolonging the coagulation or clotting process may reduce the possibility of harmful clots forming and blocking the flow of blood in an artery, a vein, or the heart itself. The formation of such clots is called *thrombosis,* and the formation of a clot (*thrombus*) in an artery to the heart (a coronary artery) can cause a *coronary thrombosis* (a "heart attack," also known as *myocardial infarction*). Clots may also form in the veins of the leg in association with inflammation; this is called *thrombophlebitis.*

Embolism
Sometimes the clots that have formed on the inner surface of an artery or vein or in the heart break loose and are carried by the blood flow to smaller blood vessels where they become wedged or trapped. This type of blockage is known as an *embolism.* For example, a clot from thrombophlebitis in the leg

can break loose and travel to the lung and cause a *pulmonary embolism,* or blood clot in the lung.

Both thrombosis and/or embolism can result in a decrease in the normal circulation of blood throughout the body, and if parts of the body do not receive the vital supply of blood they need, they will become damaged and cease to function. In the case of a pulmonary embolism, the result is damage to part of the lung. The administration of anticoagulants to reduce the possibility of obstruction or blockage of blood vessels by thrombosis or embolism is believed to help decrease the likelihood of these life-threatening developments.

In the most common situation where anticoagulants are given to prevent clots in the leg from forming or moving to the lung, the patient is usually hospitalized and placed on the drug heparin which is injected into the vein tissues or administered intravenously. After several days, the oral anticoagulant is started.

Dosage Anticoagulants need to be taken under very close medical supervision, and doses must be highly individualized and adjusted during therapy. The effectiveness of anticoagulants varies from individual to individual, and even from time to time in the same person. Laboratory blood tests measuring the time it takes for the blood to clot before and during the administration of anticoagulants are used to determine the amount of drug the person must take to produce adequate result without risking complications. These laboratory tests are extremely important and must be done on a regular basis as long as the drug is taken.

Side effects The most common complication of anticoagulation therapy is bleeding, but this can usually be treated rapidly if a physician is immediately notified of any minor bleeding. The common signs of bleeding are:

1. Red or dark brown urine, or, less commonly, excessive menstrual bleeding
2. Red or black bowel movements
3. Uncontrollable bleeding of any kind (from shaving cuts, bloody nose, or gums)
4. Unusually severe prolonged stomachache, headache, or backache
5. Sudden appearance of black-and-blue marks on the body

73

Drug interactions Many drugs taken for completely unrelated conditions can greatly increase or decrease the degree of oral anticoagulant effects. Physicians and pharmacists are aware of these interactions and they must be consulted beforehand and advised whenever *any* change in any drug regimen is planned, whether it is an over-the-counter preparation or a prescription drug that is being started, discontinued, or changed in any way. It must also be remembered that certain foods in quantity (including green leafy vegetables such as spinach, cabbage, and cauliflower) and multivitamin prescriptions containing vitamin K can affect anticoagulant therapy. Vitamin K tends to counteract the effect of the anticoagulant and this can therefore actually encourage clotting. Major changes in eating habits, especially if the above foods and multivitamin preparations are involved, should be discussed in advance with your physician.

The physician prescribing the oral anticoagulant should also be notified immediately if any other illness or injury occurs or if pregnancy is confirmed, or even suspected. Any physician, dentist, or other health professional giving treatment to a person taking oral anticoagulants should be told of this fact. If long-term therapy is planned, the person should carry a card and/or wear identification indicating that he is taking the drug.

The ability of aspirin and related drugs to prevent clotting (especially the type associated with strokes and heart attacks) by affecting one component of the blood, the small cells called *platelets,* has recently received attention, and these drugs are currently being tested for therapeutic value. The effect on clotting is much less marked than that of the Coumadin-type drugs, so the hazards relating to interaction with food and vitamin K noted above generally do not apply. The use of aspirin as well as two other drugs, Persantin and Anturane, in this way is still at an early stage. When used in low doses they appear to be relatively safe, but whether they can help prevent strokes, heart attacks, or other types of arteriosclerotic clotting remains to be proven, although recent data suggests strongly that they may be of help in this application.

Listed below are some of the commonly prescribed anticoagulants. Those with an asterisk are individually described in Part 3.

aspirin*   heparin   Persantine

Gastrointestinal Disorders

The digestive system begins at the mouth and ends at the anus. It is a dynamic, changing system, and the functions it performs in extracting vital nutrients from food and eliminating waste is so complex that it is hardly surprising it is a common site for problems, both major and minor.

Few people go through life without suffering some symptoms of nausea, vomiting, constipation, or diarrhea. Consequently, an astounding number of preparations are available by prescription or over the counter to relieve such symptoms. Usually these symptoms point to some benign and self-limiting condition, but sometimes they signal more serious problems, such as ulcers, colitis, and even cancer. Most drugs used for gastrointestinal complaints are given simply to relieve the symptoms, with varying degrees of success; they can seldom affect the underlying cause, especially if it is serious or chronic.

Sometimes dysfunction of the digestive, or gastrointestinal (G.I.), tract may be a reaction to stress—a queasy stomach or episodes of diarrhea are common symptoms of anxiety. Nonetheless, any of the gastrointestinal symptoms, if recurrent, usually requires medical evaluation to rule out serious causes. Many preparations used or prescribed for G.I. troubles act to relax the muscles of the digestive tract—the antispasmodic and antidiarrheal drugs. Many others aim to alter the actual contents of the G.I. tract: antacids (e.g., Maalox, Mylanta, Gelusil) neutralize stomach acids; laxatives and some antidiarrheals (such as Kaopectate) change the bulk of the intestinal contents and help normalize the function of the G.I. tract. Few of these drugs are for long-term use, since self-limited conditions often disappear after changes in diet or relief of stress. Specific types of disease and the drugs used for problems of the digestive tract are discussed in the next three sections.

Nausea, stomach upset, and ulcers Nausea, stomach upset, and vomiting can be due to a variety of causes. If these can be identified, they can be treated or prevented by relatively specific measures. Nausea can be due to a wide variety of problems, some as general as gastrointestinal flu. A sensation of nausea or stomach upset is often due to irritation of the stomach lining by an ulcer or by a strong, irritating medicine, such as liquid potassium, high doses of theophylline (a drug for asthma), or aspirin. In these cases, direct treatment of the ulcer with antacids (see below) or prevention of the irritation by diluting the medication with food or water may help avoid the symptoms.

Another occasional local cause of nausea or stomach distress may be overdistension of the stomach—overfilling with food or, not uncommonly, with air that has been swallowed. This seldom calls for drugs.

Vague stomach upset or vomiting is sometimes due to increased contractions of the muscles of the stomach, which often give a sensation of a knot in the stomach, hunger pangs, or nausea. These symptoms can, of course, be due to an ulcer or other local irritation, but increased stomach contractions linked to stress are often the cause. Such symptoms can often be relieved by antacids or by antispasmodic drugs such as Pro-Banthine, tincture of belladonna, or atropine. These drugs act either directly on the stomach or on the nerve supply to the stomach to decrease and slow contractions of the stomach and bowel, and they may reduce secretions, but the exact mechanism by which they work is unknown. Because these symptoms, as well as some symptoms of ulcers, are frequently associated with stress reactions, there are a number of preparations in which antispasmodic drugs are combined with tranquilizers such as phenobarbital (in Donnatal) or Librium (in Librax). Although they are in extremely wide use, there is considerable question about the advisability or effectiveness of using these fixed combinations, which are directed at two relatively different problems requiring individual attention and dosing.

Many people experience nausea after eating certain foods. People with a tendency to gallbladder disease may become nauseated after eating fatty foods, rich sauces, or butter, or sometimes corn and cabbage. Others experience symptoms of intolerance and upset in response to a wide range of foods, such as spicy foods, coffee, and dairy products. Although prevention, by avoiding the types of food responsible, is the best way to deal with this type of nausea, antacids will often, but by no means always, help to alleviate the symptoms.

Frequently nausea and vomiting are due to irritation of certain areas in the brain, including the *vomiting center,* an area called the *chemoreceptor trigger zone,* and the *vestibular apparatus* in the inner ear (which is often affected in motion sickness or in Ménière's syndrome). A number of drugs, e.g., codeine, morphine, and certain anticancer drugs, may directly affect these brain centers to cause vomiting. Fortunately, there are also a number of drugs that will stop or prevent nausea and vomiting due to these causes. Some of the most effective drugs for motion sickness are the various antihistamines (see *Antihistamines,* page 121) which act on the vestibular area. These include meclizine (Antivert, Bonine), Dramamine, Benadryl, and hydroxyzine (Atarax, Vistaril). Nausea and vomiting due to stimulation of the other areas in the brain are sometimes helped by the antihistamines, but are also prevented with major tranquilizers such as Thorazine, Compazine, or Phenergan, which are very effective, although these latter drugs in general have more potential for adverse side effects. The antispasmodic drug scopolamine is effective against most types of vomiting caused by irritation of the vomiting center and other areas. Tigan is also used, though not for nausea due to inner-ear irritation. In some cases, simple sedation with various tranquilizers is effective, but this is not usually appropriate and also entails a risk that nausea and vomiting may continue in a state of heavy sedation that can lead to aspiration—the breathing of vomitus into the lungs, which can cause serious complications.

Peptic ulcers A *peptic ulcer* is a common, specific cause of stomach upset, and occasionally of pain, nausea, and vomiting. A peptic ulcer is essentially a break in the mucus-covered lining of the stomach or of the duodenum (which connects the stomach to the intestine). This breakdown of the tissue, which can be the size of a dime or much larger, can cause pain, spasm, and hemorrhage (bleeding). Ulcers can be very serious—heavy bleeding usually requires hospitalization and sometimes surgery. For this reason, early treatment at the first sign of an ulcer is essential.

The proper treatment of ulcers has long been a subject of debate in medical circles, but at present it is felt that regular antacid therapy is of greater importance than a rigid diet in most cases. Although authorities still differ on many points, most agree that coffee, alcohol, and large amounts of spicy foods are not helpful.

Medications The stomach is essentially a muscular bag in which food begins to be broken down by hydrochloric acid and by an enzyme, pepsin, produced in the stomach lining. Any ulcer in this environment will be aggravated by the acid and enzyme; therefore, the primary goal in therapy is to neutralize the

77

acid as continuously as possible with antacids. If an antacid is given and the stomach empties slowly, acid will be neutralized longer, which may justify the addition of an antispasmodic drug, such as Pro-Banthine.

Several other aids can help achieve this goal of prolonged neutralization of acid in the stomach. First, liquid antacids are almost always more effective than tablets or chewed antacids. Second, especially in the presence of an acute ulcer, antacids may be needed as often as every thirty to sixty minutes to prevent pain, although they are usually needed at least every two to three hours. Third, antacids have a more prolonged effect when taken after food (food also neutralizes the acidity of the stomach for a while) so it is useful to take an antacid about an hour after meals, as well as every two to three hours thereafter. Fourth, acid secretions may increase at night, so a double dose of antacid and, sometimes, an antispasmodic drug at bedtime is often recommended.

Composition and side effects of antacids

Antacids come in a wide variety of compositions with different tastes and different prices. Most antacids contain one or more of the following salts: magnesium, calcium, or aluminum. Because magnesium salts usually cause diarrhea when taken alone (for example, Milk of Magnesia is an antacid, but is more commonly used as a laxative!), and calcium and aluminum salts cause constipation on their own, the majority of antacids are made up as mixtures to avoid both side effects. Often, however, this does not work and some experimenting with several antacids may be necessary to prevent constipation. Sodium bicarbonate is an effective antacid but cannot be used on a regular basis because it is absorbed and could cause problems with retention of salt and alkali.

There is some argument about using the antacid·calcium carbonate (Dicarbosil and Titralac). It is very effective in neutralizing acid, but once the effect wears off there is increased acid secretion. If taken regularly, this isn't a problem. Sometimes extra calcium from the antacid can be absorbed, although this rarely causes difficulties unless a person drinks large quantities of milk over a long period, in which case deposits of calcium may form around bones. Taking diuretics such as hydrochlorothiazide (Esidrix or HydroDIURIL) with an antacid can lead to an increase in the level of calcium in the blood.

Antacids are also used for simple gastric upset after a heavy or spicy dinner or too much alcohol (heartburn, acid indigestion), and more often than not they effectively relieve the symptoms. In conditions of hiatus hernia (where the stomach protrudes slightly through the diaphragm) and of acid reflux stomach acids often travel up into the esophagus (gullet) and can cause belching and heartburn, especially at night. These symptoms are often completely relieved by the use of antacids after the evening meal and at bedtime, along with the precaution of not reclining until at least three hours after eating and raising the head of the bed. In kidney failure, certain antacids containing aluminum, e.g., Basaljel and Amphojel, are used to prevent accumulation of phosphorus, since they bind it in the intestine and prevent it from being absorbed.

Drug interactions Because they act to protect the stomach lining and neutralize acids, many antacids prevent absorption of drugs, so that one should avoid taking other drugs at the same time—any additional medication should be taken on an empty stomach between antacid use.

New drug In 1977 a new drug was introduced which has tended to revolutionize the treatment of ulcer in several European countries as well as in the United States. This drug, Tagamet (cimetidine), is known as a *"histamine-2" receptor antagonist;* it prevents the secretion of acid after stimulation of the stomach by food, alcohol, caffeine, and other agents. It has been found to be highly effective in preventing ulcer on a short-term basis but its long-term effectiveness and its effects after its intake has been stopped are still somewhat controversial. It has been hailed as a revolution since it often frees the person suffering from ulcer from the need to take frequent antacids, which in itself has been a bothersome problem. However, in many cases, antacids are used or recommended in addition to the cimetidine therapy. One possible disadvantage of cimetidine is that experience with its use is limited and, in some cases, some serious adverse effects have been suggested including loss of white blood cells and possibly decreased sperm count. The significance of these and other effects and the long-term usefulness of this new drug remain to be established.

Antispasmodic drugs Antispasmodic drugs such as tincture of belladonna or Pro-Banthine are also useful in ulcer therapy to decrease spasm of the stomach and also to partially block the oversecretion of acid and pepsin. Antispasmodic drugs are likewise used in similar disorders where increased stomach or bowel spasm is a problem—an exception being hiatus hernia and acid reflux, which may be made worse by antispasmodics.

A large number of antispasmodic drugs are available, most of them acting as anticholinergic drugs (drugs which block the effects of the parasympathetic nervous system); they block signals to the vagus nerve, which increases acid secretion and contraction of the stomach. These antispasmodic, anticholinergic drugs act elsewhere in the body, and along with effects on the stomach they may cause dryness in the mouth, blurring of vision, and difficulty with urination at higher doses. Since a person can seldom feel the effects of medication on the stomach, the presence of a dry mouth is usually a good indication that the drug is working and is used as such. These drugs are normally taken before meals and/or at bedtime. The bedtime dose may be most useful as it slows down the stomach and can help retain the antacid over a longer period of time, decreasing the need for antacids in the middle of the night. Antispasmodic drugs may cause retention of urine in men with prostate trouble, so they are used with caution, if at all, in elderly men. They can also counteract the drugs used in glaucoma, so are likewise used cautiously in that condition.

Listed below are some of the drugs commonly prescribed for nausea, stomach upset, and ulcers. Those with an asterisk are individually described in Part 3.

Amphogel	Combid*	Mylanta
Antivert*	Compazine*	Pro-Banthine*
Basalgel	Donnatal*	Tigan*
Bentyl*	Gelusil	TUMS
Bentyl Phenobarbital	Maalox	Librax*
Bendectin*		

Constipation Constipation, commonly defined as difficult, infrequent evacuation of the bowel, has been a preoccupation of advanced societies for years. For a long time, daily evacuation of the bowels was believed to prevent virtually all disease, but we can now be absolutely certain that good health does not require regular bowel movements at fixed times. Normal bowel function can range from three bowel movements a day to three a week or even less.

The last few decades have seen a dramatic decrease in the routine administration of cathartics (purgatives) by the medical profession, but self-prescribed laxatives are still widely used by the general public, and a large majority still remain bowel conscious. This is confirmed by the availability of more than 700 different laxative products on which over $400 million is spent annually. General misconceptions about normal bowel function and extensive advertising by pharmaceutical manufacturers contribute to the overuse, misuse, and abuse of self-prescribed laxatives.

Causes   Simple constipation most frequently results from the wrong sort of diet and/or insufficient intake of liquids, sometimes from a change in habits because of travel, and perhaps from insufficient exercise. Laxatives are rarely necessary for the relief of simple constipation. Relief can be achieved by changing to a better quality diet which includes foods with a higher fiber content, drinking more liquids, and by responding promptly to the urge to evacuate the bowels.

Constipation may result from disease, e.g., hypothyroidism (decreased thyroid function), cancer of the colon, and some types of depression. It may also be caused by many drugs, including certain antacids, narcotic analgesics (such as codeine), anticholinergics, antispasmodics, some tranquilizers and antidepressants, and preparations containing iron.

Laxatives, cathartics, purgatives   The terms laxative, cathartic, and purgative are often confused: all three describe agents that act to bring about a bowel movement, but they differ in degree of action. A cathartic is slightly more active than a purgative, but the two terms are relatively interchangeable since both rapidly produce bowel evacuation and a definite change in stool consistency, the feces often becoming watery. These actions are less pronounced in the case of a laxative, although a sufficiently large dose of laxative can product a cathartic effect.

Laxatives can be classified in several groups:

1. Bulk-forming laxatives
2. Stimulant laxatives
3. Lubricants (mineral oil)
4. Stool softeners

The various frequently prescribed laxative products are discussed below in the appropriate category, although it should be noted that some products contain more than one type of active ingredient.

Bulk-forming laxatives   Bulk-forming laxatives promote bowel evacuation (bowel movement) by softening the stool and by increasing its mass through their ability to attract water and retain it in the stool.

The increased bulk of the stool usually increases the frequency of bowel movements. These laxatives are generally not absorbed from the gut and do not appear to have any influence on the absorption of nutrients from food. They are considered the safest laxatives. A bulk-forming laxative may take from one to three days to have an effect, so that to maintain a consistent result, it should be taken three or more times a week.

The major precaution to observe when taking any bulk-forming laxative is to take adequate fluid with each dose (at least eight fluid ounces of water) to ensure that the laxative does not form a hard, obstructing lump in the intestinal tract.

Bulk-forming laxatives come from two main sources. The least costly source is crude dietary fiber, including bran, whole fruits, leafy vegetables, raw carrots, and whole-grain breads. Most others are made from semisynthetic cellulose derivatives, such as psyllium (obtained from Plantago seed) and methylcellulose.

Common bulk-forming products include Dialose, Effersyllium, Hydrocil, Metamucil, and Serutan. All work in a similar way; the major differences between them lie in their cost, and selection of one or the other is a matter of personal preference.

Stimulant laxatives Stimulant laxatives increase the wavelike (peristaltic) contractions of the intestinal musculature which push the bowel content along. These drugs were so-named because it was believed that, besides having a direct effect on the muscles of the intestine, they also stimulated the nerves of the gut and irritated its lining. But stimulant laxatives also cause more fluid to enter the intestine, which in itself will provoke increased peristalsis. Therefore the exact way in which stimulant laxatives cause evacuation of the bowel is not completely known.

The potency of different stimulant laxative products varies greatly according to the response of the individual. A bowel movement usually occurs after about six hours. Stimulant laxatives should be used only occasionally and never more than daily for one week to relieve simple constipation. If stimulant laxatives are used for a long period, normal bowel function can be lost and the individual may become dependent on the drug for bowel evacuation.

Side effects Noticeable side effects of these laxatives include intestinal cramps and burning, diarrhea, and depletion of body water (dehydration). Some stimulant laxatives are eliminated by the kidneys after absorption from the gut and can produce colored urine. In general terms, these laxatives are considered the least desirable because of their unpleasant side effects and their tendency to alter bowel function after extended use.

Medications Bisacodyl (Dulcolax) is a stimulant laxative available only on prescription in either tablet or suppository form. The suppository induces a bowel movement approximately 15 minutes after insertion, while tablets usually produce an effect overnight—6 to 12 hours after being taken. To avoid irritation of the stomach lining caused by premature dissolving, Dulcolax tablets must be swallowed whole—not chewed—and should not be taken within an hour of taking antacids or milk.

Many stimulant laxative drugs are derivatives of a substance called anthraquinone, a family of natural ingredients which includes cascara sagrada (literally "sacred bark," from the buckthorn tree, *Rhamnus purshiana*), senna (dried leaflets of the cassia plant), and aloe (a leaf extract). Similar to these natural forms is a synthetic compound, danthron (Dorbane, Modane). Danthron tablets are available without prescription and, like Dulcolax, must be swallowed whole. Common anthraquinone laxatives include Black Draught, Carter's Little Pills, Cas-Evac, Fletcher's Castoria, and Senokot.

Phenolphthalein is another type of stimulant laxative compound and is a common ingredient of many products, including Ex-Lax, Feen-a-Mint, Phenocal, and Veracolate.

Saline laxatives Saline laxatives, such as Milk of Magnesia, are chemical salts that hold water within the gut, thereby indirectly stimulating peristalsis. A bowel movement usually occurs within one or two hours after a sufficient dose of the laxative has been taken. Saline laxatives can be regarded as safe and effective *only* when used occasionally. Continuous use for more than a week may cause serious side effects, mainly as a result of dehydration and/or loss of essential minerals.

The commonest saline laxatives are Milk of Magnesia (magnesium hydroxide suspension), Epsom Salts (magnesium sulfate), Fleet's Phospho-Soda (sodium phosphate), and Sal Hepatica (more than 50% sodium biphosphate). Citrate of magnesia (magnesium citrate)—often used to clear the bowel prior to x-ray examination—should be stored in a refrigerator to slow down decomposition, but in general these products are relatively stable and require no special storage.

Side effects Magnesium contained in saline laxatives can be absorbed into the blood and may produce undesirable effects. For example, in patients with kidney disease, the magnesium can build up to toxic levels in the body and cause depression of the central nervous system (sedation and confusion) and weakness of the skeletal muscles. These preparations should therefore be avoided by people with inadequate kidney function.

Sodium can be similarly absorbed, so that laxatives containing sodium chloride, e.g., Fleet's Phospho-Soda or Sal Hepatica, should be avoided by patients with any illness that requires a restriction of salt intake, including heart conditions, or any diseases involving edema or high blood pressure.

Lubricant laxatives Mineral oil, the common lubricant laxative, is a colorless, tasteless mixture of liquids that has enjoyed popular use as a laxative. Whether it lubricates the intestinal tract is not known, but the oil softens the stools and makes them easier to evacuate. Mineral oil preparations are nonirritating and absorbed only in very small quantities. The usual dose is one or two tablespoons taken at bedtime on an empty stomach.

Side effects With proper and careful use, mineral oil produces few side effects, but several problems can arise through its use, so preparations that include it should be strictly reserved for very occasional use. In theory, if lubricant laxatives are taken while there is food in the stomach the mineral oil in them could impair the absorption of fat-soluble nutrients, including vitamins A, D, E, and K. Also, a common annoyance, especially with excessive quantities, is oozing of the oil from the anus. Anal irritation may occur as well.

A significant problem can arise if mineral oil is given to someone who is prostrate: the oil may be aspirated (inhaled into the lungs) and cause the serious condition of lipid (fat) pneumonia. Aspiration is most likely to occur in very young, debilitated, or elderly bedridden people, and for such patients mineral oil is best avoided. Whenever mineral oil is used, every precaution should be taken to ensure that it is completely swallowed and is not likely to be regurgitated (a good reason for not taking mineral oil late at night).

Mineral oil is available in simple forms or as an emulsion in products such as Agoral, Haley's M-O, and Kondremul. Emulsification reduces the size of the oil droplets and enhances penetration of the oil into the feces, but at the same time it increases intestinal absorption of the oil. Emulsions are usually taken twice daily, one dose on rising and one at bedtime, but never at mealtimes. All the precautions mentioned earlier also apply to emulsions of mineral oil.

Mineral oil should not be given at the same time as stool-softening laxatives, which may enhance absorption of the oil.

Stool softeners Stool softeners are the most recently developed type of laxative. Their detergent action facilitates the penetration of intestinal fluids (primarily water) into the stool, which is thus softened and so passes out of the bowel more easily. The effects of stool softeners are apparent for only one to three days after ingestion, so for beneficial and consistent effects they should be taken at least three times a week, but not for long, continuous periods. These laxatives should be used only occasionally for simple constipation and, in any event, no more than daily for one week.

Side effects At present, only occasional, insignificant side effects have been attributed to stool softeners; however, these drugs are believed to have some action on the lining of the intestine that enhances the secretion of water. This would aid the laxative effect but might also affect the absorption of other compounds (as has been demonstrated with mineral oil). Stool softeners may well interact with other drugs and affect absorption of some nutrients.

Stool softeners are available in forms suitable for rectal or oral administration. The usual daily dose is between 100 and 250 mg, but the dose should generally be the smallest possible that produces the desired effect.

The most frequently prescribed laxatives are stool softeners. Dioctyl sodium sulfosuccinate (known by the brand names Colace, Doxinate, and Peri-Colace, or as D.S.S.) is the most popular stool-softening drug. It is marketed by numerous pharmaceutical companies in various strengths and in capsule, solution, and syrup forms. These preparations can also be bought over-the-counter from pharmacies under their generic name, with a substantial saving in cost over the better known brand preparations of the same drug. For example, Colace and Doxinate, two of the most frequently advertised and prescribed brand-name preparations of dioctyl sodium sulfosuccinate, cost about seven times as much as the same drug sold under its generic name.

Side effects Peri-Colace is a combination product that contains 100 mg of dioctyl sodium sulfosuccinate plus 30 mg of the anthraqui-

85

none stimulant laxative casanthranol (Peristim): the idea is to combine the stool-softening and stimulant properties of the two ingredients. The undesirable feature of Peri-Colace, as with most other combinations, is that both ingredients are always present and must be taken together, even if one effect is not required. The potential dangers of chronic abuse of stimulant laxatives, which have already been mentioned, apply equally strongly to casanthranol in this combination. In addition, Peri-Colace is one of the most expensive laxatives available. The rational approach is to use a stimulant or saline laxative as required and to add dioctyl sodium sulfosuccinate only when really needed.

Drugs for diarrhea Diarrhea can be defined as the passage of bowel movements with increased frequency and with increased water content. Normal bowel movements contain approximately 60 to 70% water, but in the case of diarrhea they contain as much as 80 to 95% water. When diarrhea occurs, there is usually an increase in the wavelike contractions (peristalis) of the circular muscles of the bowel walls that rush food and fluids through the gastrointestinal tract. This prevents nutrients from being properly digested and absorbed into the body and accounts for the increased fluid and undigested food particles in the stools.

Causes
Causes of diarrhea include bacterial and viral infections, parasite infestations, diseases of the intestine (e.g., ulcerative colitis), and hormonal disturbances, to name just a few. Diarrhea is often accompanied by loss of appetite, abdominal cramps due to contractions of the bowel and trapped gas, and nausea and vomiting, also due, in most cases, to increased muscle contraction. Irritants or toxins from bacteria are frequently the cause of the increased contraction, as in traveler's diarrhea or food poisoning.

Increased stress can also cause intermittent diarrhea, as can certain foods in certain people. For example, a percentage of the adult population lacks the enzyme that digests milk products normally, and this often causes diarrhea when they are consumed. In these cases, simple avoidance of milk products will prevent diarrhea. Other foods, such as coffee (in excess), or spicy or fatty foods may also produce diarrhea. Sometimes diarrhea occurs as a side effect of certain drugs as well. It can also occur due to an irritant in the bowel that may signal a serious ulcer, or even tumor. This is one of the reasons diarrhea should be evaluated if it persists for more than 2 to 3 days.

Another reason that persistent diarrhea requires medical attention is that it can cause significant loss of water and salt from the body producing dehydration. This is particularly true of infants and elderly persons. Diarrhea may also prevent absorption of certain drugs, such as oral contraceptives or anticonvulsants, so that loss of their effects can occur. The experience of diarrhea is quite uncomfortable, unsociable, and often embarrassing, so that immediate symptomatic relief is often sought.

Antidiarrheal preparations act to decrease diarrhea in two general ways. One type of product, which includes drugs such as Kaopectate, acts to increase the bulk of the stool and it may also absorb some of the toxins contributing to the increased movement or irritability of the bowel. The other type of drug, of which Lomotil is an example, tends to decrease contractions of the bowel, acting directly on the bowel muscle and thus slowing the movement of material through the gastrointestinal tract. These drugs all provide relief of symptoms but do not usually affect the cause of the diarrhea.

Side effects Prolonged use of an antidiarrheal preparation without identification of the underlying cause may result in serious complications. For this reason, taking drugs for symptomatic relief of undiagnosed diarrhea for more than two days is not recommended; after that amount of time, proper examination by a physician is advisable. All of the products listed below provide purely symptomatic relief and should not be used for more than two to three consecutive days without a physician's directions.

Listed below are some of the drugs commonly prescribed for diarrhea. Those with an asterisk are individually described in Part 3.

Donnagel*   Lomotil*   paregoric
Kaopectate*

Hormonal Drugs

A hormone is commonly defined as a substance or chemical produced in the body by organs called the *endocrine glands* (hence the name *endocrinologist* for a medical specialist dealing with gland troubles). The endocrine glands include the thyroid gland, the parathyroid glands, the adrenal glands, the pancreas, the ovaries, and the testes. The hormones produced by these glands, e.g., the thyroid hormone made by the thyroid gland, are released into the bloodstream and travel to other organs and tissues to regulate or modify their function. Thus, thyroid hormone regulates the speed of metabolism of most cells; insulin from the pancreas regulates the use of sugar by the cells; and estrogen from the ovaries helps to regulate the menstrual cycle.

The amounts of hormones released by the endocrine glands are very carefully controlled, in most instances by the so-called master gland, or pituitary. This gland is located at the very center of the head, at the base of the brain behind the nose and eyes. It releases special hormones (called *tropic* hormones) that travel to the various endocrine glands instructing them to release their own hormones in certain quantities. Some of these tropic hormones are actually used as drugs or clinicians use them as tests for gland function. An important example is ACTH (*adrenocorticotropic hormone*), the hormone that stimulates the adrenal gland to release cortisone-like hormones.

The pituitary gland, in turn, gets its signals from the *hypothalamus,* a part of the brain that monitors the hormones circulating in the blood. If the hormone level is low, signals in the form of a special type of hormone travel to the pituitary gland causing it to release tropic hormone. The tropic hormone then travels to the gland where the deficient hormone is generated, signaling it to produce more. If the level of a certain hormone is high or if a hormone is used in high doses in a drug, the pituitary gland signals the appropriate endocrine gland to decrease its production of that hormone. After prolonged periods of this condition, the gland may become less active (atrophy) and require weeks or months to recover its full function. The general scheme thus comprises a full feedback cycle and allows for very careful regulation of hormone levels.

Uses Hormones are prescribed for two general purposes. First, they are used as replacement therapy to provide normal hormone levels when a gland such as the thyroid has been removed or when a gland is malfunctioning. In diabetes, for instance, the pancreas cannot produce enough insulin. In general, hormones are given in doses similar to those normally produced in the body and at the same time they are normally secreted. Cortisone, for example, is released by the adrenal glands in the morning, so it is usually given at that time. Replacement therapy is used to make up for deficient thyroid, adrenal, ovarian (estrogen and progesterone), testicular (androgen or testosterone) and pancreatic secretions. The parathyroid hormone is not usually given because it regulates calcium metabolism, and calcium can easily be prescribed instead. The most common deficiencies are those of the thyroid, insulin, and female hormones; these are discussed further in the following essays. Deficiencies of other, much less common, hormones are not discussed here.

The second type of hormone therapy involves use of a hormone in higher-than-usual (pharmacological) doses as a drug. Synthetic hormones resembling cortisone, e.g., prednisone, are most commonly used in this way. Many uses of estrogen, including oral contraceptives, also fall into this category (see *Oral contraceptives,* page 96; *Estrogens and progestogens in hormone therapy,* page 97). This type of therapy *does* tend to interfere with normal gland function through the feedback cycle described earlier: the monitor in the brain registers high hormone levels and the pituitary generates signals to the primary glands to decrease their function. For example, when oral contraceptives are taken the ovaries get smaller, and it may take weeks or months for them to return to normal function after the hormone intake is stopped.

Drugs for thyroid disorders The primary function of the thyroid gland (located in the neck in front of the windpipe) is to produce the thyroid hormone *thyroxin*. Thyroxin is made from a simple amino acid and iodine. This is one reason why the proper amount of iodine in the diet is critical. Thyroid hormone circulates through the entire body and acts on most cells to regulate their metabolism, or turnover of oxygen and nutrients. In the fetus it may also affect the development of certain organs including the brain. Diseases of the thyroid may or may not cause changes in the amount of thyroid hormone produced.

Treatment When the body produces an excess amount of thyroid hormone, *hyperthyroidism,* a person may feel continually warm, sweaty, and shaky, and may experience diarrhea, nervousness, palpitations, and changes in the skin or hair. This is usually the result of increased function of the gland, which is often enlarged. The most usual treatments are radioactive iodine therapy or surgery to remove part of the gland. Occasionally certain drugs are used either prior to surgery or alone in an attempt to control the disease. If surgery is planned, iodine or iodide solution is sometimes used along with one of the anti-thyroid drugs, either propylthiouracil or Tapazole (methimazole). Occasionally, when the symptoms are very severe, the drugs propranolol (Inderal) or guanethidine (Ismelin) have been used for short periods of time to decrease palpitations and nervousness.

Undersecretion of thyroid hormone, *hypothyroidism,* is due either to removal of the gland or to a decrease in its function. This condition can result in slowed metabolism, causing lethargy or tiredness, increased sensitivity to cold, constipation, and dullness or dryness of the skin or hair. When this is discovered, usually by a blood test to measure levels of thyroid hormone in the blood, thyroid hormone is given as replacement therapy. If true deficiency is established, it is usually taken for life.

For many years, thyroid hormone was derived from the dehydrated thyroid glands of cows or pigs, and thyroid pills were the primary drug used. Although the amount of thyroid hormone present in the medication was tested, the actual amount tended to vary from lot to lot. Thus, when purified thyroxin (used in Synthroid) became available more recently, it quickly became the preferred form.

Side effects Thyroid therapy has unfortunately found use in many programs for weight loss since the thyroid hormone increases metabolism and the rate at which foodstuffs are used by the body. In all cases, except where true hormone deficiency has been found by blood tests, the use of such therapy is inappropriate and can cause problems, especially if there is a risk of heart disease.

Listed below are some of the drugs commonly prescribed for thyroid disorders. Those with an asterisk are individually described in Part 3.

Cytomel*   Synthroid*   thyroid*
Proloid*   Tapazole

Drugs for diabetes Diabetes mellitus is a complex disease associated with two major abnormalities. First, it is characterized by high blood sugar (hyperglycemia) and other changes in the use of foodstuffs due either to a lack of the hormone insulin or an inability to use it normally. (Insulin is manufactured in the pancreas.) Second, diabetes is usually accompanied by an abnormality of tiny blood vessels throughout the body, which over long periods of time produces abnormalities of many organs, such as the eyes, the kidneys, and nerves.

There are two very general types of diabetes that differ considerably in their severity, treatment, and the age at which people begin to be affected by them. Classic diabetes, associated with a partial or complete lack of insulin, usually starts (often abruptly) before the age of 30 or 40 and requires insulin therapy. For this reason it is often termed *insulin-dependent diabetes.* It is also called *juvenile diabetes* (or juvenile-onset diabetes) because it often starts in the teenage years. This type of diabetes is more likely to be associated with a very serious condition called *ketoacidosis* (usually requiring hospitalization) that may occur with stress, infection, or inadequate insulin therapy.

The other, much more common, type of diabetes is due not necessarily to an absolute lack of insulin, but rather to a dysfunction of the pancreas in releasing insulin and/or an inability of the body to use the insulin properly. It is often termed *maturity-onset* or adult-onset diabetes because it is more often seen in people over the age of 40, particularly in people who are overweight. Only 10 to 20% of the people with this type of diabetes actually require insulin, and sometimes only when they become ill from another cause. In most cases diabetes can be treated by diet and weight loss, although for certain people oral antidiabetic drugs may be required. People suffering from this type of diabetes seldom get out of control with ketoacidosis and seldom require hospitalization for their diabetes, except when there are late-stage complications such as foot ulcers and arteriosclerosis.

Treatment   The treatment of diabetes has several goals, some readily achieved, others more difficult. The two major objectives are to allow a person to live a relatively normal life and to live a normal life span with few complications. There is considerable controversy among experts in diabetes as to which goal is more important, since there is a potential conflict. Normalization of activity and diet may or may not prolong life. Conversely, procedures such as a strict diet, which are aimed at control of diabetes, are believed to prolong life and prevent complications but they may interfere with what we think of as a normal life. Actually, most regimens address both goals and try to achieve a happy medium, however, each individual's situation needs to be discussed with a physician.

Most specific treatment of diabetes attempts to prevent the following:

1. The "spilling" of excess sugar into the urine, accomplished by regulation of the diet, and/or the use of insulin, and/or the use of antidiabetic drugs
2. Infection, prevented by adequate vaccination, avoidance of people with infectious diseases, and special regard to hygiene
3. Excess lowering of blood sugar, or hypoglycemia
4. Arteriosclerosis and vascular changes associated with many of the longer-term problems, such as foot disorders and arterial blockage

There is considerable argument over whether or not there should be close control of the amount of sugar in the blood, although most experts agree that continual spillage of sugar in the urine is not desirable. After food is eaten, it is converted in part to sugar that travels throughout the body to the cells where it provides energy. But this sugar cannot easily enter a cell without help from the hormone insulin, released from the pancreas shortly after food is eaten. If the amount of insulin in the system is inadequate, or if the cells are unable to make use of the sugar, it will remain in the blood and its level will be higher than normal for several hours after eating. The presence of high levels of sugar in the blood is known as *hyperglycemia*. When the blood sugar level becomes very high, excess sugar will spill over into the urine, where its presence is usually a good indication of a diabetic problem. Only rarely is sugar in the urine a sign of a "leaky" kidney.

Sugar that goes into the urine is accompanied by a certain amount of body water that dilutes it. But if the blood sugar stays high and sugar and extra water continue to be excreted in the urine, a person can lose too much water and thus become dehydrated. This extra water loss can result in increased thirst and intake of fluids and, consequently, increased urination. If this cycle continues, a person's body metabolism changes to get energy from other foodstuffs, sometimes resulting in the beginnings of ketoacidosis—one of the most serious complications of diabetes. Therefore, it is usually agreed that the amount of sugar spilled in the urine should be kept to a minimum.

Urine testing To avoid excessive spilling of sugar, most diabetics are taught to check their urine for sugar with tablets (Clinitest) or paper strips (Diastix or Tes-Tape). In the presence of certain drugs, such as vitamin C in high doses (more than one gram per day) or the antibiotic Keflex, Clinitest tablets can give a false positive result, so Tes-Tape or Diastix must be used. Sometimes they are also asked to check for acetone (an early sign of developing ketoacidosis) with Ketostix, Acetest, or Keto-Diastix. In people with insulin-dependent diabetes, urine testing may be done frequently; it is usually checked less often in most adult-onset diabetics. The testing and the expected results should be thoroughly understood by the patient. Most physicians ask the diabetic to keep a chart to monitor therapy, as this is the best way to establish correct doses of insulin or other drugs.

It is not known how helpful it is to lower blood sugar that is higher than normal but not high enough to cause spillage into the urine. Regulating the diet, the mainstay of all diabetic therapy, will often prevent blood sugar from becoming excessively high, but in insulin-dependent diabetics, insulin is also required. When insulin is used to regulate the blood sugar, there is a danger that the blood sugar will drop too low (hypoglycemia) and cause an insulin reaction. Most physicians prefer to regulate the diet and to use insulin or oral drugs in doses sufficient to prevent the spilling of large amounts of sugar into the urine (the majority of diabetics do occasionally spill sugar) without lowering the blood sugar level so far as to cause frequent hypoglycemic attacks.

Diet therapy Because diabetes is a disease of metabolism and limits the flexibility of the body in handling various foodstuffs, the base of all therapy and a prerequisite for either insulin or oral antidiabetic therapy is a well-rounded controlled diet. The specifics of diet therapy are discussed in many books on the subject and should be well understood by the diabetic. Suffice it to say that diabetic diets aim to maintain optimum body weight (which usually entails reducing for adult-onset diabetics, who are frequently overweight) and to provide the necessary carbohydrates, fat and protein while preventing the development of hyperglycemia, ketoacidosis, or hypoglycemia.

Insulin therapy Before the 1920s, the outlook for people with insulin-dependent diabetes was very bleak. The discovery that this protein hormone could be extracted from the pancreases of pigs and cows and used in treatment was a great medical advance. There have been many refinements since and insulin is now available in several forms, primarily differentiated by their speed of onset and length of action. The short-acting "regular" insulin is commonly used when treatment is first started and during stress or illness, usually in the hospital. For chronic or long-lasting therapy, intermediate-acting forms of insulin are used (e.g., NPH or Lente), which often require only one injection a day. Longer-acting insulins are infrequently used. Insulin is measured by units—a unit standing for a certain amount of a biological activity (its capacity to lower blood sugar levels).

Because insulin is destroyed in the stomach it must always be given by injection, usually into the fatty (subcutaneous) tissue of the arms or legs. Local itching and redness may occur when insulin injections are first started, but this usually disappears within a few weeks. The patient is taught to rotate injection sites to prevent damage to the skin.

Insulins are available in three concentrations: U-40, U-80 and the newer, more concentrated U-100. To help avoid errors or confusion over the various concentrations of insulin, it is now generally being recommended that all diabetics convert to U-100 insulin, which has specially measured syringes.

Dosage In prescribing insulin, the physician must determine the best type of insulin for that individual (i.e., intermediate-acting or "regular," short-acting insulin) as well as establish the proper dose and schedule for use. With three meals a day, the blood sugar will rise three times a day, the level depending on how much is eaten and how much insulin is available. Frequently, a person is put on a dose of intermediate insulin, such as NPH, which is injected in the morning. It begins to act in two hours on the blood sugar produced by digestion of breakfast and has its peak of action eight to ten hours later, near the time of the evening meal. If a person eats no lunch, then the blood sugar may get so low that a *hypoglycemic reaction,* with symptoms of shakiness, dizziness, lightheadedness or sweating, may occur. This is always treated by taking some type of readily available sugar—a sugar cube, orange juice, or a candy bar—the only instance where such high-sugar food is permitted for a diabetic. A diabetic on insulin is usually advised by his physician to carry some source of readily available sugar for this purpose. In some cases, a shorter-acting, regular insulin is given in the morning to cover the effects of breakfast and lunch. Occasionally, good control is obtained only when insulin is given twice daily. *This must always be determined individually,* usually using urine testing as a guide. The requirements of any individual tend to stabilize, but may change with diet, exercise and the presence of infection.

Oral therapy   In the early 1960s the introduction of a new group of drugs, some chemically related to sulfa drugs and thiazide diuretics, promised the potential of oral therapy for diabetics that would eliminate the need for insulin. Two general types of drugs were introduced: the *sulfonylurias,* such as Orinase (tolbutamide), Tolinase (tolazamide), Diabinese (chlorpropamide), and Dymelor (acetohexamide), which act to enhance the action or secretion of insulin; and the *biguanides,* including phenformin (DBI), which act on the metabolic processes to decrease resistance to insulin action. These agents were used very widely in the 1960s, especially in older patients, before it was generally recognized that elevation of blood sugar is often part of the aging process and does not always need treatment. In many cases it was found that these drugs were not useful for true insulin-dependent diabetics, but only for maturity-onset diabetics.

In the 1960s a large study of these drugs was undertaken to see if they were more effective and safer than diet alone or insulin with a diet. The results have been the source of great controversy. The study suggested that the drugs were no more, and possibly less, effective in preventing the long-term complications of diabetes—stroke, heart attack, and arteriosclerosis—than other traditional therapy. Many have criticized the design of the study and its findings are still debated, but it did cause many physicians to look critically at their prescription of these drugs and generally to limit use to a select group of persons who could not or would not control their diet, or who could not take or did not require insulin. The biguanides (phenformin or DBI) have been particularly criticized. Although they are effective in lowering blood sugar, they are also associated with producing a special complication called *lactic acidosis* that requires careful surveillance by the physician. A well-regulated diet must usually accompany their use. In the absence of food, they can also cause excessively low blood sugar levels (hypoglycemia). Recently the

95

government asked for an orderly withdrawal of DBI from the market, since it was felt that the risks involved outweighed its potential benefits, particularly in the light of other alternatives.

Listed below are some of the drugs commonly prescribed for diabetes. Those with an asterisk are individually described in Part 3.

Diabinese*   regular insulin*
NPH Insulin*   Tolinase*
Orinase*

Oral contraceptives Oral contraceptives have been taken by women in the United States since 1960. Although there are several types of contraceptive pill, the most common and most reliable is the type containing a combination of two synthetic female hormones, an *estrogen* and a *progestogen*. This combination-type pill, if taken regularly as directed, is almost 100% effective in preventing pregnancy.

The estrogen-progestogen pill The female menstrual cycle is regulated by several hormones and by interactions among these hormones. Estrogen and progesterone (to which the synthetic progestogens are related) are produced in the ovaries. The production of these hormones is stimulated by hormones from the pituitary gland, located at the base of the brain. Once the supply of hormones secreted by the ovary reaches a certain level, the supply of the stimulating pituitary hormones is depressed, working in a feedback system.

The minute amounts of additional estrogen supplied by oral contraceptives inhibit the production by the pituitary of the hormone that stimulates the growth, in the ovary, of the follicle containing the egg. The progestogen inhibits another pituitary hormone that triggers ovulation—the release each month of an egg from an ovary. With no ovulation taking place, conception is impossible.

If by some remote chance an egg is produced, additional safeguards will stop a pregnancy. The progestogen contained in the pill causes a thickening of the mucus in the cervical canal so that sperm cannot enter the uterus. Yet another effect of the pill is to alter the lining of the uterus so that it would not be receptive to a fertilized egg in any case.

The estrogen-progestogen pill is taken for 21 days (sometimes a day more or less, according to the brand), starting on the fifth day of the menstrual cycle. (The first day of bleeding is counted as day 1.) The pill is then stopped for a week. Within a few days of stopping the pill, menstruation begins. The amount of bleeding may be less than in a normal period, a fact which explains why women on the pill are less likely to suffer from iron deficiency than women who do not take the pill. Many women who have had irregular periods in the past may experience an improvement in regularity, and some women with acne find that the condition improves after they begin taking the pill.

Side effects Women taking the combined estrogen-progestogen pill have reported a variety of side effects, including increased weight, depression, reduced sexual desire, cramps in the legs, and dryness in the vagina. Women who wear contact lenses after using the pill for several months may find that their eyes become dryer and more sensitive to the lenses. Each individual may react differently to different contraceptives. A woman's doctor may need to change the prescription once or twice to find one that minimizes the side effects. However, the body often needs a couple of months to adjust to this almost daily administration of extra hormones. Therefore, if side effects are present but not severe, it may be worthwhile to try a product for at least three cycles before changing to a different product.

More serious adverse effects are also possible. The most serious is the risk—a relatively low risk—of *thrombosis*. Thrombosis is the formation of a blood clot, usually in the deep veins of the leg or in the pelvis. If a clot forms and moves to the lungs, where it could cause a blockage called a *pulmonary embolism,* death may result. In rare cases, another type of thrombosis may occur in the blood vessels supplying the brain to produce a stroke. A variety of other dangerous side effects have now been reported. They include high blood pressure, serious eye changes, diabetes, hyperglycemia (high levels of sugar in the blood) and vascular tumors of the liver. In women over the age of 35, the risk of adverse side effects is sufficiently large for many doctors to recommend alternative methods of contraception. These adverse effects include gallbladder disease and heart attacks (especially in heavy smokers).

Although the theory has not been conclusively proved, it is now believed that the estrogen in the pill may be the cause of these risks. Accordingly, doctors now tend to prescribe contraceptives containing the minimum effective dose of estrogen—50 micrograms or less. Whether this dose does in fact decrease the risk is not yet known.

The progestogen pill Some women, however, are at risk from taking any amount of additional estrogen. For women who have had a thrombosis, or who have some heart conditions, liver disease, or a history of liver disease, another kind of oral contraceptive may be prescribed. One alternative is a pill containing only progestogen. This pill is taken every day, instead of just for three weeks of the cycle, and it must be taken at the same time every day (whereas the estrogen-progestogen pill is effective even if 36 hours elapse between taking one pill and the next). The progestogen-only pill works mainly by building up the sperm-deflecting mucus in the cervical canal; it apparently does not prevent ovulation. Even if the pill is taken every 24 hours, there is still a slightly greater risk of pregnancy than with a pill containing estrogen and progestogen. There are also some side effects, notably irregular and heavy periods.

A third type of oral contraceptive, the sequential type, is no longer prescribed in the United States. Each packet of sequential contraceptives contained some estrogen-only pills, to be taken on the first 15 days of the cycle, and some combined estrogen-progestogen pills to be taken on the following five to seven days.

Precautions All women should have a complete physical examination before starting the pill so that subsequent measurements, such as blood pressure, can be compared with the original ones. The leaflets provided with packets of pills ("patient package inserts") explain the symptoms that you may observe while taking the pill and distinguish between those that are minor and those that should be reported to your doctor. For example, any increase in the frequency of headaches or pains in the legs or chest should be reported. The pill will be stopped if your blood pressure rises, if vision becomes disturbed, or if migraine or jaundice develops.

Although many women become pregnant soon after stopping the pill, a few have experienced difficulty. This difficulty is unrelated to the length of time the pill has been taken; it seems rather to be more common among women who started menstruating relatively late and had irregular periods. After a few months the reproductive organs and the pituitary gland will, in most cases, have adjusted to the loss of the extra hormones and will begin once more to function normally.

Listed below are some of the commonly prescribed oral contraceptives. Those with an asterisk are individually described in Part 3.

Brevicon
Demulen 21*
Enovid
Loestrin
Lo-Ovral*
Micronor
Modicon
Norinyl 1/50 21*
Norinyl 1/80 21
Norlestrin 21*
Nor-Q.D.
Ortho-Novum*
Ortho-Novum
  1/50 21*
Ortho-Novum
  1/80 21*
Ovral*
Ovral 28*
Ovulen 21*

Estrogen and progestogen therapy In the last 15 years or so, female hormones also have been widely used for reasons other than contraception, the most common example being estrogen for the treatment of postmenopausal symptoms. Premarin, an estrogen preparation marketed almost exclusively for this purpose, is one of the most frequently prescribed drugs of any type. The wisdom of this widespread use is now being questioned, due to increased awareness of potential problems with long-term use of the estrogens. Clearly written brochures (patient package inserts) on the benefits and risks of such medication have been ordered by the government to be given with each prescription. These leaflets should be carefully read. If you have any further questions, discuss them fully with your doctor.

Menopausal symptoms The female menopause or "change of life" is a period of time usually occurring between the mid-40s and early 50s when the ovaries begin to lose their ability to produce estrogens

99

and progesterone. As a result, ovulation and menstrual periods usually become irregular, less frequent, and finally cease. The decrease in the level of female hormones is registered by the feedback system and, in an attempt to compensate, the pituitary gland releases increased amounts of the tropic (stimulating) hormones, FSH and LH, in order to stimulate the unresponsive ovaries more strongly. This process may occur over months to years. The same situation takes place, but more abruptly, when ovaries are removed surgically. The menopausal symptoms, which may or may not occur, are believed to be related to those changing levels of hormones in the blood.

The symptoms experienced in the menopause vary considerably in frequency, severity, and duration. In addition to changes in menstrual periods, there are often "hot flashes" or flushing, depression or irritability, and mood changes, especially in the early stages. As the menopause progresses, a reduction in vaginal secretions may produce irritation during intercourse and predispose to bladder irritation. Approximately 25% of women (usually white women) experience loss of bone (called osteoporosis) and may be more susceptible to fractures, especially of the spine.

Estrogen therapy It has been common practice in the United States until very recently to give estrogen to almost all women with menopausal symptoms. This practice has recently been strongly challenged by the findings that use of estrogens in this way increases the risk of cancer of the uterus, and a considerable controversy has arisen.

The proponents of continued therapy contend that estrogens can markedly improve the quality of life of a woman beset with hot flashes and mood changes, and most importantly, prevent spinal and other fractures that may be crippling.

The opponents of estrogen therapy primarily cite the fairly well-established increased risk of cancer of the uterus, the potential for adverse cardiovascular effects such as thrombophlebitis (inflammation of the veins associated with blood clotting), and the risk of heart attack or stroke that have been reported in older oral contraceptive users. It is also noted that the risk of osteoporosis is limited to only a certain proportion of women.

As yet, no simple answer has emerged from this controversy, but it has served to stimulate more individualized therapy, which is desirable in any case. For example, many women, especially later in the menopause, will have essentially no symptoms except dryness of the vagina. This is most easily relieved by local hormone therapy, an estrogen-containing vaginal cream. This treatment can entirely remove the symptoms, while introducing only small amounts of estrogen into the body.

It is generally felt that estrogen therapy in the menopause should be directed at relieving specific symptoms such as hot flashes or preventing specific problems such as osteoporosis. In young women whose ovaries have been removed surgically, estrogen therapy is usually begun and continued until the usual time of menopause. Both in normal women and in those who have had their ovaries removed, the goal is to gradually decrease the dose and eventually discontinue the drug. An exception may be those predisposed to osteoporosis, but this also remains controversial. It should be considerably clarified when better methods are found of measuring the bone changes indicative of early osteoporosis.

Estrogen therapy for postmenopausal symptoms is usually given in a cyclic fashion, that is, for three to four weeks, followed by a week off the drug, since this somewhat resembles a normal cyclic sequence and may be less likely to predispose to uterine cancer. Common estrogen preparations used include Premarin, conjugated estrogens, and Estinyl. Some physicians will add a progesterone-like drug at the end of the cycle, to more closely imitate the normal cycle, but the real value of this remains unclear.

Estrogens are also used for other purposes. For example, they can be used to regulate irregular menstrual cycles, to treat a disease called endometriosis and to prevent pregnancy after rape (DES has been approved for this use). They are also used in two specific types of cancer therapy: cancer of the breast in certain postmenopausal women and cancer of the prostate in men.

Side effects Estrogens may have a variety of side effects, which are discussed in detail in the section on *Oral contraceptives,* page 96. They may cause weight gain, breast enlargement, and some gastrointestinal distress. On a longer-term basis, they may predispose to gallbladder disease, blood clots in the legs, and other circulatory problems. Because of the many side effects, the pros and cons of estrogen therapy should always be discussed with the doctor and a regular exam, including a breast check and Pap (Papanicolou) smear should be done every six to twelve months after stopping therapy.

Progesterone Progesterone is the other major female hormone, but it has been much less in the public eye than the estrogen hormones. Progesterone and progesterone-like drugs, called progestogens, are similar in chemical structure to estrogens, but they have somewhat different actions and are thought to have many fewer side effects than estrogens. This fact has stimulated some interest in the progestogen-only birth control pills (Micronor, Nor-Q.D., and Ovrette), but they are somewhat less effective in preventing pregnancy and have caused bleeding between cycles ("breakthrough bleeding"). Progesterone has also been incorporated into an intrauterine device (IUD), the Progestasert, but, although it may be more effective than an ordinary IUD, the fact that it must be reinserted periodically has limited its use.

Other, relatively specialized, uses of progesterone are to treat abnormalities of the menstrual cycle or cancer of the breast or uterus. Very rarely, because it stimulates breathing, progesterone is used to treat severe lung disease. Preparations commonly used include progesterone, hydroxyprogesterone (Delalutin), medroxyprogesterone (Provera), and norethindrone (Norlutin).

Listed below are some of the commonly prescribed estrogens and progestogens used in hormone therapy. Those marked with an asterisk are individually described in Part 3.

DES   Premarin*   Provera*
Estradiol

Steroids, or cortisone-like drugs Cortisone and related steroids resembling the hormones produced by the adrenal gland were introduced as "miracle drugs" for arthritis over 20 years ago. Subsequent experience reveals that the miracle carried a very high price in the form of severe side effects. The cortisone-like drugs (called corticosteroids, or simply steroids) have now gained widespread use, but their proper role remains a subject of much controversy.

Properties The paired adrenal glands, located one on top of each kidney, are stimulated by a hormone from the pituitary gland, ACTH (adrenocorticotropic hormone), to secrete several steroid hormones: cortisone, hydrocortisone, and small amounts of male and female hormones, as well as other hormones. The corticosteroid hormones are classified according to two types of activity: *glucocorticoid activity,* the ability to affect the metabolism of sugar (glucose); and *mineralocorticoid activity,* the ability to affect levels of the minerals sodium and potassium. Cortisone and hydrocortisone each exhibit some of both properties, and this double activity not only accounts for their usefulness as medication, but also explains their side effects. many synthetic steroid hormones have properties similar to the natural hormones cortisone and hydrocortisone, and some, such as prednisone, are more frequently used.

Uses The corticosteroid hormones are used both for replacement therapy when the adrenal glands are not functioning (as in Addison's disease) and in higher doses for drug therapy in a variety of diseases. In replacement therapy, the naturally occurring hormones are most commonly used. In drug therapy, such synthetic corticosteroids as prednisone, methylprednisolone (Medrol) or triamcinolone (Kenalog) are used, partly because their less pronounced mineralocorticoid effect results in fewer problems of salt retention, edema, and potassium loss.

Corticosteroids have a broad spectrum of effects on the body, some very powerful in treating diseases, and some equally powerful in causing severe unwanted side effects and reactions. The primary useful effects are associated with the glucocorticoid activity. They include suppression of inflammation (redness and swelling of an area), useful in such diverse conditions as poison ivy and poison oak; ulcerative disease of the colon (ulcerative colitis); and various types of acute arthritis. Other effects include a decrease in scar formation and a decrease in immunity to infection, which although normally hazardous, also has a use in suppressing rejection by the body's immune system of a transplanted organ. In many cases, corticosteroids are used without a clear understanding of exactly how they work, although they are clearly known to be successful. They have been used in a very wide variety of acute and chronic diseases. The list is long: rheumatoid arthritis; certain collagen diseases such as lupus erythematosus; certain types of chronic hepatitis; serious skin diseases such as psoriasis; acute severe bronchial asthma; and blood diseases such as leukemias. In addition, they have been used to treat shock and certain neurological diseases such as multiple sclerosis, where their effectiveness is a matter of debate.

Adverse effects The many significant adverse effects of these hormones when used in high doses are clearly related both to the dose and to the duration of treatment. For example, a few days of even relatively high-dose therapy will rarely cause problems. But if therapy extends beyond one to two weeks, problems invariably begin to appear. The glucocorticoids, in excessive doses, usually cause a variety of metabolic changes. The blood sugar often increases, bringing out diabetes in those predisposed to it. The body fat deposits become gradually redistributed: the face often becomes rounded into a "moon face," a "buffalo hump" may appear on the back of the neck, and fat may accumulate in the abdominal area. There is usually a weight gain, although this is partly due to the mineralocorticoid effects of salt and water retention. The decreased immunity, although useful in preventing rejection of transplants, can also increase susceptibility to many types of infection, e.g., tuberculosis and fungal infections. The suppression of scar formation, useful in some situations, can also cause easy bruising and thin tissues that heal poorly. Corticosteroids make the protective mucus lining the stomach thinner, predisposing it, many experts believe, to peptic ulcers and bleeding. For this reason antacids are frequently given along with steroid therapy. Because corticosteroids also affect calcium metabolism, high dosages over a long period of time will weaken the bone structure and predispose to fractures, especially in the spine. There are also effects on the brain, so that persons receiving moderate doses (e.g., 15 to 25 mg of prednisone a day) may feel in a better mood. High doses often produce mental symptoms such as hallucinations, but these are reversed by decreasing the dose.

Those corticosteroids with mineralocorticoid effect—hydrocortisone and prednisone, for example—can also cause salt and water retention (and thus swelling of the hands and feet) and loss of the mineral potassium, bringing about weakness. The frequent practice of treating the edema or swelling with diuretics (see *Diuretics,* page 63) may compound the problem as they too may cause potassium loss.

It is apparent that because of these adverse effects, corticosteroids used other than locally or for short periods (less than 7–10 days) are ideally used only when less toxic drugs are ineffective and/or therapy is life-saving. A final condition further emphasizes this need for caution.

Adrenal arrest As is the case with other hormones, a high level of adrenal corticosteroid hormone will cause the master gland, the pituitary, to decrease its secretion of ACTH (adrenocorticotropic hormone), the hormone that stimulates the adrenal gland to produce the corticosteroid hormone (see *Hormonal drugs,* page 87). If a steroid is given at high levels for a long time, the adrenal glands gradually shrink owing to lack of stimulation, and after a time stop working. Therefore, once corticosteroids have been taken for longer periods (greater than two to three weeks) they must be withdrawn gradually to allow the adrenal gland to recover. If steroids such as prednisone have been taken for months or years, it may take several months to completely discontinue the drug safely. A person on corticosteroids for long periods should wear appropriate identification since in a time of stress, such as an auto accident or surgery, he may need extra steroids to prevent serious complications.

Fortunately, it was discovered several years ago that in many cases it is possible to give certain corticosteroids every other day and get almost the same beneficial effects while avoiding, not only most of the side effects noted above, but also the shrinkage and loss of function of the adrenal glands. This method offers obvious advantages and has been very useful in certain diseases, especially in children. In other types of diseases, however, such as some cases of severe rheumatoid arthritis, this method has not been successful.

Ways of administering steroids

Corticosteroids can be given by mouth, by injection, as enemas (for ulcerative colitis), in the eyes (for inflammation), or applied to the skin (steroid creams and ointments are one of the most frequently used dermatological drugs). Recently, they have been used as aerosols (Vanceril, or beclomethasone) in the treatment of chronic asthma. They are used locally by injection into joints or into other inflamed areas such as large acne lesions. The overall principle has been to use corticosteroids locally when possible, and in high doses for short periods. The pituitary gland hormone ACTH, which stimulates the adrenal gland to produce steroids, is sometimes administered by injection in place of the corticosteroid hormones although usually the corticosteroids are preferred. More often, ACTH is used to test the adrenal gland for its level of functioning. In summary, corticosteroid hormones have occasional use in replacement therapy but extremely wide use as drug therapy for many ailments of many organs. The problems corticosteroids can cause emphasize the critical

105

need for careful cost/benefit analysis whenever their long-term use is considered.

Listed below are some of the commonly prescribed steroids, or cortisone-like drugs. Those marked with an asterisk are individually described in Part 3.

Decadron   Medrol*   prednisone*

Weight Loss

Obesity—excess body fat—is a common problem in our over-fed Western society. Most of us eat more and exercise less than we should, and the result is often excess pounds. Severe obesity, besides being unattractive, may be dangerous. Many doctors now believe that the obese person has a decreased life expectancy and a greater than average chance of contracting diabetes, gallstones, cardiovascular disorders and orthopedic problems—although the extent to which obesity contributes to these disorders is debated.

The possible health hazards of obesity and the desire to be more attractive induce millions of overweight people to try reducing techniques of various kinds. A seemingly endless number of treatments for obesity have been announced in the popular press, each heralded as the ideal method. These include radical diets consisting of only a few specific foods or liquids; various kinds of psychotherapy, including aversion therapy and hypnosis; medical treatments using hormones and other drugs; and even surgical procedures such as wiring the jaw shut, removing part of the intestine, or actually removing the fatty tissue in certain areas.

Some overweight people believe that their problem has a glandular (endocrine) cause. In fact glandular disorders account for only a small fraction of all cases of obesity. A sudden increase in appetite or weight is sometimes associated with decreased function of the thyroid gland, a disorder of the adrenal glands, or some other endocrine disturbance. But the great majority of overweight people acquire their excess pounds gradually through habits of overeating that often begin in childhood. The overeating may have a psychological cause, and in such cases some form of psychotherapy may help the person to get at the root of his problem.

The only method of losing weight safely and maintaining the reduced weight is to reduce one's intake of calories by eating less and adhering to a balanced diet low in starches, sweets, and fats. "Crash" diets or radical diets may achieve a sudden weight loss, but they fail to establish a healthy pattern of food intake needed for maintaining the reduced weight. This kind of diet is almost invariably followed by an eating spree and, consequently, a weight increase.

Many drugs have been used in the treatment of obesity. None have been shown to be consistently effective in producing lasting weight loss. Some are very hazardous.

Bulk fillers Among the most widely promoted weight-loss products are the *bulk fillers* and *expanders*. These are available over the counter, usually in the form of cookies or candies. They generally contain methyl-cellulose, a compound which expands in the stomach to give a sensation of fullness. These drugs are safe and do help to prevent constipation. They also help to curb appetite by creating a feeling that the stomach is full. They are customarily taken before meals with water. Whether their success is due to a decrease in appetite or to the psychological effect of simply "doing something" is not clear—possibly it's a combination of both.

Anorexiants A group of drugs frequently prescribed in reducing programs comprises the *anorexiants*. They include amphetamines and other similar drugs. The name anorexiant is derived from the medical term *anorexia,* which means loss of appetite; they can cause a loss of appetite for a period of a few days to several weeks. The drug itself has no direct effect on body weight; what it does is stimulate the central nervous system in such a way as to make you want less food. Soon, however, the body will develop a tolerance for the drug, and as the appetite-suppressing effect wears off, the person taking the drug will resume his or her former eating habits—unless he or she has, in the meantime, resolutely established a restricted diet. In other words, an anorexiant might help to launch a diet, but it will *not* do the work of dieting for the person hoping to lose weight.

Hazards of anorexiants The use of these drugs has more serious drawbacks. Because they tend to make the user feel alert and full of energy (although they make some people nervous and jittery), he or she may be tempted to increase the dose as time goes on, in order to regain the original euphoric effect that the original dose no longer provides. A habit of dependence is quickly established. Side effects of the anorexiants include rapid heartbeat and increased blood pressure. These characteristics make them especially hazardous for people suffering from heart ailments or hypertension.

The amphetamines are particularly dangerous in terms of their addictive potential. Widespread abuse of drugs in recent years has led to their being classified by Federal law as restricted drugs. The number of amphetamines prescribed by doctors and the number kept in stock by pharmacists must be reported and must not exceed certain limits. By law, package inserts on amphetamines must bear the following warning:

Amphetamines have a high potential for abuse. They should thus be tried only in weight reduction programs for patients in whom alternative therapy has been ineffective. Administration of amphetamines for long periods of time in obesity may lead to drug dependence and must be avoided.

Diuretics Diuretics are drugs that rid the body of excess water, and in the process cause it to lose some weight. Women who have been prescribed a diuretic to relieve premenstrual swelling and discomfort sometimes use the drug to help them reduce, and some doctors prescribe a diuretic in the first few weeks of a weight-reducing program. However, a diuretic has no effect on fat, and the long-term use of diuretics in reducing programs can be hazardous, because they deprive the body of necessary minerals such as potassium. They have no place in legitimate weight-reducing programs.

Thyroid hormone Preparations containing the thyroid hormone are often prescribed inappropriately by weight-control clinics to promote weight loss. When there is an excess of thyroid hormone (which occurs when the thyroid gland is overactive) the body's metabolism is speeded up, causing it to burn up more calories; despite an increase in appetite, weight loss will occur. Other effects of this condition (called *hyperthyroidism*) are nervousness, irritability, diarrhea, and increased heart rate. The same symptoms may be produced if a large dose of the hormone is taken. If someone has been taking a thyroid preparation and suddenly stops taking it, he or she may experience a temporary state of *hypothyroidism,* or abnormally low thyroid activity, with its accompanying symptoms of fatigue, sleepiness, and sluggishness. Thus, weight reduction with thyroid preparations can be hazardous. These drugs should be used only when the person is suffering from hypothyroidism and not simply for weight control. (See *Thyroid disorders,* page 89.)

HCG   Another hormone often used in reducing clinics in the U.S. is human chorionic gonadotropin (HCG) which is produced during pregnancy by the placenta and is similar to a pituitary hormone. Its weight-reducing properties—if any—have not been clearly established. Most clinics giving HCG injections also put their patients on a very strict low-calorie diet, which will in itself cause weight loss. When the treatment is stopped the patient often quickly regains the lost weight.

To sum up, drugs have very limited usefulness in weight reduction programs. A balanced, low-calorie diet is the only sure, safe way to lose weight.

Listed below are some of the drugs commonly prescribed for weight loss. Those with an asterisk are individually described in Part 3.

amphetamines	Fastin*	Tenuate*
Dexedrine	Ionamin*	
Dexamyl	Ritalin*	

Asthma and Lung Disease

To understand how drugs for lung disease work, we must first look at the way the lungs themselves work. Each lung contains a system of tubes called *bronchi* and smaller tubes called *bronchioles* that branch out from the *trachea,* or windpipe. The bronchioles end in clusters of tiny sacs called *alveoli.* The thin walls of the alveoli contain minute blood vessels that absorb the oxygen in the air we breathe into our lungs. Red blood cells carry the oxygen to other parts of the body and bring back to the lungs the waste product carbon dioxide, which is released when we breathe out. Because this oxygen-carbon dioxide exchange is essential for life, the airways of the lungs must always be kept open.

Bronchial constriction   In some respiratory diseases—notably asthma, but also some cases of "reactive" bronchitis and emphysema—constriction of the muscular walls of the bronchioles causes them to contract and so restrict the passage of air. The reason for this constriction varies. It may be inhalation of cold air, of an irritant such as cigarette smoke, or of a substance to which the person is allergic, such as pollen or cat fur; or it may be emotional stress. The resulting bronchoconstriction is indicated by the symptom of wheezing—a high-pitched whistling sound caused by the air trying to get through narrowed airways.

Narrowing of the airways also occurs in bronchitis, a disease in which repeated infection causes scarring that constricts the bronchial tubes. In emphysema the lung tissues lose their elastic quality, so that when the person breathes out, some bronchioles may close, trapping air in the lungs. Unfortunately, because both emphysema and chronic bronchitis bring about a permanent change in the small bronchial tubes, neither condition responds as effectively to drug therapy as does asthma, in which the constriction of the bronchial tubes is due to temporary spasm.

Bronchodilators Most drugs used to open the airways of the lungs act on the muscles in the bronchial tubes. Called *bronchodilators,* they include epinephrine (adrenaline), theophylline, Tedral, Marax, and Isuprel. It is believed that most of these drugs achieve their results by regulating the amount of a hormone-like substance called *cyclic AMP* in the bronchial muscles. An increase of cyclic AMP causes the muscles to relax; when the substance is used up, the muscle tends to constrict again.

One group of bronchodilators relaxes the muscles by increasing the production of cyclic AMP. These are drugs related to epinephrine (adrenaline), such as ephedrine, Brethine, Bricanyl and Alupent. If these drugs are used continually, the body may develop resistance, or tolerance, to their effects, and they will become less useful. They can also have adverse effects: an increased heart rate, palpitations, high blood pressure, trembling, and dizziness.

Another group of bronchodilator drugs acts in a preventive way by inhibiting the breakdown of cyclic AMP in the bronchial muscles. This preventive action has the same result as the increased production of cyclic AMP caused by the first group of drugs; by maintaining the level of cyclic AMP, it helps the muscles to relax. This second group of drugs includes theophylline and other similar drugs. Adverse effects of these drugs are rapid heart rate, loss of appetite, nausea, and vomiting.

Bronchodilators can be taken in a number of ways. Most of them are available in inhalers, which permit small droplets of the drug to be inhaled through the mouth into the bronchial tubes. This is probably the quickest, but not necessarily the most efficient, way to get the drug where it is needed.

Bronchodilators are also given orally, by injection, and, in the case of theophylline, even as rectal suppositories.

A third group of drugs acts by preventing bronchoconstriction from occurring in the first place. For example, in cases of asthma caused by an allergic reaction, some antihistamines and other drugs such as Aarane and Intal (cromolyn) will block the constrictive action of histamine on the muscles and reduce the severity of an attack. However, they are not effective against all substances causing an allergic reaction.

Steroid therapy In cases of severe asthma one of the cortisone-like drugs such as prednisone may be prescribed. These drugs are thought to act to increase the effectiveness of the bronchodilator drugs and also possibly to prevent recurrent attacks of the disease. They belong to a group of drugs called steroids (see *Steroids, or cortisone-like drugs,* page 102). Prednisone is usually taken orally, either for a short period with the dose tapering off gradually or for a longer term in a low dosage. Another type of steroid recently put on the market is administered by inhaler and is called Vanceril.

It is important to remember that the immediate causes of bronchoconstriction can vary considerably. A person can be breathing completely normally, and then come in contact with something that causes his bronchial airways to close suddenly. Naturally, the wheezing and difficult breathing that result can be alarming, and he must be prepared for it—by learning from his doctor how to use the drugs that have been prescribed for him, how long they take to act, and exactly how much should be used and how often. Excessive use of either inhalers or oral drugs may cause more harm than good and make subsequent therapy more difficult.

Listed below are some of the drugs commonly prescribed for asthma and lung disease. Those with an asterisk are individually described in Part 3.

Aarane	Bronkosol	Quibron*
Alupent	Elixophyllin*	Tedral*
Aminophyllin*	Intal	theophylline
Bricanyl	Marax*	Vanceril

Infections

Simply stated, an infection is the invasion of the body by disease-producing microorganisms, such as bacteria, viruses, protozoa, and fungi. Infections can be local, as a boil on the skin or pneumonia in the lungs, or general, as is common with typhoid, mumps, or malaria, which affect many parts of the body. The symptoms of and the damage caused by an infection are the result of both the microorganism's invasion of tissue and the response of the body's defense system. The most common signs of infection are inflammation (pain, heat, redness, swelling, and pus production) and fever.

Not all microorganisms produce infections, and even those that can, called *pathogenic* (disease-causing) microorganisms, do not do so all the time. Those bacteria better at breaching the body's defense mechanisms are more likely to cause disease and are described as *virulent*. Most virulent are the bacteria that cause cholera and typhoid fever; they almost always bring on severe infection if they enter a person who has not been immunized. Other types of bacteria are completely harmless and may even be beneficial, such as certain ones that live in the gastrointestinal tract or those that rarely cause infection, like the *Lactobacillus bulgaricus* strain found in yoghurt.

The fewer bacteria present, the lower the likelihood of infection. This is why it is advisable to cleanse and cover open wounds or cuts. The location of the bacteria also affects their ability to cause infection. Under normal circumstances, with good standards of hygiene, the bacteria in the air and those that colonize the skin, the mouth, and the intestines are harmless. The response of each individual to potential invaders differs according to the state of the body's defense mechanisms—the *immune system*, comprised of natural antibodies, antibodies that result from vaccination, and white blood cells called *phagocytes* that "eat" foreign organisms. When infection occurs, more phagocytes are produced and sent through the bloodstream to the site of the problem.

Resistance to infection may be decreased by frequent bouts of disease or by certain drugs that reduce the effectiveness of the immune system. People who have received kidney or other organ transplants and those taking anticancer or cortisone-like drugs may become infected on exposure even to small numbers of pathogenic organisms.

In summary, whether infection occurs depends on the balance among these factors: the virulence, numbers, and location of the microorganism, and the resistance of the individual. All of these factors should be kept in mind when a specific treatment or prevention plan is developed.

Prevention of infection

Prevention of infection may involve a variety of measures:

1. Lowering the numbers of microorganisms by keeping the skin clean, using antiseptics (agents to prevent the growth of microorganisms), and administering antibiotics before surgery
2. Decreasing exposure to pathogenic organisms through quarantine, isolation, or avoidance of infected people
3. Increasing the individual's immunity by vaccination

Treatment

Treatment of infection through medication aims to decrease the number of microorganisms or to eliminate them without significantly harming the host (the infected person). By this means, the host can recover or continue to fight the few remaining organisms. Treating infections in people with very low resistance is much more difficult, and direct aids to the body's defenses, such as a transfusion of extra white blood cells, may be necessary.

Some infections are easier to treat than others. Those caused by bacteria, e.g., "strep throat" (a streptococcal infection), bladder infection, and bacterial pneumonia, are often readily treated with antimicrobial drugs. In contrast, most viral infections, e.g., measles, mumps, herpes simplex (cold sores), encephalitis, and the common cold, are either difficult or impossible to treat, although some symptoms, such as fever, can be treated. Between these extremes are infections caused by fungi and parasites, which are sometimes easily treated and sometimes not; these are discussed later.

Antibiotics Infections caused by microorganisms (microbes) are treated with *antimicrobial drugs,* among them antibiotics and sulfa drugs (discussed later). Antibiotics are themselves produced by microorganisms; they can be obtained from molds or other microorganisms and are then purified or modified for therapeutic use. For centuries it was known that certain moldy materials were useful in treating local infections such as boils. But not until 1928 did Alexander Fleming discover that the mold *Penicillium notatum,* which was growing accidentally in a bacterial culture, could kill bacteria. Following this chance observation, the active substance was identified and called penicillin. But penicillin was not tested in humans until 1941. This date marks the beginning of the present antibiotic era of drug treatment.

After sedatives and tranquilizers, antibiotics are today among the most frequently prescribed drugs; they account for up to one-third of some hospital pharmacy budgets. They can be used both to treat and to prevent infections caused by bacteria, but they are essentially ineffective against viruses and effective against only certain parasites and fungi. Antibiotics may be *bactericidal* (they kill the bacteria) or *bacteriostatic* (they stop bacterial multiplication). They act in conjunction with the body's defenses to overcome infection. In serious infections, their timely help is essential to redress the balance in favor of the host and provide a chance for him to recover.

Some antibiotics are very specific: they kill some kinds of organisms, but not others. These antibiotics are classified according to the type of bacteria they affect; bacteria, in turn, are classified according to whether they can be dyed with a particular microscopic stain, Gram stain. Those that take up the blue dye are called Gram positive (one example is *Streptococcus,* which causes strep throat); those that do not and appear red under the microscope are called Gram negative (e.g., *Salmonella,* which causes food poisoning). Bacteria are also classified according to shape into, for example, *cocci* (round) and *bacilli* (rod-like). An antibiotic that is effective against more than one such category, for instance, an antibiotic that kills both Gram-positive and Gram-negative bacilli, is described as a *broad-spectrum antibiotic.*

Many common infections, such as strep throat, local infections of the hands and feet, and gonorrhea, are known to be sensitive to particular antibiotics. Strep throat is almost always treated with penicillin, except in people who are sensitive to penicillin, for whom erythromycin is usually substituted. Bacteria may also be collected from an infected area or from the urine, cultured, and tested for their sensitivity to a range of antibiotics (a procedure often abbreviated to C & S). In this way, the antibiotics most likely to be effective can be identified. In chronic infections, as those in the bladder, sensitivity testing is very helpful because the bacteria may have become resistant to the antibiotic normally used.

Administration Antibiotics are given systemically by injection and by mouth, as well as locally on the skin, in the eye and elsewhere. Because many common antibiotics, such as tetracycline, are not well absorbed into the bloodstream if taken with food, most oral antibiotics should be taken on an empty stomach. Many oral antibiotics, however, may cause diarrhea, because the drug kills some of the beneficial bacteria in the gut. This side effect is not usually a major problem, but in certain cases, for instance with clindamycin (Cleocin), diarrhea can be a serious problem and any occurrence should be brought to the doctor's attention.

Antibiotics for treating infections are usually taken for at least five days, and more often for eight to ten days. Completion of the course of treatment is extremely important, even though the patient may often feel better, with a normal temperature, after two or three days. If the medication is not all taken, any surviving but temporarily subdued bacteria may later cause a recurrence of the infection. Worse, the bacteria may develop a partial immunity to that particular antibiotic, making future treatment more difficult.

Antibiotic groups   Specific antibiotics and their characteristics are discussed under their individual names in Part 3, but the common antibiotics can usefully be considered in groups, for several reasons:

1. Antibiotics in the same group often act in a similar way.
2. If an allergy or immunity exists to one antibiotic in a group, it will often transfer to other antibiotics in the same group.
3. In some cases, the major difference within a group may be cost; if this consideration arises, checking with your physician may be worthwhile.

The major, most commonly prescribed antibiotics are described in this book, although in some cases only the generic forms have been fully dealt with since the brand-name preparations are identical.

Other Antimicrobial Drugs

Sulfonamides (sulfa drugs)   Certain antimicrobial drugs cannot be obtained from molds or other organisms. But, although the means of production are different, the reasons for using these drugs, their mode of action, and the duration of therapy are the same as for antibiotics. Sulfa drugs (properly called *sulfonamides*), first used clinically in 1935, were derived from dyes produced in Germany in the early 1900s.

Sulfa drugs were once widely used against bacterial infections and provided the first effective method of treating certain diseases, such as gonorrhea and bacterial meningitis.

But, for a variety of reasons, their use declined with the advent of penicillin and the subsequent development of other antibiotics such as chloramphenicol (Chloromycetin) and chlortetracycline (Aureomycin). Nevertheless, many sulfa drugs (notably Gantrisin), are still widely used in treating bladder and urinary-tract infections.

Sulfa drugs, including the combination preparation co-trimoxazole (discussed below), are usually taken in the form of rather large pills washed down with lots of water to counteract the drug's slight tendency to recrystallize, which could damage the kidney. This precautionary measure is always important, although the problem is less likely to occur with some newer sulfonamides.

Other antibacterial agents
In the late 1960s it was discovered that an unrelated antimicrobial agent, trimethoprim, increased the effectiveness of sulfonamides. Accordingly, a combination called co-trimoxazole (Bactrim, Septra), consisting of trimethoprim plus a sulfonamide, has recently been introduced. This combination drug reduces the chance that bacteria will become resistant to the antimicrobial action, a problem that has been quite common with sulfa drugs. This ability to overcome resistance makes co-trimoxazole especially useful in treating chronic bladder infections, but the product seems to have a broad range of other uses, too. Most recently, efforts are being made to market trimethoprim alone. Another frequently prescribed major antibacterial drug is the antiseptic nitrofurantoin, or Macrodantin. It is used to treat protracted urinary diseases that do not respond to other medication.

Antiviral drugs
Very few drugs are effective in treating viral infections. The only antiviral preparation with any wide use is idoxuridine (Stoxil), and that is used only for a particular type of eye infection. Amantadine (Symmetrel), a drug used for Parkinson's disease and as an antiviral agent, has been found to be useful in preventing the severity of symptoms of certain types of influenza. Considerable research is being carried out to find clinically useful antiviral agents, and hundreds of chemicals, both naturally produced and synthetic, are being tested. Unfortunately, doctors often come under pressure to "prescribe something" when patients come in with valid complaints, such as chest colds. Antibiotics are sometimes prescribed, *but they have absolutely no effect on the virus.*

Antifungal drugs
Fungal infections within the body are fortunately uncommon, for they are extremely difficult to treat, but those on the

skin or nails, or in the vaginal region, are susceptible to direct treatment. Such local fungal infections tend to persist or recur, and, in many cases, treatment must continue for lengthy periods. For example, griseofulvin, the oral antibiotic used to treat fungal nail infections, often needs to be taken for six months to a year. Tolnaftate (Tinactin), one of several antifungal drugs applied locally to treat common fungal infections of the skin (e.g., athlete's foot), commonly needs to be used regularly for 10 to 14 days to assure success. Other antifungal drugs, including the antibiotic nystatin (Mycostatin), are discussed further in the chapter on *Skin and local disorders,* page 125.

One other often-prescribed antimicrobial drug deserves mention. Since its usefulness was discovered in 1960, metronidazole (Flagyl) has found an established place in the treatment of vaginal infections caused by the common protozoan *Trichomonas.* This is discussed further in the chapter on *Skin and local disorders,* page 125. More recently, metronidazole has been found effective in other parasitic and bacterial infections.

Listed below are some of the drugs commonly prescribed to treat infections. Those with an asterisk are individually described in Part 3.

Achromycin-V*	Gantanol*	Pediamycin*
Amcill*	Gantrisin*	penicillin G*
Ampicillin*	Garamycin*	penicillin VK*
Amoxil*	Ilosone*	Pentids*
Ancef	Keflex*	Pen-Vee-K*
Azo Gantrisin*	Keflin	polycillin
Bactrim	Laratid*	Principen
Cefadyl	Macrodantin*	Robitet*
Chloromycetin	Minocin*	Septra*
E.E.S.*	Mycolog*	sulfasoxisole
E-Mycin*	Mycostatin	Sumycin
Erythrocin*	Mysteclin-F*	tetracycline*
erythromycin*	Omnipen	V-Cillin-K*
		Vibramycin

Coughs and Colds

The common cold is undoubtedly man's most widespread affliction, a source of general inconvenience and loss of work. Unfortunately, partly due to the fact that colds are caused by viruses—and for most viral illnesses, no effective drugs are available—the successful prevention, cure, or even shortening of the duration of colds, is somewhere in the future. The alleged (and much publicized) ability of vitamin C to prevent or cure colds, still a matter of controversy,and the role of antibiotics such as penicillin, which have no effect on the true common cold, will not be discussed here. For the present, therapy is aimed at relieving the very typical symptoms, which may vary in severity from person to person or from one episode to another.

Literally hundreds of drugs are available by prescription or over-the-counter for the treatment of colds and related problems such as hay fever and sinusitis. Many of the drugs, especially combination products, are aimed at several or all of the symptoms. Therefore, it will be useful to define the symptoms and see how they can be relieved by this multitude of remedies.

Characteristically, the symptoms of a cold start with either the fairly sudden onset of sneezing and a runny nose or a tickling or a soreness at the back of the throat. Fever, headache, general aching, a husky voice or laryngitis, sore throat, and a few days later, a cough are apt to follow. The symptoms may continue for as long as 7 to 14 days. A closer look at these symptoms will reveal why certain drugs are included in the medications commonly used.

Congestion Certain other disorders—especially hay fever—have many similar symptoms and often are treated with the same drugs. Sneezing and a runny, stuffy nose, blocked ears and congested sinuses are characteristic of colds, hay fever (allergic rhinitis), and sinusitis. These symptoms are due to increased production of fluid and mucus and to swelling of the lining of the nose, the Eustachian tubes (which extend from the back of the throat to the ears), and the sinuses—hollow cavities that branch out from inside the nose above and below the eyes. Three kinds of drug relieve these symptoms: (1) decongestants, (2) anticholinergic drugs, and (3) antihistamines.

Drugs to relieve congestion The swelling of mucous membranes in the nose, sinuses, and Eustachian tubes is caused by the dilation of blood vessels in reaction to the viral infection or an allergen. Sometimes blood vessels will dilate from other causes, but the symptoms are the same. Decongestants decrease the swelling by constricting the blood vessels. These blood-vessel-constricting drugs, or *vasoconstrictors,* are found both in nasal sprays such as Afrin or Neo-Synephrine and in many of the cough/cold medicines such as Actifed, Sudafed, Allerest, Dimetapp, or Ornade. The common decongestant component of these mixtures includes such drugs as ephedrine, pseudoephedrine, phenylephrine, phenylpropanolamine, napthazoline, and oxymetazoline, to name a few. Although they are effective, these decongestants have some drawbacks. Used repeatedly, they begin to lose their effectiveness and greater amounts may be needed. Also, since they cause constriction of all blood vessels in the body, they often raise the blood pressure and increase the heart rate, a hazard for the person who has high blood pressure or is taking drugs for high blood pressure. These individuals should consult a physician before using decongestants.

If the runny nose and congested sinuses are due to an allergy, the release of a substance called histamine may be contributing to the overproduction of fluid and mucus. For this reason, antihistamine drugs such as methapyrilene, doxylamine, pyrilamine, brompheniramine, chlorpheniramine, and diphenhydramine found in a varity of cough/cold medications may be helpful in drying the secretions; however, they also reduce natural bacteria barriers and cause drowsiness. Secretions caused by a cold can be decreased if an anticholinergic drug—one which blocks the activity of the parasympathetic nervous system—such as atropine or belladonna alkaloid is used. But since most antihistamine drugs also have anticholinergic effects, making them effective for both colds and allergies, they are the drugs usually preferred. The majority of cough/cold preparations do contain either antihistamines or anticholinergic drugs.

Cough medications: suppressants and expectorants

Most people with a cold develop a cough, often several days later. A cough, essentially the rapid expulsion of air from the lungs, is a protective reflex intended to clear the bronchial tube of any foreign material, including mucus. In some cases, the airways are simply irritated and the cough is a reflex response. Drugs for coughs may act in two different ways: (1) simply to suppress coughing, or (2) to loosen or help liquefy the mucus in the lungs (an expectorant effect). Thus, an expectorant may either decrease or increase coughing! On the one hand, it stimulates coughing by loosening the mucus, on the other, it reduces the cough by decreasing the irritation caused by drying mucus. Cough suppressants, for their part,

119

can act either locally in the bronchial tubes to prevent irrita-tion or in the brain to suppress the cough reflex. Codeine is one of the most effective cough suppressants known; others include the non-narcotic drugs dextromethorphan (Romilar) and diphenhydramine, which is the antihistamine Benadryl. Although these medications are effective, it is not advisable to take cough suppressants unless coughing becomes repetitive and very bothersome, for a cough is a valuable protective re-flex which helps to get rid of mucus and prevents obstruction. In any case, cough suppressants should be taken for short pe-riods only.

The majority of cough medicines contain one or more drugs intended to help eliminate thick mucus or phlegm, among them terpin hydrate, glyceryl guaiacolate, benzoin, camphor, menthol, and iodides. Unfortunately, although the theory of expectorant action is good, it has been difficult to determine whether any of these drugs really functions in quite this way. The issue may be clarified in the near future, however, when the FDA completes its review of cough and cold medicines. In the meantime, it is likely that most cough syrups containing expectorants will continue to be used with the hope that they relieve some symptoms—although simply drinking adequate fluids may be sufficient to give the same expectorant effect. Whether the extra drug is worth the ex-pense remains to be seen.

A patient afflicted with a cold will usually experience one or two days of feeling tired, and may have headache, muscle aches, or back pains, which are also fairly typical of most other infectious illnesses. A drug that reduces these pains is therefore useful. The most common, aspirin and acetaminophen (Tylenol), reduce both pain and fever. One or the other of these may be included in cough/cold medica-tions, e.g., Phenaphen with codeine. Frequently, aspirin or acetaminophen, taken with lots of fluids and adequate rest, is the best medication for colds.

Listed below are some of the drugs commonly pre-scribed for coughs, colds, and sinus allergies. Those with an asterisk are individually described in Part 3.

Actifed*	Benylin Cough	Neo-Synephrine
Actifed-C Ex.*	Syrup*	nasal spray
Afrin*	Drixoral*	Novahistine-DH*
Ambenyl Ex.*	Naldecon*	Novahistine Ex.*

Ornade*	Phenergan VC Ex.*	Sudafed*
Phenergan Ex.*	Phenergan VC Ex. with	Tuss-Ornade*
Phenergan Ex.	Codeine*	
with Codeine*	Singlet*	

Antihistamines

Antihistamines, which are available over-the-counter or by prescription, have a variety of uses. First, they counteract congestion caused by allergic reactions, e.g., a stuffy nose or congested sinuses due to hay fever or other allergy (often, however, they are not very effective in allergic asthma). Second, they help relieve itching in skin eruptions, especially those due to an allery such as hives. Third, since they cause drowsiness, these preparations are also often used as tranquilizers or mild sleeping pills. Finally, antihistamines can act to decrease nausea and vertigo due to motion sickness and certain disorders of the inner ear.

Various applications The numerous applications of antihistamine drugs stem from the variety of pharmacologic effects that they share. The most important is their ability to block the effects of histamine, a substance released by the body in allergic reactions. Histamine can cause nasal stuffiness, itching and redness of the skin, and local swelling. Antihistamines are most effective when used prior to, or in anticipation of, an allergic reaction, or when used in a continuing allergic reaction such as hay fever or allergic sinusitis.

Antihistamines also cause varying degrees of drowsiness. This reaction is so common that certain antihistamines such as Atarax, Vistaril, and Benadryl are used as anti-anxiety or sleeping medication. In other situations, however, drowsiness may be undesirable, as it can interfere with the concentration needed for driving or operating machinery. Another unwanted effect of antihistamines in cough and cold remedies is that in drying up excess nasal secretions they may harm the lining of the nose and respiratory tract. Not only can this drying lower the body's defenses against infection, it can actually lead to increased congestion.

Antihistamines, especially Dramamine and Antivert, can be taken to overcome nausea and vertigo associated with motion sickness and certain disorders of the inner ear (e.g., Meniere's syndrome). They achieve this effect by acting directly on the brain.

121

In spite of their many effects, antihistamines are relatively safe drugs; however, it must always be borne in mind that they can themselves cause allergic reactions, that the drowsiness may be bothersome or even dangerous, and that the sedation is additive to other sedatives, tranquilizers, and alcohol. Antihistamines are generally inexpensive, especially in single generic ingredient forms. Combinations such as Ornade or Dimetapp are more expensive.

Listed below are some of the commonly prescribed antihistamines or antihistamine-containing drugs. Those with an asterisk are individually described in Part 3.

Actifed*	Dimetane Ex.*	Phenergan Ex. with
Actifed-C Ex.*	Dimetane Ex. DC*	Codeine*
Ambenyl Ex.*	Dimetane Tabs.*	Phenergan
Antivert*	Dimetapp*	VC Ex.*
Atarax*	Dramamine	Phenergen
Benadryl Cap./	Drixoral*	VC Ex. with Codeine
Tabs.*	Naldecon*	Polaramine Tabs.*
Benadryl Elixir*	Novahistine-DH*	Singlet*
Benylin Cough	Novahistine Ex.*	Teldrin*
Syrup*	Ornade	Tuss Ornade*
chlorpheniramine	Periactin*	Vistaril*
Chlor-Trimeton	Phenergan Ex.*	
Tabs.*		

Vaccines

Vaccines are not medicines, but a discussion of vaccines has nevertheless been included in this book since they are given to almost every individual in the United States at one time or another and play a vital part in maintaining good health.

Vaccines and antiserums are used to build immunity against infectious diseases caused by bacteria or viruses.

Active and passive immunity Two kinds of immunity can be produced. In *active immunity*, the vaccine stimulates the body to make antibodies against the bacteria, the toxins produced by bacteria, or the virus. If a person is then exposed to the infection, a protective mechanism already exists in the body to fight the disease. Such immunity will vary in duration, depending on the type of infection being prevented. It can last for many years (for example, seven to ten years with tetanus toxoid) or for a very short time (from weeks to months as with influenza vaccines).

Passive immunity is obtained when blood serum (the pale yellow fluid remaining after certain blood cells, clotting factors, and other elements, are removed from whole blood) containing antibodies (called an *antiserum*) is taken from another person or animal and given to the individual *after* he has been exposed to the infectious disease. For example, a course of injections of rabies antiserum is given if the patient has been bitten by an animal likely to be infected; tetanus antitoxin is given after the patient has received a potentially contaminated wound. Passive immunity serves either to prevent severe effects of the disease (as in rabies) or to counteract the toxin (as in botulism or tetanus). It lasts a very short time.

There are several types of vaccines. Some bacterial vaccines are made from small amounts of killed whole bacteria or from the toxins produced by bacteria (in which case the vaccine is called a *toxoid*). Vaccines for viral infections are commonly made from live viruses, which have been greatly weakened or modified in a laboratory so that they do not produce disease but do signal the body to produce antibodies capable of fighting the harmful virus. This is why, in certain cases, mild symptoms of the disease are experienced, as when measles or mumps vaccine is given.

Some very general facts about vaccines or antiserums should be fully understood. First, personal records of immunizations are important. In recent years, because some people have neglected to receive certain vaccines unnecessary outbreaks of measles and polio have occurred.

The majority of virus vaccines—including measles, mumps, rubella, polio, and smallpox vaccines—are made from modified viruses that cause no disease. However, people who have low immunity, for example, those suffering from cancer, those being treated with anticancer drugs for tumors or other diseases, and those taking cortisone, prednisone or related drugs, generally should not be immunized.

Vaccines are usually grown in chicken or duck eggs; if you have an allergy to eggs, vaccines from another source may be needed; alternatively, desensitization should be accomplished before the vaccine is given.

Common vaccines The majority of common vaccines are given in early infancy and childhood according to a recognized schedule. These include: diphtheria and tetanus toxoid and pertussis (whooping-cough) vaccine, usually given in a combination known as

123

DPT; the vaccine for all three polio viruses, taken orally (but not to be taken when the child is suffering from diarrhea); and measles, rubella (German measles), and mumps virus vaccines. Since most of these diseases are primarily childhood diseases, the only common vaccine that needs renewal in adulthood is the tetanus toxoid, which should probably be renewed with a booster every 10 years. Further, if a person has a cut or wound associated with obviously dirty material such as rusty metal, passive immunization with tetanus antitoxin or tetanus immunoglobulin may be needed, depending on the number of previous tetanus immunizations and the type and age of the wound. The only other vaccinations necessary in adulthood are those required when traveling to areas where contagious diseases are endemic (see below) and those required when a person, such as a hospital worker, is exposed to a particular disease, e.g., polio.

Several vaccines or antiserums are given in special circumstances. The requirements for the once-common smallpox vaccination are changing because of the almost complete elimination of this dreaded disease, although immunization is still required for travel to a few countries. Also required for certain countries are typhoid, plague, cholera, typhus, and yellow fever vaccines.

Influenza vaccines　Influenza vaccination is generally recommended only for those likely to be severely affected by the illness, such as the elderly, people with severe lung disease such as emphysema or chronic bronchitis, or diabetics. This is because first, there is often a high incidence of reactions to influenza vaccines (although they are usually mild, e.g., fever for several hours), and second, the immunity is variable and of short duration. Influenza viruses, moreover, change in character frequently, necessitating new vaccine strains. The swine influenza vaccine was generally recommended in 1976 in part because it was strongly felt that this particular influenza virus would be very likely to seriously affect younger people. But, in most instances, the previous practice of giving influenza vaccine only to susceptible people still applies.

The principle of preventive therapy in stimulating the body to create its own immunity is old, but continues to be a very promising area of medical research. In the future we may well see vaccines or other drugs which will provide greater immunity against the hepatitis virus, the common cold, and other common viruses. The usefulness of immunotherapy in treating cancer is also being studied, but its value is not yet known.

Skin and Local Disorders

External or local problems may be conspicuous or disfiguring (and therefore embarrassing) as well as uncomfortable, and a wide variety of preparations is available for application to ailing skin or body orifices, most of them designed to produce a local (topical) effect. Literally hundreds of drugs, several ranking among the most commonly prescribed medicines, are used for local disorders.

Steroid preparations   The most widely used topical medications are the corticosteroid creams and ointments such as Valisone, Synalar, Cordran, Lidex, T.A.C. (triamcinolone), and hydrocortisone. These have a cortisone-like effect (see also *Steroids, or cortisone-like drugs,* page 102), and are prescribed for many skin disorders with symptoms of inflammation and itching, e.g., eczema, neurodermatitis, and psoriasis. Because of their rather dramatic effect on some skin ailments, these products have tended to be used indiscriminately on every skin lesion, on occasion leading to the problems that can occur with long-term use of steroid drugs. Some of the corticosteroids applied to the skin are the same as those given orally or by injection, for example, hydrocortisone and triamcinolone. In other preparations, fluorine has been added to the steroids to increase their strength and potency, as in Synalar and Valisone. After long use, these fluorinated steroids can produce shrinkage and other changes in the skin.

Because topical corticosteroids seem to work better on moist skin, moistening the skin is advisable before application. In some cases an occlusive dressing is used: steroids that must be applied for many days are more effective if the area is covered with plastic wrap to seal in the moisture. This procedure is regularly used in psoriasis treatment. Long-term use of topical corticosteroid creams often results in absorption of the drug in sufficient quantities to cause corticosteroid side effects and to decrease normal activity of the adrenal gland. The cost of many brand-name preparations is very high, but equally effective preparations are available by generic name.

Steroid compounds   A related group of locally applied drugs consists of steroid creams compounded with such antibiotic or antifungal drugs

125

as Cortisporin, Mycolog, NeoDecadron and Vioform-Hydro-cortisone. These combinations attempt simultaneously to reduce local inflammation and to eliminate the infection. In some cases this approach may be effective, but it is difficult to know which component has the effect; it may be that in some instances the steroid prevents normal healing. The answer is probably to use both ingredients, but separately and only as needed.

Topical antibiotics Topical antibiotics such as Neosporin and Bacitracin ointment find frequent use on small wounds and cuts. The effectiveness of these preparations has been questioned, since it is not certain whether the antibiotic in an ointment can really be active against skin bacteria, or whether that action is any more effective than simply keeping a wound clean and protected. Certain new topical preparations containing antibiotics such as tetracycline and erythromycin do appear to be effective in treating acne. Preparations containing the antibiotic neomycin (e.g., Neosporin, Cortisporin) have a fairly high incidence of skin sensitization, producing an allergic reaction.

Antifungal preparations In contrast with antibiotic creams and ointments, antifungal preparations such as nystatin (Mycostatin), candicidin (Candeptin), miconazole (Monistat), and Tinactin (tolnaftate) appear to be relatively effective when applied locally. Because fungi are very persistent, it is extremely important when taking medication for a fungal infection to use the preparation regularly for the prescribed period, usually 10 days or more. Allergic reactions to these preparations are relatively infrequent.

Vaginal medications A specialized group of local antimicrobial preparations comprises creams or suppositories for vaginal infections. Infections of the vagina frequently occur in association with the use of oral contraceptives, the use of antibiotics such as ampicillin or tetracycline, and in diabetes. They may also occur without any obvious cause, in which case they are usually due to changes in the vaginal pH (degree of acidity or alkalinity) affecting the normal bacteria residing in the vagina. Under these conditions there is often a white discharge, with itching and burning. Vaginal discharge may also be due to fungal infections, bacteria, Trichomonas (a protozoan) or certain venereal diseases, e.g., gonorrhea. The cause should be diagnosed by a physician or at a family planning clinic. If a fungal or Monilia (Candida) infection is diagnosed, it is usually treated with antifungal creams such as Mycostatin (nystatin), Candeptin (candicidin) or Monistat (miconazole). If it is due to Trichomonas, treatment will be with an oral drug, Flagyl, sometimes with treatment of the woman's sexual partner if it is recurrent. If the problem is due to neither Trichomonas nor a fungus, the infection is probably bacterial. If this is the case, and gonorrhea has been ruled out, vaginal creams containing sulfa drugs (e.g., AVC Cream, Sultrin Cream, and Vagitrol) are frequently prescribed—although failure to use them for the prescribed course is a common mistake. Many gynecologists believe that wearing cotton underwear and normalizing the acidity of the vagina with simple vinegar douching may eliminate the problem.

Local anesthetics An unrelated local problem is pain caused by cuts, sunburn, or other minor superficial wounds. A common treatment is to use drugs called *local anesthetics*. The Novocain (procaine) and Xylocaine used by dentists to prevent pain are examples. Benzocaine is a common local anesthetic sold for relief of pain such as sunburn (for example, Solarcaine). Many of these local anesthetics do not act on intact skin but may do so on burned skin or abrasions. The major concern about their use is the tendency for some local anesthetics—benzocaine, for example—to cause allergic reactions. The general rule is to discontinue use if the condition worsens.

Eyedrops A large number of medicines are used directly on the eye. The effects of such preparations are usually local, on the pupil, cornea or lids, but sometimes they can be absorbed into the system and produce side effects. A variety of preparations are used. Antibiotics, alone or in combination (e.g., Neosporin eyedrops), are often used for local infections or corneal scratches. Corticosteroids, with or without antibiotics, are also used. These, however, are controversial, because, although in some cases they are essential to prevent corneal scarring, when applied to virus lesions, as in a Herpes infection involving the eye, they can worsen the condition. If used for long periods, they can also predispose to fungal diseases of the eye.

Another common use of eyedrops is for glaucoma. Glaucoma, a hereditary disorder, causes a block of normal fluid flow in the eye and can lead to a buildup of pressure in the eye. The increased pressure on the retina and optic nerve may result in blindness. Topical drugs such as pilocarpine (Isopto Carpine) can relieve the pressure. Oral drugs, especially the diuretic Diamox, are also used to decrease the pressure.

When using eye medicines, it is essential to keep the droppers sterile to prevent infections. If different medicines are applied to each eye, it is very important to have all of them clearly marked to avoid confusion.

Eardrops The ear canal is a specialized area where a few drugs are applied only to treat local infections or skin disorders. Since the eardrum closes the canal and forms a barrier, medicines do not usually reach the middle or inner ear by this route. If the eardrum is not intact, eardrops should generally be avoided. The most commonly used ear preparation is Cortisporin, a mixture of steroid and antibiotics; it is discussed in Part 3.

Listed below are some of the commonly prescribed drugs for skin and local disorders. Those marked with an asterisk are individually described in Part 3.

Aristocort Derm.*	Isopto Carpine*	Synalar
AVC Cream	Kenalog Derm.*	TAC Cream
Cordran*	Lidex*	Triple Sulfa
Cortisporin*	Mycolog*	Cream
Flagyl*	Mycostatin*	Valisone*
hydrocortisone	Neosporin Eyedrops*	Vioform-
cream	Sultrin Cream	Hydrocortisone*

Neurological Problems

Many neurological and neuromuscular disorders (that is, those that involve the brain and nerves and/or the muscles) are due to gradual destruction of nerves or muscles. The cause of the destruction (or degeneration) is sometimes unknown—as for example in multiple sclerosis and certain types of muscular dystrophy. In other cases, destruction is due to loss of blood supply to the brain, as in a stroke. Medical science has not yet developed medicines that halt or reverse degenerative diseases, or reverse the effects of a stroke.

Thus, the use of medication in these diseases is limited to treating their symptoms, which may include muscle spasm, thought disorders, or depression. There are some neurological disorders that do not respond to drugs, the most common of these being migraine headaches (actually a disorder of the blood vessels to the brain), convulsions or seizures, and Parkinson's disease. These disorders are briefly discussed in the following sections.

Migraine True migraine headaches are often confused with other types of severe headache, which are due to stress or tension. Tension also appears to precipitate true migraine in some people. Migraine is a specific kind of headache, which may be preceded by a feeling (called an aura) that the headache is about to occur. Migraine often occurs on one side of the head and may be accompanied by a loss of appetite, nausea and vomiting, and transitory visual changes. It may last for hours or days. Migraine appears to result from constriction of some of the arteries to the head (which may produce the aura), followed by relaxation of the arteries, which produces the severe pain. However, the reason this occurs is not known. Symptomatic treatment of mild migraine often involves the same analgesics or pain-relieving medicines used for other headaches, such as aspirin or Darvon. But if the migraine is severe, narcotics may be required to relieve the pain. The regular use of narcotics, even codeine, should be avoided because of the potential for addiction with recurrent use.

Ergotamine The most specific drug treatment for true vascular or migraine headache is ergotamine (Ergomar, Gynergen), taken at the first warning sign of an attack. It may be given by injection, taken by inhaling, dissolved under the tongue, or swallowed; if nausea or vomiting is present, it can be administered effectively as a rectal suppository. Ergotamine (which is derived from ergot, a fungus disease of rye plants) acts to constrict the arteries and possibly prevents the relaxation (pain) stage. Ergotamine is also combined with caffeine (in Cafergot) as well as with other sedative, anti-nausea, or pain-relieving drugs (Cafergot P/B, Midrin, Bellergal, Wigraine, Migral). Caffeine appears to increase the absorption of ergotamine from the stomach, but the value of such ingredients varies from individual to individual and has been questioned. Because there is a tendency for resistance (tolerance) to develop, regular use of ergotamine to prevent attacks may hinder effective treatment of an acute attack.

If taken regularly, Sansert (methysergide) has been found to prevent recurrent attacks of migraine. It is usually discontinued at intervals, however, due to serious side effects, which can result in extensive scar-tissue formation around the kidneys, lungs or heart. It is always used under careful medical supervision.

Listed below are some of the drugs commonly prescribed for migraine.

Bellergal   Cafergot   ergotamine

Seizures (convulsions) When certain parts of the brain are disturbed by injury, high fever, or damage from a stroke, a tumor, or a congenital defect, a seizure may occur. The seizure results from a brief disorganization of the brain's electrical impulses, which can be measured by an electroencephalograph (EEG). Physically, seizures range from localized twitches or arm movements to rigidity of one side, or of the entire body (grand mal seizure), or take the form of a sudden fall to the floor (akinetic seizure). The most common type of seizure has no known external cause, and is called *idiopathic epilepsy.* The majority of people with seizure disorders can, with proper treatment, function quite normally.

Only a few drugs are suitable for treating epilepsy, and they are geared to preventing seizures from occurring. In rare cases, seizures persist and must be treated with intravenous drugs such as Valium or Amobarbital.

The drugs used to treat epilepsy include drugs from three chemical groups: the *barbiturates,* e.g., phenobarbital, methylbarbital (Mebaral), primidone (Mysoline); the *hydantoins,* Dilantin (phenytoin), mephenytoin (Mesantoin); and the *succinimides,* Zarontin, Celontin, and Milontin. Other drugs are used much less commonly, but include a new agent, sodium-valproate (Depakene).

Anticonvulsants   By far the most commonly used anticonvulsant drugs are Dilantin and phenobarbital. Treatment for epilepsy is often started with one of these two drugs, and the dose adjusted to prevent seizures. If a normal dosage of one drug alone is not effective, the other may be taken at the same time, depending on the type of seizure. Although childhood idiopathic seizures do not require lifelong therapy, those occurring in adulthood (after a head injury, for example) may. Initial physical and psychological adjustment to therapy is needed, but once stability has been achieved, treatment should present no major problems. Long-term use of both drugs mentioned can lead to adverse effects (discussed in Part 3). In most cases, the drugs are well tolerated, but sudden stoppage, especially of phenobarbital, may bring on a seizure *status epilepticus* (a series of fits in unconsciousness), requiring the intravenous administration of diazepam.

Listed below are some of the drugs commonly prescribed for seizures or convulsions. Those with an asterisk are individually described in Part 3.

Clonazepam	Mesantoin	Valium*
Dilantin*	phenobarbital*	
Mebaral	primidone	

Parkinson's disease Parkinson's disease is a brain disorder with a characteristic set of symptoms, all or some of which may be present. These symptoms include tremor (which is greater at rest) of the hands, feet, and head; rigidity of the arms and legs; slowness of movement; loss of facial expression; a tendency to drool; and mental deterioration. Often these symptoms may be very mild and progress very slowly. This set of symptoms (Parkinsonism) may be seen not only with Parkinson's disease but also commonly as a side effect of therapy with major tranquilizers such as Thorazine.

The symptoms seem to be due to damage or to degeneration of a very specific part of the brain. In cases not related to drugs, Parkinsonism is due to deficiency of a substance in the brain called *dopamine.* This substance and another, called *acetylcholine,* balance each other, making body movement smooth and coordinated. When there is not enough dopamine, acetylcholine is assumed to cause the symptoms. These facts form the basis for drug therapy in Parkinson's disease: either to increase dopamine levels or to block the effects of acetylcholine.

Anticholinergic drugs Until the last few years, only one group of drugs was available, the acetylcholine-blocking or anticholinergic drugs, the most commonly used being Artane (trihexyphenidyl) and Cogentin (benztropine). These are prescribed for certain types of Parkinson's symptoms and are the only drugs effective in cases due to major tranquilizer usage. They are also used to treat mild Parkinsonism, although their effect tends to grow weaker with continued use.

Levodopa Treatment of Parkinson's disease was changed considerably several years ago with the introduction of levodopa, or L-Dopa (Dopar), which is converted into dopamine by the body. Initially hailed as the therapeutic answer to Parkinson's disease, levodopa is now reserved for more difficult cases owing to its side effects that include severe movement disorders, heart palpitation, low blood pressure, and mental changes. Nonetheless, it has considerably widened the possibilities of treatment, allowing many people to function normally, despite some side effects, for much longer. A refinement to levodopa therapy was the addition of carbidopa to form a combination product called Sinemet, which has less marked side effects.

Amantadine A third useful drug, called amantadine (Symmetrel), was introduced as an antiviral agent. It is now used alone in mild cases of Parkinson's disease, or in combinations with the other two types of drugs mentioned above, although it is only effective in some cases.

Treatment of mild cases frequently is initiated with an anticholinergic drug (e.g., Artane or Cogentin) or amantadine, often in conjunction with therapy aimed at exercising muscles to maintain function, and decreasing stress or tension. Levodopa or Sinemet is later added or substituted after gradual withdrawal of other drugs.

There is still much to be desired in the therapy of Parkinson's disease, particularly with respect to the frequency with which drugs must be taken and their side effects. But the fact that drugs for Parkinson's disease are able to correct very minute biochemical abnormalities in the brain brings some hope for development of more specific medication for this and related disorders in the future.

Listed below are some of the drugs commonly prescribed for Parkinson's disease. Those with an asterisk are individually described in Part 3.

Artane*   Cogentin   L-dopa

Gout

Gout is an arthritis-like disease that can cause very painful, red, and swollen joints; the first manifestation is often an acute attack affecting the big toe. Chronic gout can cause degeneration of joints, in addition to the formation of characteristic crystalline deposits of uric acid salts, called *tophi,* around the joints and cartilage and in the kidney. Gout is caused by an excess of uric acid in the blood. There appears to be a genetic predisposition to gout, although it can arise in association with certain blood diseases, tumors, or cancer therapy. Men are more likely than women to suffer from gout.

Uric acid is formed from the breakdown of nucleic acids (DNA and RNA) which are present in every cell in the body. In addition, a small quantity of uric acid is derived from the diet, especially from such foods as brain, heart, liver and sweetbreads and certain seafood, including anchovy, lobster and sardines. Some people with gout are therefore advised to avoid such foods. Alcohol, particularly in excess, may also increase uric acid levels. These facts suggest that there is an element of truth in the notion that gout was an affliction of the wealthy, brought on by rich foods and large quantities of wine.

Medication for acute attacks Drugs for gout are used to treat an acute attack and to prevent recurrent attacks. Those used to treat an acute attack include colchicine, oxyphenbutazone (Tandearil), phenylbutazone (Butazolidin), and rarely, indomethacin (Indocin). These medications reduce inflammation, but have little effect on the primary disease. Colchicine is quite specific for acute attacks of gout, providing striking relief—and proof that the diagnosis is correct—in an authentic attack. As detailed below, colchicine is sometimes taken in small does together with other drugs to prevent recurrent attacks.

Preventive therapy Medication taken to prevent recurrent attacks acts to decrease the amount of uric acid in the body. Two commonly used older drugs, probenecid (Benemid) and sulfinpyrazone (Anturane), promote the elimination of uric acid by the kidneys. (Probenecid is also available combined with colchicine as Colbenemid.) Allopurinol (Zyloprim), often more effective than the older drugs, acts by inhibiting an enzyme that is essential to the breakdown of body cell constituents into uric acid.

When treatment is started with any of the three preventive drugs, there is a risk that an acute attack of gout may occur. Consequently, colchicine or another anti-inflammatory drug is also given for a few weeks.

Precautions Although diet restrictions are no longer necessary when taking anti-gout medication, many diuretic drugs (see *Diuretics,* page 63) tend to raise uric acid levels by reducing its elimination by the kidneys. These small increases do not usually cause gout, but it is necessary to monitor the level of uric acid

133

in the blood and sometimes to discontinue the diuretic. Aspirin and other salicylates should not be taken in large doses or continually with most drugs used for gout (although this does not apply to allopurinol), but acetaminophen can be taken if an analgesic is required. In order to avoid kidney damage, or the possibility of stone (calculus) formation, plenty of liquids should be drunk—about three quarts daily.

Listed below are some of the drugs commonly prescribed for gout. Those with an asterisk are individually described in Part 3.

Anturane	Colbenemid	Zyloprim*
Benemid	colchicine	

Vitamins and Minerals

Vitamins and minerals are nutrient substances essential for human body growth and function. The amounts required are often very tiny compared to the amount sold and taken by the American public.

The subject of vitamins and minerals—as well as other substances termed "nutritional supplements," e.g., lecithin, kelp, garlic, and so on—is surrounded by a good deal of debate and controversy, leading to much confusion for the layman. A vast amount of material has been written on the subject—some in scientific journals, but the majority in the form of personal testimonials about the value of particular vitamins or specially formulated mixtures of these substances. The whole controversial issue cannot be addressed here but a few useful facts may be presented.

Most experts do not view vitamins and minerals as drugs, yet in many respects they have some similarities to drugs and also to hormones. For example, vitamins travel essentially the same route as drugs: from the stomach to the liver to the bloodstream, to their place of action, and finally to the kidney, where they are eliminated. Taken in high doses, vitamins, especially fat-soluble vitamins, can cause adverse effects, and they can interact with medicines. Like drugs, they affect many tissues and organs; in the case of some vitamins, we are only now beginning to understand their important actions. Vitamin D is felt by some to be more properly called a hormone, since it is produced in the body after exposure to the sun and has some resemblance to cortisone; however, because it is not produced by a gland it is not a true hormone.

The normal varied diet of an adult usually contains adequate amounts of most of the required vitamins and minerals. It has never been shown that a healthy person on a well-rounded diet benefits in any way from vitamin or mineral supplements. In fact, rarely is the average person who feels run down or tired actually suffering from a lack of vitamins or minerals, especially if a normal diet has been followed.

Uses of vitamin and mineral supplements Despite the fact that a balanced diet precludes the need for vitamin and mineral supplements, in most cases,there are situations where additional vitamins may be essential. In determining needs, however, it should be noted that many foods, e.g. milk, margarine, and bread, are supplemented with vitamins so that requirements even for additional vitamins may often be met through diet, rather than by taking pills. Recent food labeling laws require vitamins and minerals to be listed to allow calculation of intake.

Supplementary vitamins and minerals are needed when there is an increased demand for vitamins, for instance, during growth (in infancy and childhood), pregnancy, and lactation. Occasionally vitamins are necessary in prolonged, severe illnesses, especially where there has been fever. An inadequate supply of vitamins can result from a poor diet—either from consumption of excessive amounts of carbohydrate and fat and few vegetables, or from certain fad diets. A decreased supply to the body can also result if vitamins in food are not absorbed owing to chronic diarrhea or diseases causing malabsorption. Supplies of vitamins and minerals can become exhausted, but once they are replenished and a normal diet is resumed, supplements are not always necessary.

Vitamins and minerals are sometimes prescribed in situations where their action is essentially that of a drug. For example, vitamin C (ascorbic acid) has the ability to make the urine acid. Because bacteria do not grow well in acid urine, vitamin C is sometimes given, often in relatively large doses, to help prevent urinary infections. The mineral calcium in the form of a salt (calcium carbonate) is used in some antacids to neutralize stomach acid. Finally, the mineral potassium chloride is often taken to replace the potassium lost when a diuretic is given.

There are some basic differences between the two major

types of vitamins—fat-soluble and water-soluble—as well as between vitamins and minerals.

Fat-soluble vitamins

The *fat-soluble vitamins*—A, D, E and K—are so called because they are more soluble in fat than in water, and their absorption from the intestines is similar to the absorption of fat. These vitamins are stored in the liver and eliminated very slowly, so that excessive doses can accumulate and cause serious problems and illness (especially vitamins A and D). Deficiencies of the fat-soluble vitamins may occur when there is poor absorption in the intestine owing to diseases of malabsorption, chronic diarrhea, or excessive use of laxatives. These vitamins are measured in units of activity called international units (IU). In general, an IU represents a specific amount of biological activity in a biological test system.

Water-soluble vitamins

The *water-soluble vitamins,* which include vitamin C (ascorbic acid), the B complex (B1-thiamine, B2-riboflavin, B6-pyridoxine, B12-cyanocobalamin), niacin, folic acid, pantothenic acid, and biotin are found in many plants and animals. They act at sites throughout the body and are rapidly eliminated in the urine. Accumulation is unlikely if the kidneys are functioning normally, and adverse effects of excessive doses are not common, except in the case of niacin. Amounts of these vitamins are usually expressed in terms of weight in milligrams.

Minerals

Minerals are simple elemental substances which occur as organic and inorganic complexes or "salts" that are necessary to the makeup of all tissues and fluids. Common table salt (sodium chloride) is the most well-known and essential mineral; it is present on both the inside and the outside of all living cells. Minerals are sometimes subdivided into *macrominerals* and *trace minerals.* The macro-minerals—calcium, sodium, potassium, magnesium, phosphorus, sulfur, and chlorine—are present in the body in relatively large amounts and occur in most cells. Requirements are expressed in milligrams. The trace minerals—zinc, iron, iodine, copper, cobalt, chromium, fluorine and manganese, and others—are present in much smaller amounts and are often complexed with proteins to affect their structure or function (as in enzymes). The amounts usually required are much smaller and less is known about the actual function and essential nature of many, such as manganese and zinc. Iodine and iron, on the other hand, are well understood and their function is known to be quite essential.

Recommended Daily Allowances

The Food and Nutrition Board of the National Research Council has studied the available data and established Recommended Daily Allowances (RDA) for dietary supplements. These are *not the same* as the United States Recommended Daily Allowances (USRDA) which is a set of values for labeling purposes. The RDA have been established as amounts necessary to maintain good nutrition in most healthy persons. They have been established for various age groups and for pregnant and lactating women.

It is important to understand that if certain vitamins are taken in excess, they may create relative deficiencies of other nutrients. For example, B-complex vitamins often occur together in nature and are best taken in balanced amounts, except in special cases where it is known that only one is depleted. Furthermore, since vitamin and mineral deficiencies are more often multiple than isolated, it is sensible to use multivitamin preparations in the treatment of general nutritional deficiency. It is currently thought by some authorities that an appropriate multivitamin should contain only the substances specified in the RDA, and only in amounts proportional to those given in the RDA. Those containing other substances such as choline, bioflavonoids, or inositol are of unknown value.

Multivitamins

There are at least four different types of multivitamin preparation, each of which has different uses. First are the dietary supplements or "prophylactic vitamins," which contain no more than one to one-and-a-half times the RDA and may be useful in preventing mild deficiencies during dieting or short illnesses. Second are the therapeutic multivitamins, which may contain three to five times the RDA (except in the case of vitamins A, D and folic acid: excess A and D can cause poisoning, while excess folic acid can mask pernicious anemia). These are recommended for true nutritional deficiency associated with alcoholism, malabsorption, or gastrointestinal surgery. Their use for any length of time should be supervised by a physician.

A third type of multivitamin is formulated to suit the requirements of pregnant and lactating women, but its composition varies considerably from brand to brand. In general, a pill containing more than five times the RDA of any ingredient, more than 10,000 IUs of vitamin A or 4,000 IUs of vitamin D, is not as appropriate as a combination containing recommended amounts.

The fourth category of multivitamins is that which also contains mineral supplements. Except for calcium, iron, and possibly fluoride, the specific need for and usefulness of the added minerals is not very well known. Calcium may be useful in pregnancy and lactation, iron in conditions where there is blood loss (most commonly in women with heavy menstrual periods; healthy men who have no bleeding problems almost never need iron), and fluoride where the local water contains none. Much is being written about the value of the other trace minerals, but generally they are obtained in very adequate amounts in the diet.

Vitamin preparations vary considerably in cost, and higher cost does not necessarily assure greater benefit. If it meets RDA requirements, a generic multivitamin at lower cost may be essentially equivalent to high-priced preparations. Except in cases of true deficiency, a good varied diet should eliminate the need for any expenditure on vitamins and minerals.

Listed below are some of the commonly prescribed vitamins and minerals. Those with an asterisk are individually described in Part 3.

Feosol*	potassium	Tri-Vi-Flor Drops*
Poly Vi-Flor	chloride*	
Chewable*	Slow-K*	

An Alphabetical Guide to Over 200 of the Most Frequently Prescribed Drugs

Acetaminophen

Trade names

Tylenol, Nebs, Tempra, Datril

Action and uses A popular mild pain reliever used as an alternative to aspirin. Like aspirin, it can also reduce fever. Unlike aspirin, it has no anti-inflammatory effects, but it also has fewer side effects and drug interactions. It is present in a large number of pain-relieving combination drugs. Another common pain reliever, phenacetin, is actually converted to acetaminophen in the body.

Adult dosage Two 325 mg tablets every four to six hours as needed for pain or fever.

Adverse effects In usual doses, there are few adverse effects, although excessive doses can cause liver damage. In contrast with the similar drug phenacetin, acetaminophen does not cause kidney damage.

Precautions Excessive doses over long periods may cause liver damage. This very popular drug is a very common cause of accidental and often *untreatable* overdosage in children. It should always be kept well out of their reach.

Drug interactions Rarely, this drug may increase the effects of anticoagulants or major tranquilizers, but this is of questionable significance.

See *Non-narcotic pain relievers,* page 42.

Acetazolamide (generic name). See DIAMOX ORAL.

Achromycin-V

Generic name

tetracycline (available by generic name)

Action and uses One of the most commonly used oral antibiotics. In the generic form (tetracycline), it was the fourth most frequently prescribed drug in 1976. There are a number of tetracycline drugs available, and most are comparable in their actions and side effects (with the exceptions of Minocin and Vibramycin). Tetracycline is known as a "broad-spectrum" antibiotic because it can be used in a wide variety of different infections, although it is the first choice drug in very few common infections. It acts by stopping the production of proteins in sensitive bacterial cells with little effect on human cells. Tetracycline is currently very commonly prescribed in low doses to inhibit the bacteria on the face which are believed to contribute to acne. It is also frequently used by those with chronic bronchitis or other lung disease. Less frequently, it is used to treat urinary tract infections or venereal disease in cases where penicillin allergy is present. It has no effect on viral illnesses, including colds, or on fungal infections.

Adult dosage The usual oral dose is 250 or 500 mg every six hours for a prescribed number of days as specified by the physician. It is very important to take this on an empty stomach. The dose may vary in some cases; for instance, when prescribed for acne it may be lower.

Adverse effects Tetracycline often causes various gastrointestinal symptoms, including nausea and vomiting, burning stomach or belching, cramps, and diarrhea. The last symptom is often due to the fact that tetracycline inhibits some bacteria in the lower intestine and elsewhere and allows overgrowth of other bacteria (normally held in check) and minor fungi. This can also result in vaginal infection, anorectal itching, and a fungal infection of the mouth, causing soreness (thrush). These symptoms tend to disappear when the drug is discontinued. Less commonly, tetracycline can cause rashes or other allergic reactions and sensitivity of the skin to sunlight (photosensitivity) which may cause rashes. It also tends to worsen certain types of kidney disease and rarely causes liver damage or blood-cell abnormalities.

Precautions Tetracycline should not be taken by pregnant or potentially pregnant women or nursing mothers, and should be used with caution when significant liver or kidney disease is present. This antibiotic, like all others, should be taken for the full period as directed by the physician, and every dose should be taken. Failure to do this can result in inadequate treatment of the infection, leading to recurrence or development of resistant infections.

Drug interactions The most common interaction occurs with antacids or milk products; the tetracycline binds to these and does not get absorbed into the body. Tetracycline can potentially increase the effect of the anticoagulant Coumadin to increase the hazard of bleeding.

See *Infections,* page 111

Actifed

Actifed C Expectorant

ACTIFED

Generic ingredients

> antihistamine : tripolidine hydrochloride
> decongestant : pseudoephedrine hydrochloride

ACTIFED C EXPECTORANT

Generic ingredients

> antihistamine: tripolidine hydrochloride
> decongestant : pseudoephedrine hydrochloride
> narcotic : codeine phosphate
> expectorant : glyceryl guaiacolate

Action and uses Actifed is a combination drug used to control seasonal or perennial allergic rhinitis (hay fever—characterized by runny nose, watery eyes, and sneezing). Allergic rhinitis may be due to specific irritants, such as the pollen of trees or grass, or may even be caused by emotional stress or worry, grief, or other upsetting experiences (vasomotor rhinitis). The decongestant ingredient in Actifed shrinks the linings of the nose and respiratory passages. The antihistamine blocks histamine—the substance which causes the breathing passages to swell and discharge mucus. Actifed C Expectorant contains in addition codeine phosphate, used here not as a painkiller but to control coughing, and the expectorant glycerol guaiacolate, which helps to liquefy the mucus blocking up the

141

breathing passages. (These effects might counteract each other.) Actifed C Expectorant thus provides cough-suppressant, expectorant, decongestant, and antihistamine effects.

Adult dosage Actifed: One tablet three times a day or two teaspoonfuls (10 ml) of the syrup three times a day. Actifed C Expectorant: the usual dose is two teaspoonfuls (10 ml) four times a day. For severe cases the above dosages may be reduced by half and given every three hours.

Adverse effects Side effects may include drowsiness (due to the antihistamine) and possibly palpitation (due to the decongestants). Although the amount of codeine is small, it may cause nausea and vomiting, and, if used for several days, constipation. The expectorant may cause nausea.

Precautions These drugs should be avoided by pregnant or potentially pregnant women and nursing mothers. Driving or operating heavy equipment may be hazardous if sedation is an effect of this medication. People taking medicine for high blood pressure or heart ailments should check with their physicians before using these preparations, since the decongestants may elevate the blood pressure. Repeated use for any period of more than two to four days should be avoided in most cases.

Drug dependence The codeine in this compound can cause habituation if taken for prolonged periods.

Drug interactions The sedative effects of the antihistamine, and to a lesser extent the codeine, can be additive to any other sedating drug, e.g., tranquilizers or alcohol. The decongestants can raise the blood pressure and thus counteract the effect of any drug used to treat high blood pressure. Like most drugs of this type, Actifed may add to the effects of antispasmodic drugs used for stomach disorders, such as Pro-Banthine and Librax. This can cause excessive mouth dryness and difficulty in urinating.

See *Coughs and colds,* page 117.

Afrin

Generic name

oxymetazoline hydrochloride

Action and uses A nasal decongestant used to relieve congestion of the nasal passages, sinuses, and throat. Afrin reduces the flow of blood to the tissues lining these areas, and thereby relieves congestion. It is used to counter the symptoms of a variety of allergies and infections including the common cold. Afrin may lose its effectiveness after prolonged use.

Adult dosage Usually two or three squeezes of the nasal spray in each nostril, twice a day. Afrin also comes as a liquid with a dropper. The usual dosage is one dropperful in each nostril, not more than twice a day.

Adverse effects Side effects include burning, stinging, and dryness of the nasal passages. Some individuals may experience nervousness, headache, lightheadedness, and sleeplessness, and some may suffer from pounding of the heart (palpitations) and elevation of the blood pressure.

Precautions Afrin should be avoided by people who have heart disease or high blood pressure or are taking medicines for these conditions.

Drug interactions Afrin can cause elevation of the blood pressure and other reactions in people taking drugs for depression (MAO inhibitors or tricyclic antidepressants) or for high blood pressure, such as reserpine.

See *Coughs and colds,* page 117.

Aldactazide

Generic ingredients

diuretics: spironolactone; hydrochlorothiazide

Action and uses A fixed-dose combination of two diuretics ("water pills"), used in the treatment of disorders that cause excessive retention of salt and water and high blood pressure. One component is spironolactone, a drug which, by blocking the hormone aldosterone, causes the body to eliminate excess water and salt, but not potassium. Most other diuretics tend to eliminate this essential mineral along with salt and water.) The second, somewhat stronger, diuretic is hydrochlorothiazide. Although the diuretic effects of its two ingredients are additive, Aldactazide, like other fixed-dose combinations, has several disadvantages: the dosage of one component cannot be adjusted without affecting the dosage of the other; it has an increased number of side effects; and it is more expensive than other equally effective products.

Adult dosage Usually two to four tablets per day in divided doses. (Each tablet of Aldactazide contains 25 mg of spironolactone and 25 mg of hydrochlorothiazide.)

Adverse effects Possible side effects of spironolactone include the retention of waste products by the kidney, headache, drowsiness, skin rash, breast enlargement, and in women, irregular menstrual periods. Possible side effects of hydrochlorothiazide include a rise in the blood sugar level, which can precipitate diabetes, and a rise in the body's uric acid level, which can precipitate gout. Both drugs can cause allergic reactions.

Precautions Aldactazide should not be used by pregnant or potentially pregnant women, or by patients with kidney disorders.

Drug interactions Because of the spironolactone in Aldactazide, a dangerous rise in the body's potassium level is possible if supplementary potassium (KC1 or Slow-K) is taken concurrently.

See *High blood pressure,* page 58; *Diuretics,* page 63.

Aldactone

Generic name

> spironolactone

Action and uses A mild diuretic ("water pill") used to treat the excessive water retention caused by certain heart, liver, and kidney diseases and by some types of high blood pressure. A major factor in these disorders tends to be the overproduction of aldosterone, a hormone which encourages the body to retain its salt and water and eliminate the mineral potassium. Aldactone works by blocking this hormone—thus making it possible for the body to eliminate excess salt and water and retain potassium. (Most other diuretics do not prevent the loss of this essential mineral. However, although this effect may be advantageous when there is a need to prevent excess potassium loss, the advantage must be weighed against the problems and expense of using Aldactone.)

Adult dosage Usually 50–300 mg per day, divided into several doses. Often Aldactone's effect will not be felt until the effects of the hormone aldosterone have worn off—which can take as long as three days.

Adverse effects Aldactone has a high incidence of side effects. The major adverse effect is a dangerous, even life-threatening increase in the body's potassium level, particularly if supplementary potassium is being taken (a common practice when other, stronger diuretics are also in use). For this reason, blood tests should be made at intervals to check the body's potassium level. Another side effect that should be checked by occasional blood tests is a decrease in the kidney's ability to eliminate waste products. Other side effects may include headache, drowsiness, skin rash, breast enlargement, and in women, irregular menstrual periods.

Precautions Aldactone should not be used by pregnant or potentially pregnant women and should be used with caution by patients with a kidney disorder.

Drug interactions Dangerously high levels of potassium may accumulate in the blood if Aldactone is taken along with supplementary potassium such as Slow-K or KCl.

See *High blood pressure,* page 58; *Diuretics,* page 63.

Aldomet

Generic name

methyldopa

Action and uses A drug used to treat high blood pressure. It works by blocking the sympathetic nervous system to cause relaxation of the muscular walls of the blood vessels. Usually it is prescribed with a diuretic ("water pill") to enhance its effect. Aldomet is, in fact, often the second drug tried when a diuretic alone has not succeeded in lowering the blood pressure.

Adult dosage The usual daily dose is 500 mg two to four times per day. Initially, the dose may be 250 mg two or three times per day, with a dosage adjustment at intervals until the desired effect is produced or a daily total of 2 grams is reached.

Adverse effects Initially, most patients experience drowsiness or lethargy, but these effects usually wear off within two or three weeks. Less common side effects may include dry mouth, stuffy nose, lightheadedness on moving suddenly, skin rash, depression, nightmares, joint and muscle pain, nausea, and changes in sexual function. Some of these effects may decrease with time. More rarely, abnormalities of blood cells or the liver may occur.

Precautions When first started Aldomet can cause marked drowsiness and driving and operating heavy equipment should therefore be avoided. If possible, pregnant or potentially pregnant women and nursing mothers should not take Aldomet.

Drug interactions Aldomet can interact with many other drugs, and the doctor's advice should be sought before taking *any* other prescription or over-the-counter drug. Drugs that can seriously impair Aldomet's effectiveness and lead to a rise in blood pressure include antidepressants such as Elavil, Tofranil, and Sinequan; major tranquilizers such as Thorazine; MAO inhibitor drugs such as Nardil; amphetamines such as Dexedrine and Benzedrine; appetite suppressants such as Preludin; nasal sprays such as Neo-Synephrine and decongestant drugs for coughs, colds, asthma, and allergy, such as Actifed.

See *High blood pressure,* page 58; *Diuretics,* page 63.

Aldoril

Generic ingredients

diuretic : hydrochlorothiazide
antihypertensive : methyldopa

Action and uses One of several popular fixed-combination drugs used to treat high blood pressure. Aldoril contains two types of ingredient: methyldopa, an antihypertensive drug, which acts on the sympathetic nervous system to relax the walls of the blood vessels; and hydrochlorothiazide, a diuretic, which causes the kidneys to eliminate salt and water, thus reducing the amount of fluid in the blood and the body tissues. Like other fixed-combination drugs, Aldoril has several disadvantages: its dosage is inflexible (the amount of one ingredient cannot be altered without affecting the amount of the other); it increases the number of side effects; and it is more expensive than equally effective single-ingredient products.

Adult dosage Usually two to six tablets per day in divided doses. The drug comes in two strengths: Aldoril-15, which contains 15 mg of hydrochlorothiazide and 250 mg of methyldopa; and Aldoril-25, which contains 25 mg of hydrochlorothiazide and 250 mg of methyldopa.

Adverse effects The hydrochlorothiazide in Aldoril may cause an excessive loss of the mineral potassium, which may result in dizziness, unusual tiredness, muscle cramps, and/or tingling in the extremities. Fortunately, it is easy to replace lost potassium by adding to the diet high-potassium foods, such as dried fruits, bananas, citrus fruits, and orange or tomato juice; by using salt substitutes such as Lite-Salt; or with a supplement of potassium chloride liquid (KC1). The amount of loss and the need for potassium replacement can be ascertained by regular blood tests. Other side effects from hydrochlorothiazide may include an elevation of the blood sugar level in patients predisposed to diabetes and a rise in the body's uric acid level, which may predispose to gout. Both these effects can be watched for and rarely produce problems. Finally, some people are allergic to hydrochlorothiazide and develop reactive skin rashes.

The methyldopa in Aldoril may cause drowsiness or lethargy, dry mouth and nasal stuffiness, and lightheadedness on changing position suddenly, but these effects tend to disappear in two to four weeks. Less frequently, the methyldopa in Aldoril can cause skin rash, nausea, depression, nightmares, joint and muscle pain, liver or blood abnormalities, and changes in sexual function.

Precautions Aldoril can cause marked drowsiness when first started, and driving and operating heavy equipment should therefore be avoided. If possible pregnant or potentially pregnant women and nursing mothers should not take Aldoril. If digoxin (digitalis) is also being taken, the blood potassium level should be checked or potassium supplements taken.

Drug interactions Cortisone and cortisone-like drugs such as prednisone can interact with the hydrochlorothiazide in Aldoril to cause excessive potassium loss. Potentially serious interactions may also occur with digitalis drugs for the heart; if too much potassium is eliminated from the system by the action of the hydrochlorothiazide, the heart becomes sensitive to the toxic effects of digitalis. Drugs that may impair the blood-pressure-lowering effect of the methyldopa in Aldoril include antidepressants such as Elavil, Tofranil, and Sinequan; major tranquilizers such as Thorazine; MAO inhibitor drugs such as Nardil; amphetamines such as Dexedrine and Benzedrine; appetite suppressants such as Preludin; nasal sprays such as Neo-Synephrine; and decongestant drugs for coughs, colds, asthma, or allergies, such as Actifed. Finally, alcohol, barbiturates, sedatives, and pain relievers may be additive to Aldoril's sedative effect. The doctor should be consulted before *any* prescription or over-the-counter drug is taken by a patient on Aldoril.

See *High blood pressure,* page 58; *Diuretics,* page 63.

Ambenyl Expectorant

Generic ingredients

antihistamines : diphenhydramine, bromodiphenhydramine
expectorants : ammonium chloride, guiacolsulfonate
miscellaneous : chloroform, menthol, alcohol
narcotic cough suppressant : codeine

Action and uses A widely prescribed cough mixture containing two anti-histamines which are also believed to have a mild cough-suppressant effect, and expectorants, which are believed to help liquefy bronchial secretions. In fact, the effectiveness of this and other similar cough syrups is difficult to establish. Codeine is included in the mixture because it suppresses coughing, which is often desirable, but the presence of codeine, which is a narcotic, means that use of the mixture must be restricted.

Adult dosage Usually two teaspoonfuls every four hours, not to exceed 12 teaspoonfuls in 24 hours.

Adverse effects The antihistamines can cause drowsiness, and, less frequently, dizziness. The expectorants can sometimes cause nausea. The codeine, although present in small amounts, may also cause nausea and constipation.

Precautions If drowsiness occurs, it may interfere with driving and operating machinery. Ambenyl should be avoided by pregnant or potentially pregnant women and nursing mothers.

Drug dependence The codeine, if taken for prolonged periods in excessive doses, may cause habituation.

Drug interactions The antihistamine and codeine in Ambenyl can add to the effects of alcohol, tranquilizers, and sleeping pills, as well as those of antispasmodic anticholinergic drugs such as Pro-Banthine or Librax. Because of its alcohol content, Ambenyl can cause a hazardous interaction if Flagyl or Antabuse is also taken.

See *Coughs and colds,* page 117; *Antihistamines,* page 121.

Amcill

Generic name

ampicillin (available by generic name)

Amcill is a trade name for ampicillin and is described fully under that heading below.

Aminophyllin

Trade names

Amesec, Aminodur, Mudrane, Quinamm,
Somophyllin (available by generic name)

Action and uses Aminophyllin is a drug for the treatment of acute and chronic asthma. It is available as various oral preparations, as rectal suppositories and solutions, and for intravenous injection. Together with other related drugs (see Elixophyllin and Choledyl), aminophyllin represents the mainstay of asthma treatment, although it is frequently used in conjunction with other anti-asthma drugs. It is often given intravenously for severe attacks and orally at other times. Rectal administration is controversial—its effect is often unpredictable because absorption is variable and,if used frequently, it can cause irritation—so it is usually reserved for occasional use. Recently, it has been found that the effect of aminophyllin varies greatly from individual to individual due to a variety of factors including the patient's sex, smoking, and the presence of liver or heart disease. Thus, therapy may be monitored by measuring the level of the drug in the blood.

Adult dosage Oral forms: initially usually 200 mg three or four times daily, the dose being adjusted subsequently according to symptoms and blood levels. Dose requirements may be lower or considerably higher (up to 1600–2000 mg per day).

Adverse effects The most common side effect is gastric irritation from the direct effect of the drug in the stomach, as well as nausea and vomiting, which are related to indirect effects of the drug. The nausea and vomiting may be decreased by lowering the dose. Other dose-related effects include headache, muscle cramps, palpitations, and occasionally nervousness or insomnia.

Precautions The use of aminophyllin by people with irregular heart rhythms or other types of heart disease should be carefully supervised.

Drug interactions Aminophyllin is additive to other drugs used to treat asthma, and its side effects can also be additive. It is important that the prescribing physician be aware of all prescription and over-the-counter drugs being taken for this condition. Aminophyllin has effects on the clotting system which can alter the effects of blood-thinning drugs such as heparin or Coumadin.

See *Asthma and lung disease,* page 109.

Amoxil

Generic name

amoxicillin

Action and uses

Amoxil is almost identical to ampicillin in its actions, uses, and side effects, except that it can be taken without regard to meals, while ampicillin must be taken on an empty stomach. See the detailed discussion on ampicillin below.

Amoxicillin (generic name). See AMOXIL, LAROTID.

Ampicillin

Trade names

Amcill, Omnipen, Pen A, Penbritin, Pensyn, Polycillin, Principen, Supen, Alpen, Totacillin

Action and uses

An antibiotic used to treat many infections, including those of the urinary tract, ear, nose, and throat. It is one of several so-called "semi-synthetic" penicillins which is made by both chemical and biological manipulation of penicillin produced by the mold *penicillium*.

Ampicillin, like penicillin, acts by preventing bacteria from forming their cell walls. They therefore break up. It has no effect on human cells since they have a different structure. Though basic penicillin (penicillin G) is still one of the most important of all the antibiotics, it has several disadvantages. One is its somewhat limited effectiveness against certain types of bacteria—the "gram-negative" organisms. Another disadvantage is that it is not totally effective when taken by mouth because penicillin G is broken down by stomach acid. Ampicillin, however, is highly effective when taken by mouth on an empty stomach because it is not broken down by stomach acids. Because it is active against many kinds of bacteria, it is called a "broad-spectrum" antibiotic. It is less effective than penicillin G against "gram-positive" cocci (found in abscesses and ear infections), but more effective against gram-negative bacteria (which cause urinary tract infections). It is not effective against fungal or viral diseases. Antibiotics should not be used for trivial infections or to treat nonsensitive bacteria (those against which they are not effective); such use only produces resistant bacteria, which are difficult to eliminate.

Adult dosage The average adult dose is 250 mg or 500 mg every six hours on an empty stomach (or at least two hours after a meal). The dose should always be established by a physician and will vary with the type and severity of infection.

Adverse effects Many people develop allergic reactions to the penicillin group of drugs. Once sensitization develops *all* forms of penicillin, including ampicillin, can produce a reaction. An allergic reaction may be manifested by any of the following symptoms: skin rashes, hives, itching, fever, difficulty in breathing, and swelling of the lips and tongue. Persons who have infectious mononucleosis often develop rashes in response to ampicillin and should not take it while they have the disease. Ampicillin can also produce stomach upset, due to the killing of certain normal bacteria in the intestine, and may cause diarrhea. It may also cause mild fungal infections of the anorectal area or the vagina.

Precautions This antibiotic should not be used if there is a history of allergy to any type of penicillin. It should not be taken by people with infectious mononucleosis, because it is accompanied by a high incidence of rashes. Once treatment with ampicillin is begun, the prescribed course of not less than five to seven days should be completed (unless, of course, side effects occur). It should *not* be stopped when the infection seems to be gone, since despite the disappearance of symptoms the bacteria may not be entirely eliminated and the infection could recur. The frequent starting and stopping of any antibiotic only leads to the development of resistant bacteria which are much more difficult to treat. Nursing mothers should ask the physician's advice before taking ampicillin.

Drug interactions The effectiveness of ampicillin may be hindered if used at the same time as the antibiotics erythromycin and chloramphenicol. Food and antacids may interfere with the absorption of this drug.

See *Infections*, page 111.

Antivert

Generic name

meclizine (available by generic name)

Action and uses An antihistamine prescribed for the control of the nausea, vomiting and dizziness associated with motion sickness. It is also used to treat Ménière's syndrome and other disorders that affect the center of equilibrium in the inner ear and produce vertigo (the sensation that one's surroundings are spinning). It has the other actions of antihistamines and is sometimes used for allergies or itching.

Adult dosage For the prevention of motion sickness, the usual dose is 25–50 mg one hour before embarkation. The dose may be repeated every six to eight hours for the duration of the journey, as needed. For the control of the dizziness caused by disorders affecting the inner ear, the usual dose is 25–100 mg per day in divided doses. It is advisable to begin with a low dose and adjust as needed until the dizziness is controlled or a maximum of 100 mg per day is reached. This drug may also be purchased without a prescription.

Adverse effects Antivert may cause drowsiness, blurred vision, or dryness of the nose, mouth, or throat. Rashes may rarely occur.

Precautions Antivert must not be taken during pregnancy because tests have shown that it causes birth defects in animals. It should be used with caution by those planning to drive a car or operate heavy machinery while under the effects of the drug.

Drug interactions Oversedation may result if Antivert is taken in combination with alcohol, sleeping pills, tranquilizers, antidepressants, pain relievers, drugs containing narcotics, and other antihistamines.

See *Antihistamines,* page 121; *Nausea, stomach upset, and ulcers,* page 75

Anusol-HC Suppositories & Cream

Generic ingredients

anti-inflammatory steroid : hydrocortisone
miscellaneous ingredients : bismuth subgallate
bismuth resorcin
benzyl benzoate
pervian balsam
zinc oxide

Action and uses Anusol-HC is a hydrocortisone-containing preparation used for symptoms of itching, pain, and discomfort due to inflammation and other disorders of the anorectal area. The hydrocortisone in the preparation can act to decrease inflammation, but the precise action of the remaining mixture of ingredients in this preparation is essentially unknown. The preparation is often prescribed for limited time periods for the treatment of hemorrhoids, anal fissures, and following anorectal surgery.

Adult dosage One suppository or application of cream in the morning and at bedtime for three to six days or as directed by the physician. Use beyond seven to ten days is seldom necessary.

Adverse effects One common cause of anorectal discomfort is yeast or minor fungal infections and the hydrocortisone may make this worse rather than better. Likewise, some of the other ingredients may cause burning or stinging and/or allergic reactions which can also cause an increase of symptoms.

Precautions Prolonged use of topical corticosteroids such as hydrocortisone can delay normal healing and weaken tissues. If the preparation is used in excess and/or for long periods, the hydocortisone can be absorbed into the body and may cause other effects. Finally, it can aggravate certain infections caused by yeasts or fungi. Accordingly, Anusol-HC should be used for short periods of time only. It should also be used only with caution during pregnancy.

Drug interactions None are known and are unlikely under proper conditions of use.

See *Skin and local disorders,* page 125.

Apresoline

Generic name

hydralazine (available by generic name)

Action and uses A drug used to lower blood pressure; it acts by relaxing, and therefore dilating (widening) arterial blood vessels. It is used in the treatment of mild to moderate hypertension, and is usually used in conjunction with a diuretic ("water pill") and/or a drug that prevents the sympathetic nervous system from constricting the blood vessels, e.g., Aldomet or reserpine.

Adult dosage

As response to this drug varies considerably, it is usually started at a dose of 10 mg taken three to four times per day and gradually increased, according to individual requirements, up to a maximum of 100–300 mg per day. Occasionally, under supervision, the drug can be taken twice a day rather than four times a day.

Adverse effects If Apresoline is taken along with a sympathetic-blocking drug such as Aldomet or Inderal, it has relatively few side effects apart from a sensation of lightheadedness on moving suddenly. In the absence of a sympathetic-blocking drug, Apresoline can, because of its dilating effect on the blood vessels, cause an increase in heart rate. This can be a problem in the presence of other heart conditions, e.g., angina pectoris, because of the extra work required of the heart. Other side effects may include occasional headache, nausea, and flushing. At high doses, some patients develop *lupus erythematosus,* an arthritis-like disorder characterized by a facial rash and joint and muscle pain, which usually necessitates the discontinuation of the drug. Allergic reactions may also occur.

Precautions   Apresoline should not be taken by pregnant or potentially pregnant women or nursing mothers and should be used with caution by people with angina pectoris or previous stroke.

Drug interactions   Other drugs for high blood pressure; diuretics like Aldactone, Lasix, and hydrochlorothiazide; and MAO inhibitor drugs like Marplan, Nardil, and Parnate, can all increase Apresoline's effect on blood pressure.

See   *High blood pressure,* page 58; *Diuretics,* page 63.

Aristocort Cream & Ointment

Generic name

triamcinolone (available by generic name)

Action and uses   A commonly used preparation of a synthetic corticosteroid (cortisone-like drug) for local (topical) application. It is used primarily for its anti-inflammatory effects in the treatment of many types of skin disorders such as psoriasis, certain types of neurodermatitis (inflammation of the skin associated with emotional factors), and a variety of other conditions where no infection is present. In many cases, the effects are dramatic. Because it also retards formation of scar tissue, Aristocort can prevent scarring.

Adult dosage   The 0.025–0.5% preparation is applied sparingly three or four times daily. It is available as an ointment and as a cream in several strengths, the choice depending on where it is used.

Adverse effects   If the preparation is not used for long periods or on infected areas, there are virtually no important adverse effects; however, if the preparations are used for long intervals on the face, they can cause eruptions and redness. If Aristocort preparations are used for long periods on a large area of the body, the corticosteroid can be absorbed into the body through the skin. This can cause weight gain, ulcers, or stomach upset, decreased resistance to infection and stress, and can be quite dangerous. If used on an infected area of the skin it can help the infection spread, and it can be very hazardous if used for any viral skin lesions such as those of herpes simplex ("cold sores"), shingles, or chicken pox.

Precautions Do not use without a physician's specific instructions, and use only on affected areas. Do not use on a skin area which appears infected without consulting a physician.

Drug interactions No significant interactions will occur although other topical preparations placed on the same area of skin as Aristocort may interfere with its effects.

See *Steroids, or cortisone-like drugs,* page 102; *Skin and local disorders,* page 125.

Artane

Generic name

> trihexyphenidyl

Action and uses A drug used to treat tremor and rigidity of muscles, particularly in Parkinson's disease. Parkinson's disease is thought to be caused by an imbalance of nervous activity in the brain. It is presumed that Artane helps correct this imbalance by blocking the activity of cholinergic nerves; thus, the drug is said to be an *anticholinergic.* It may also relax muscles directly. It is only moderately effective in some people, and a newer drug, levodopa, is now far more widely used to treat Parkinsonian symptoms. If the two different drugs are used together in lower doses, fewer side effects are often experienced. Artane and a similar drug, Cogentin, are also used to treat Parkinsonian symptoms which arise as a side effect of certain drugs, particularly the major tranquilizer Thorazine.

Adult dosage The dose varies according to the response of the patient. Initially, the dose is 1 mg daily. This is increased every three to five days by 2 mg to a daily total of 10 mg, or sometimes even 15 mg. High doses are best taken in three or four divided doses with meals. When optimum dosage has been established, Artane may be replaced by the long-acting Sequels, which are taken usually as a single dose after breakfast.

Adverse effects These are common to all anticholinergic drugs (e.g. atropine) and include dry mouth, constipation, and retention of urine. Blurring of vision, nausea, dizziness, or nervousness may also occur.

Precautions Artane may increase visual problems in people with glaucoma, bladder difficulties in those with prostate trouble, and make expectoration difficult in those with chronic lung disease.

Drug interactions Artane adds to the effects of other anticholinergic drugs such as antihistamines, antispasmodics, cough/cold medicines, and tricyclic antidepressants. This can cause dry mouth, difficulty in urinating, constipation, and blurred vision.

See *Parkinson's disease,* page 131

Aspirin (acetylsalicylic acid)

Trade names

ASA, Ecotrin, Measurin

Action and uses Aspirin is still one of the most effective drugs for the relief of mild to moderate pain. It is also useful in bringing down fever, and because it reduces inflammation, has proved itself a most effective drug in the treatment of arthritis. Recently, aspirin has also been prescribed for its anticoagulant effects: it helps prevent blood clotting by reducing the stickiness of certain blood cells called *platelets.* Its primary use, however, is as a pain reliever and anti-inflammatory agent.

Originally, the word "Aspirin" (based on the German word for salicylic acid, *Spirsaure*) was used only by the Bayer Drug Company as a brand name for their product. Since then, the drug has become so popular and widely used that "aspirin" has become virtually synonymous with the acetylsalicylic acid it stands for.

Today, aspirin is marketed not only on its own, but also in over a hundred different combination drugs for everything from headaches and hangovers to strained and aching muscles and heavy colds. Alka-Seltzer, APC, Anacin, Ascriptin, Bufferin, Cope, Coricidin, Darvon Compound, Dristan, Empirin Compound, Equagesic, Excedrin, Fiorinal, Norgesic, Percodan, Phenaphen, and Vanquish are just a few of the aspirin-containing compounds in popular use. It is important to be aware of the aspirin content in all these and many other cold and headache remedies available over-the-counter, because, however commonplace and "harmless" aspirin may seem, it *is* a drug and can produce side effects, allergic reactions, and harmful interactions with other drugs.

It is also interesting to note that, despite all the claims made by the various "name brands," plain ordinary aspirin has often proved itself, for the relief of any type of pain, to be as good as or better than any other non-narcotic pain reliever on the market. Many of the combination drugs are a good deal more expensive, the extra cost being for various additions or refinements of dubious value. In the case of Ascriptin, Bufferin, and similar drugs, you may be paying for the addition of "buffers" or antacids to prevent stomach irritation, despite the fact that the antacids are present in quantities too small to be very helpful in preventing irritation. Some aspirin-containing pain relievers are "coated" to keep them from irritating the stomach: unfortunately, this also means that they usually take considerably longer to take effect, or are never absorbed into the body! Alka-Seltzer gets around the problem of gastric irritation by including sodium bicarbonate (a well-known antacid) with aspirin. The presence of sodium bicarbonate, however, limits Alka-Seltzer's all-round usefulness (for example, the sodium can cause fluid retention) and, of course, also raises the price of the preparation.

Adult dosage Customarily available in 300 mg (5-grain) tablets, aspirin is usually taken with lots of water in doses of 600 mg (10 grains), or two tablets' worth, every three to six hours as needed for pain. For the treatment of arthritis, it is taken in somewhat higher doses (frequently two to four tablets every four hours) on a regular basis under a doctor's supervision. Aspirin may deteriorate if it becomes damp and should be discarded if it develops a strong acid or vinegar odor.

Adverse effects Aspirin may irritate the stomach lining, causing nausea, vomiting, pain, and even bleeding, especially when taken frequently or in higher doses. Even when taken on an occasional basis, aspirin should always be taken with plenty of fluid to help prevent stomach irritation. Too much aspirin can also produce dizziness, mental confusion, and a ringing in the ears. Some people are allergic to aspirin, and may develop skin rashes or symptoms like those of asthma or hay fever.

Precautions Aspirin and drugs containing it should be avoided by people with peptic ulcer and by anyone taking anticoagulants, except under the specific instructions of a physician. Those who have allergic sinusitis or asthma may have an allergy to aspirin. Because this common drug is a major cause of accidental overdose in children, it should always be kept out of their reach.

Drug interactions Aspirin adds to the effects of anticoagulant drugs such as Coumadin and dicumarol to increase the risk of bleeding. Taken in conjunction with cortisone-like drugs, it increases the chances of developing ulcers. It may interact with Diabinese and other drugs for diabetes to cause a dangerous fall in blood sugar.

See *Pain with inflammation,* page 43.

Atarax

Generic name

> hydroxyzine

Action and uses An antihistamine which is promoted primarily for its antianxiety and sedating actions. It has a chemical structure similar to other antihistamines which are used for motion sickness (e.g.,Marezine), and it is essentially identical to the drug Vistaril. It is also used on occasion as an antihistamine and in the treatment of conditions which cause itching of the skin.

Adult dosage Because sensitivity to its effect varies, the dose ranges from 25 to 100 mg two or three times a day.

Adverse effects Excessive sedation or decreased mental alertness may create a significant problem. Other side effects are relatively uncommon.

Precautions Atarax may interfere with driving or operating machinery. It should not be taken by pregnant or potentially pregnant women, or by nursing mothers.

Drug interactions Atarax is additive to other drugs causing sedation, for example, sleeping pills, tranquilizers, alcohol, and narcotics such as morphine; these combinations should be avoided unless greater sedation is required.

See *Antihistamines,* page 121; *Minor tranquilizers,* page 45.

Ativan

Generic name

> lorazepam

Action and uses A minor tranquilizer used to treat the symptoms of anxiety and nervousness by producing calm and a decreased sense of anxiety. Ativan is one of a group of chemically similar drugs (which include Valium, Librium, Serax, and Tranxene) which are the drugs most frequently prescribed in the United States. All of these drugs are prescribed to relieve the symptoms rather than the cause of a condition in the same way that narcotics are used to relieve pain. In general, they have no effect on the cause of the symptoms. Ativan can also be used as a sleeping medication in a similar way to Dalmane, another chemically related drug. It is recommended only for short-term use.

Adult dosage The usual dose of Ativan is from 0.5–2 mg two to four times a day, sometimes with the larger proportion of the total daily dose at bedtime. The doses for older people are usually lower and all doses require individual adjustment.

Adverse effects The most common side effect is sedation, but dizziness, unsteadiness, and depression are not uncommon. These symptoms can interfere with driving and operating machinery but may disappear at lower doses. Other side effects are relatively uncommon. When Ativan is taken in combination with alcohol the two drugs act together and marked sedation or dizziness may occur.

Drug dependence Ativan is not addictive in the same way as narcotics, but, like other sedatives, it can be habit forming to a certain extent, if taken for long periods of time (months to years), possibly even at normal doses. If it is then stopped suddenly, some withdrawal symptoms may occur, especially after large doses. These can include anxiety, insomnia, and nightmares.

Precautions There is a possibility that minor tranquilizers may cause birth defects and the manufacturers therefore warn against the use of Ativan by pregnant or potentially pregnant women and nursing mothers.

Drug interactions Ativan can enhance the sedative effect of alcohol, antihistamines, sleeping pills, and narcotics, sometimes to a dangerous extent. Unlike many sedatives, it does not interfere with the actions of the anticoagulant Coumadin.

See *Minor tranquilizers,* page 45.

159

Atromid-S

Generic name

> clofibrate

Action and uses A drug used to lower high levels of cholesterol (a fatty substance) in the blood. It is believed to help prevent coronary heart disease and other circulatory disease by reducing the accumulation of fatty deposits that line the walls of the arteries and endanger the normal flow of blood to the heart and elsewhere. However, it is probable that a program of exercise and weight reduction, a balanced low-fat diet, and giving up smoking may be more effective than this or other currently available drugs in the battle against the build-up of fat in the arteries.

Adult dosage Usually 1–2 grams per day in divided doses.

Adverse effects Atromid-S may cause a wide variety of adverse effects, the most common being gastrointestinal upset, including reactivation of ulcers. Less frequently, it can cause (reversible) liver damage, blood-cell abnormalities, irregular heart rhythms, various skin rashes, and flu-like symptoms.

Precautions Atromid-S should not be taken by patients with impaired liver or kidney function. It should not be taken by pregnant or potentially pregnant women.

Drug interactions Atromid-S may markedly increase the effects of the anticoagulant drug Coumadin, thus increasing the risk of bleeding. It can also increase the effects of oral antidiabetic drugs and possibly other drugs.

See *Poor circulation,* page 68.

AVC Cream & Suppositories

Generic ingredients

> antibacterials : sulfanilamide, aminacrine
> miscellaneous : allantoin

Action and uses AVC preparations are used to treat vaginal infections not due to yeast or to the protozoan *Trichomonas.* Although the effectiveness of such sulfonamide vaginal creams has been questioned, it has been generally conceded that they are probably effective for certain types of infection. Because of the diversity of vaginal infections, however, the effectiveness of such preparations (see also SULTRIN) has been difficult to prove.

Adult dosage	One application of cream or one suppository once or twice daily for seven to ten days, or through one menstrual cycle, as directed.
Adverse effects	Local sensitivity or burning may occur, and sensitivity to the sulfonamide may occur locally or throughout the body. If so, the preparation should be discontinued.
Precautions	This preparation should not be used by women who are allergic to sulfonamide drugs. Safety in pregnancy and during nursing has not been established.
Drug interactions	Drug interactions are unlikely to occur with the local preparation.
See	*Skin and local disorders,* page 125.

Azo Gantrisin

Generic ingredients

```
antibacterial : sulfisoxazole
painkiller : phenazopyridine hydrochloride
```

Action and uses	A fixed-combination drug used to treat infections of the kidney, bladder, and urinary tract, including cystitis. It combines a sulfonamide (or "sulfa" drug) with phenzopyridine, a painkiller which acts specifically on the urinary tract. Azo Gantrisin is therefore particularly suitable for treating painful urinary infections.
Adult dosage	Usually four to six tablets initially, followed by two tablets four times per day for three days. Treatment is usually continued with Gantrisin tablets.
Adverse effects	This drug may sometimes cause nausea, vomiting, or other gastrointestinal symptoms, and also headaches or dizziness. Like all sulfa drugs, Azo Gantrisin may cause allergic reactions ranging from rashes to very serious, life-threatening reactions with fever, severe rash, and kidney failure. The most common but harmless side effect is the change in the color of the urine to an orange-red, due to the "azo" dye. This is harmless (though it can stain underwear) and disappears when the drug is stopped. Rashes or other allergies may also occur due to this dye.
Precautions	It is always important to drink plenty of water while taking this drug to prevent crystal formation in the kidney. If any fever, nausea, or rash occurs after starting the drug, it should be discontinued and the doctor notified. It should be avoided

161

by people with severe kidney disease or G6PD deficiency (a congenital enzyme deficiency). As in the treatment of all infections, it is important to take the drug for the full course prescribed to prevent recurrence of the infection. Pregnant or potentially pregnant women and nursing mothers should avoid the drug if possible.

Drug interactions As with many sulfa drugs, Azo Gantrisin may increase the effect of oral antidiabetic drugs to cause low blood sugar and may interact with Dilantin, Butazolidin, and phenobarbital to increase the likelihood of toxic effects of these drugs.

See *Infections,* page 111.

Bactrim DS

Generic ingredients

antibacterials : sulfamethoxazole, trimethoprim

Action and uses A fixed-combination drug used to treat infections of the urinary tract. It is the same drug as Septra, another trade-name preparation. Bactrim combines a sulfonamide ("sulfa" drug), which is particularly effective against the bacteria that commonly affect the bladder and kidney, with a chemical antibacterial drug which acts against the same bacteria. Together the two drugs are more effective than either one alone, since each inhibits a separate enzyme in the bacteria; this decreases the likelihood of resistance developing. This combination is also finding use in certain other common diseases, such as typhoid fever.

Adult dosage Usually one double-strength tablet, or two ordinary tablets, or four teaspoonfuls of liquid every 12 hours for 10 to 14 days. It may be used for longer periods in chronic urinary-tract infections.

Adverse effects This drug may sometimes cause nausea, vomiting, or other gastrointestinal symptoms, and also headaches or dizziness. Like all sulfa drugs, Bactrim may cause allergic reactions ranging from rashes to very serious, life-threatening reactions with fever, severe rash, and kidney failure. Abnormalities of the blood cells may also occur.

Precautions It is always important to drink plenty of water while taking this drug to prevent crystal formation in the kidney. If any fever, nausea, or rash occurs after starting the drug, it should be discontinued and the doctor notified. It should be avoided by people with severe kidney disease and G6PD deficiency (a congenital enzyme deficiency). As in the treatment of all infections, it is important to take the drug for the full course prescribed in order to prevent recurrence of the infection.

Drug interactions As with many sulfa drugs, Bactrim may increase the effect of oral antidiabetic drugs to cause low blood sugar, and may interact with Dilantin, Butazolidin, and phenobarbital to increase the likelihood of toxicity to these drugs.

See *Infections,* page 111.

Benadryl
Benadryl Elixir

Generic name

> diphenhydramine (available by generic name)

Action and uses A popular drug used to treat allergies, rashes, and itching of the skin. Benadryl is also sometimes used as a sedative. It is an antihistamine which blocks the effects of histamine—a substance released in the body during allergic reactions. When histamine is released it causes itching, swelling, and redness. Benadryl is useful in hay fever, hives, redness of the eyes, or allergic conjunctivitis. It is not generally used in allergic asthma. It is sometimes used as a sleeping pill, particularly for older people, and when effective it is relatively useful and safe.

Adult dosage Usually 25–50 mg every six to twelve hours for allergic problems. The dose varies according to the sedative effects on the individual. For nighttime use the usual dose is 50 mg. The drug comes in tablet, capsule, and elixir form.

Adverse effects The most common side effect of Benadryl is drowsiness; it occurs in some people but not in others. Other side effects are not common.

Precautions When drowsiness occurs it is advisable to avoid driving or operating fast-moving machinery. Benadryl should be avoided by pregnant or potentially pregnant women and nursing mothers.

Drug interactions Benadryl is additive to (i.e. it compounds the effects of) any other sedative or tranquilizer, and to alcohol, especially in those people who are more susceptible to its sedative effects. It also interacts with drugs such as Pro-Banthine and Librax to increase the likelihood of side effects such as blurred vision, dry mouth, and difficulty in urinating.

See *Antihistamines,* page 121; *Sleeping pills,* page 47.

Bendectin

Generic ingredients

antihistamine/antinauseant : doxylamine
vitamin : pyridoxine (vitamin B_6)

Action and uses A combination of an antihistamine and vitamin B_6 promoted for morning sickness (the nausea often experienced in early pregnancy). Although it has not been clearly demonstrated that Bendectin can produce any harmful effects on the unborn baby if taken during pregnancy, there has recently been a great deal of controversy over this possibility. Like many antihistamine drugs, Bendectin has a prominent antinauseant effect, but it also has other antihistamine effects. The vitamin B_6 is present to help correct any existing vitamin deficiency, but it is doubtful whether this is of any practical value.

Adult dosage Usually, two tablets at bedtime. In severe cases or when nausea occurs during the day, one additional tablet in the morning and, sometimes, another in mid-afternoon.

Adverse effects Bendectin has the same side effects as other antihistamine drugs—namely sedation and occasionally dry mouth, blurring of vision, wheezing, and possibly difficulty in passing urine. Some people feel restless rather than drowsy, and find it difficult to sleep.

Precautions Because of the possible sedative effect, driving or operating hazardous machinery should be avoided when taking Bendectin. In those who suffer from asthma or glaucoma, Bendectin may be contraindicated.

Drug interactions The effects of Bendectin are additive to those of sedative drugs, sleeping tablets, and alcohol, and to the antispasmodic effect of drugs such as Pro-Banthine and Librax.

See *Nausea, stomach upset, and ulcers,* page 75; *Antihistamines,* page 121; *Vitamins and minerals,* page 134.

Bentyl

Generic name

antispasmodic : dicyclomine hydrochloride
(available by generic name)

Action and uses A drug used to relieve spasm, or tightness of the muscles, of the stomach and intestines. Bentyl is an antispasmodic-anticholinergic drug which acts to produce a relaxing effect directly on the stomach. It is used in the treatment of stomach and duodenal ulcers and other gastrointestinal spasm. It is also available combined with phenobarbital; this preparation is like many similar products which combine an antispasmodic with a minor tranquilizer on the assumption that the relief of anxiety will relieve the symptoms as well. Single antispasmodic drugs are likely to be as effective.

Adult dosage Usually 10–20 mg three or four times a day.

Adverse effects The antispasmodic component may cause a dry mouth, difficulty in urinating (particularly in the elderly), blurred vision, and constipation. It can also cause drying of bronchial secretions.

Precautions Bentyl should be used with caution by people who have glaucoma, prostate trouble, hiatus hernia, or chronic lung disease.

Drug interactions The effects of Bentyl can be additive to those of antihistamines, cough/cold medicines, and tricyclic antidepressants, causing excessive dry mouth, constipation, and occasional bladder problems.

See *Nausea, stomach upset, and ulcers,* page 75.

Benylin Cough Syrup

Generic ingredients

antihistamine : diphenhydramine
expectorants : ammonium chloride, sodium citrate
miscellaneous : chloroform, menthol, alcohol

Action and uses A widely prescribed cough mixture containing an antihistamine, which is also believed to have a mild cough-suppressant effect, and expectorants, which are believed to help liquefy bronchial secretions. In fact, the effectiveness of this and other similar cough syrups is difficult to establish.

Adult dosage Usually two teaspoonfuls every four hours, not to exceed 12 teaspoonfuls per 24 hours.

Adverse effects The antihistamines can cause drowsiness, and less frequently, dizziness. The expectorants can sometimes cause nausea.

Precautions If drowsiness occurs, it may interfere with driving and operating machinery. Benylin should be avoided by pregnant or potentially pregnant women and nursing mothers.

Drug interactions The antihistamines in Benylin can add to the effects of alcohol, tranquilizers, and sleeping pills, as well as antispasmodic anticholinergic drugs such as Pro-Banthine or Librax. Because of alcohol content, Benylin can cause a hazardous interaction if Flagyl or Antabuse is also taken.

See *Coughs and colds,* page 117; *Antihistamines,* page 121.

Brethine

Generic name

terbutaline

Action and uses Brethine, like Bricanyl (another trade name for terbutaline), is a drug used to treat asthma. It is either taken orally or applied as an aerosol spray. It acts to relax the muscles which close off the bronchial tubes in an asthma attack. It represents a refinement in therapy since it has the same beneficial effects on the bronchial airway as Adrenalin (epinephrine), its therapeutic predecessor, but it lacks some of Adrenalin's adverse effects. It is sometimes used alone, but more frequently it is used along with other drugs such as theophylline (see AMINOPHYLLIN, ELIXOPHYLLIN). It is also available in injections for use in acute attacks.

Adult dosage Usually, 2.5–5 mg orally three times daily at six-hour intervals during waking hours.

Side effects Common side effects include nervousness and trembling, which may lessen at lower doses. Rapid heartbeat or palpitations, headaches, nausea and vomiting, and muscle cramps may also occur.

Precautions Brethine should not be used with other drugs with a similar action, e.g. ephedrine (in Sudafed), epinephrine, and Isuprel, except in special circumstances prescribed by your physician. It should not be taken during pregnancy without very careful supervision since it can affect the function of the uterus.

Drug interactions Brethine can add to the effects of any epinephrine-like drug to increase its toxicity.

See *Asthma and lung disease,* page 109

Brompheniramine (generic name). See DIMETANE.

Butabarbital (generic name). See BUTISOL.

Butazolidin

Generic name

phenylbutazone

Butazolidin Alka

Generic ingredients

anti-inflammatory drug : phenylbutazone
antacids : aluminum hydroxide, magnesium trisilicate

Action and uses A drug used to reduce inflammation, especially in the joints. Butazolidin relieves the painful symptoms of inflammation but does not cure the disease which causes the inflammation. It is not known how it works. It is not a steroid hormone and is not related to steroids, although its anti-inflammatory actions are similar. Because it has very serious side effects, it is used only when milder drugs, such as aspirin, do not relieve the symptoms of inflammation. It is useful in treating isolated severe joint pains of inflamed tendons and joints, occasionally for acute gout, and for the acute flare-ups of rheumatoid arthritis.

Adult dosage The dosage of Butazolidin varies from person to person and must be determined by the physician for each individual case. It is available in 100 mg tablets, and the daily dose ranges from 300–600 mg, usually taken in divided doses with meals or milk.

Adverse effects While Butazolidin is an effective and useful drug it is also a dangerous and poisonous one. Many severe reactions occur, particularly if it is used for longer than seven days, especially by people over the age of 60. It may poison the bone marrow and prevent the body from producing both red blood cells, thereby causing anemia, and white blood cells, thereby causing loss of resistance to infection. If such a reaction occurs the effects may be irreversible unless the drug is stopped immediately. Hives, skin rashes, itching, and sores in and around the mouth can be signs of serious reactions to the drug and should be reported to the physician immediately. Butazolidin also may cause stomach upsets, nausea, vomiting, and indigestion, though this may be avoided by taking it with meals. It can also cause liver damage and fluid retention.

Precautions Butazolidin should not be be used by children under the age

167

of 14 or by pregnant or potentially pregnant women or nursing mothers. It should never be used for more than seven days by anyone over the age of 60 unless specifically ordered by and discussed with a physician, and its administration should be followed with regular blood counts. It should be used cautiously by people who have stomach or intestinal trouble or ulcers.

Drug interactions Butazolidin interacts with many drugs, including antidiabetic drugs, other anti-inflammatory drugs such as Motrin, sulfa drugs, Dilantin, and Coumadin, increasing the risk of toxicity of each.

See *Pain with inflammation,* page 43.

Butisol

Generic name

butabarbital (available by generic name)

Action and uses A barbiturate similar to Seconal and Nembutal. Butisol is chiefly used as a sleeping pill, although it is occasionally used as a daytime sedative to relieve anxiety and tension. It takes effect 15–30 minutes after being taken and this effect lasts for five to six hours. When used as a sleeping medication Butisol decreases the time it takes to fall asleep, but suppresses dreaming. After a few days, tolerance can develop and it is necessary to increase the dosage to produce the same sleep-inducing effect. Some of the effects of Butisol may last longer than five to six hours; for example, a "hangover" may occur the morning after taking the drug.

Adult dosage For sleep the usual dose is 50–100 mg at bedtime. If used in the daytime for relief of anxiety and tension the usual dose is 30 mg, two to four times a day.

Adverse effects When used as a sleeping pill, Butisol may cause a hangover effect the following morning. It may also cause a feeling of depression and tiredness, together with nausea, vomiting, and diarrhea. If Butisol is withdrawn after several weeks of use, withdrawal symptoms may appear. There is often a tendency for increased dreaming and even nightmares. There may be insomnia (difficulty in sleeping) and nervousness. If the dose has been high (over 400 mg per day) seizures may occur. All these effects are prompted by withdrawal of the drug. Other mild side effects to the drug include allergic skin reactions, upset stomach, and muscular aches. Butisol can suppress breathing in people with severe lung diseases.

Precautions Butisol and other barbiturates have long been a major cause of suicidal and accidental drug overdose and death. If taken in high doses they can be lethal. Barbiturates can be particularly dangerous if taken with alcohol or other tranquilizers.

Drug dependence If taken for longer than seven to ten days, tolerance to Butisol may develop. If this occurs, dependence on the drug may develop and if it is suddenly stopped withdrawal symptoms may occur. Therefore, if it has been used for a long time its use must be discontinued gradually. Because of this problem, as well as its potential for abuse, the prescribing of Butisol is restricted.

Drug interactions Butisol can interact with many other drugs, particularly with the anticoagulant Coumadin to decrease its effect.

Barbiturates add to the effects of other tranquilizers, sleeping pills, and alcohol. Combining them with any of these drugs can be very hazardous, causing suppression of breathing and even death.

See *Minor tranquilizers,* page 45; *Sleeping pills,* page 47.

Catapres

Generic name

clonidine

Action and uses A drug used to treat moderate or severe high blood pressure, usually given only if other drugs (e.g., Aldomet or Inderal) are ineffective. It acts in the brain to block the sympathetic nervous system and cause relaxation (dilation) of the arteries. Most commonly it is used with a diuretic ("water pill").

Adult dosage Initially, 0.1 to 0.2 mg twice daily, with gradual dosage adjustments until the desired blood pressure response is obtained. The maintenance dose from then on is usually 0.2 to 0.8 mg daily in two or three divided doses. The drug's effect on blood pressure will be felt 30–60 minutes after it has been taken, and lasts for six to eight hours. The last dose of the day is usually taken just before retiring to ensure adequate overnight blood-pressure control.

Adverse effects Catapres may cause dry mouth, constipation, sleepiness, dizziness, headache, and fatigue. These side effects tend to disappear as therapy with the drug continues. The major problem with Catapres is that sudden discontinuation of the drug can cause an equally sudden, often severe rise in blood pressure, which may be accompanied by headache, nervousness, and agitation as well as by more severe symptoms. Discontinuation of Catapres should therefore be done slowly and cautiously under a doctor's supervision.

Precautions The sedation caused by Catapres may interfere with driving or operating machinery. Catapres should be used with caution by pregnant or potentially pregnant women.

Drug interactions Oversedation can result from combining Catapres with alcohol, sedatives, sleeping pills, tranquilizers, antihistamines, or pain relievers, whether narcotic or non-narcotic.

See *High blood pressure,* page 58; *Diuretics,* page 63.

Chloral Hydrate

Trade names

Noctec, Somnos, Kessodrate

Action and uses A common sleeping pill. It is often prescribed for elderly people since it is believed to be better tolerated and less likely to cause excitement than other sleeping pills. In lower doses, it does not suppress dreaming (REM sleep) as most sleeping pills do. The value of this is unknown, but lack of REM sleep has been shown to cause irritability and anxiety. The effectiveness of the drug in producing sleep decreases with time as tolerance develops.

Adult dosage 0.5 to 1.0 gram at bedtime, taken with water or milk to reduce the risk of stomach irritation.

Adverse effects Like other sleeping pills, chloral hydrate can cause a morning hangover. It can also cause dizziness, depression, and very occasionally excitement. It can also cause stomach irritation. Allergic reactions can occur in rare instances.

Precautions This drug should not be used by pregnant or potentially pregnant women or nursing mothers. The sedating effect may interfere with driving or operating machinery.

Drug dependence Chloral hydrate can cause psychological and physical dependence and withdrawal symptoms can occur if it is discontinued after prolonged use.

Drug interactions Chloral hydrate can add dangerously to the sedative effects of alcohol and minor tranquilizers. It can also alter the effects of the anticoagulant Coumadin.

See *Sleeping pills,* page 47.

Chlordiazepoxide (generic name). See LIBRIUM.

Chlorothiazide (generic name). See DIURIL.

Chlorpheniramine (generic name).
See CHLOR-TRIMETON, POLARAMINE, TELDRIN.

Chlorpromazine (generic name). See THORAZINE.

Chlor-Trimeton

Generic name

chlorpheniramine (available by generic name)

Action and uses A commonly prescribed antihistamine which is used to treat allergic conditions, especially allergic rhinitis, sinusitis, or conjunctivitis (redness of the eye). In common with most other antihistamines, it acts by blocking the effects of histamine and thus can decrease itching of the skin caused by allergies, hives, or rashes. It also can sometimes have a sedating effect, although it is not customarily used for this. It is not useful for the treatment of asthma. It is usually much less expensive in generic form as chlorpheniramine.

Adult dosage Chlor-Trimeton is available in oral tablets and liquids and for injections. The usual oral dose is 4 mg two to six times daily, or one 8 mg Repetab twice daily as needed for treatment of allergic conditions.

Adverse effects Chlor-Trimeton may cause significant sedation in some people, although possibly less frequently than some other antihistamines. Other side effects are relatively rare, but can include dry mouth, blurred vision, or difficulty in urinating, especially in older people or those with glaucoma or prostate trouble.

Drug interactions Chlor-Trimeton is additive to other sedative or tranquilizing drugs and alcohol. It is also additive to other antispasmodic drugs used to treat ulcers or stomach problems, such as Pro-Banthine or Librax, causing excessive dry mouth, constipation, and difficulty in urinating.

Precautions The sedative effects may interfere with driving or operating machinery. This drug should be used with caution by those with glaucoma or prostate trouble. It should be avoided by pregnant or potentially pregnant women and nursing mothers.

See *Antihistamines,* page 121.

Choledyl

Generic name

oxtriphylline

Action and uses Choledyl is a drug used to treat asthma. It is a methylxanthine drug very similar to theophylline (Elixophyllin) and aminophyllin. The methylxanthine drugs are frequently the mainstay of asthma treatment; they act to open up the constricted bronchioles (airways) of the lungs. Choledyl is more costly than other related drugs such as theophylline and its promotion has claimed that it is less irritating to the stomach. This effect, however, has not been clearly demonstrated in most cases.

Adult dosage The usual adult dose is 200 mg of the tablets or 2 teaspoonfuls of the elixir, three or four times daily, but the dose will be adjusted individually for each patient. Choledyl can cause stomach upset and nausea in some people. It can also cause palpitations or, less commonly, irregular heart rhythms and muscle cramps. Rarely, if doses are excessive, it can cause anxiousness, tremors, and convulsions.

Precautions The dosage should be adjusted individually for each patient, often by means of measurements of the amount of the drug in the blood. Lower doses may be required for people with heart disease or liver disease. Use in pregnancy or during nursing should be carefully supervised and discussed with the physician.

Drug interactions Choledyl is additive in effect to other drugs used to treat asthma, including aerosols (e.g. epinephrine) and oral medication such as Brethine or ephedrine. The additive effects include the therapeutic effects as well as most side effects, particularly rapid heartbeat and nervousness.

See *Asthma and lung disease,* page 109

Cleocin

Generic name	clindamycin

Action and uses An antibiotic used to treat infections caused by specific bacteria. Cleocin is particularly effective in treating infections caused by the bacterium *Bacteroides,* which most commonly causes serious pelvic and abdominal infections. It can cause serious adverse reactions and should only be used for infections for which other drugs are not effective. It is not used to treat infections such as colds and bronchitis.

Adult dosage Usually 150–300 mg every six hours.

Adverse effects The most common side effect of Cleocin is diarrhea. This may be mild, but in some cases may be severe and may result in a serious inflammation of the large intestine, which can even result in death. Some people may develop skin rashes when taking the drug.

Precautions Pregnant or potentially pregnant women and nursing mothers should be cautious about taking this drug. Use of Cleocin requires careful medical supervision. If diarrhea occurs, the physician should be notified.

Drug interactions Clindamycin and erythromycin may be antagonistic to one another and thus should not be used together.

See *Infections,* page 111.

Codeine

Action and uses A very common oral narcotic for the treatment of moderate to severe pain. It is frequently combined with other pain relievers such as aspirin, acetaminophen and/or phenacetin in preparations such as Empirin with codeine or Tylenol with codeine. Its use alone requires special restricted prescriptions.

Adult dosage This varies with severity of pain and need. It is usually 15–30 mg every four to six hours for severe pain.

Adverse effects A certain number of people suffer nausea when taking codeine, although this is not a true allergy. Constipation almost always occurs if use continues for more than one or two days. Some experience dizziness or unusual dreams.

Precautions Codeine should be used only when less potent pain relievers are not effective. It must be used with caution in persons with chronic lung disease.

Drug dependence Codeine can cause physiological dependence,and,if it is discontinued after prolonged use, withdrawal symptoms can occur.

Drug interactions Codeine can add to the sedative and breathing depression effects of sedatives, tranquilizers,and alcohol. It can also add to the constipating effect of many antispasmodic drugs and antihistamines.

See *Narcotic pain relievers,* page 41.

Combid

Generic ingredients

> antispasmodic : isopropamide
> major tranquilizer : prochlorperazine

Action and uses A fixed-combination drug used in the treatment of stomach and intestinal disorders. Combid is widely used to treat ulcers, irritable and spastic colon, and colitis. Like many similar drugs it combines an antispasmodic anticholinergic drug (which reduces secretions from the stomach and decreases tightness—spasm—of the stomach muscles) with a major tranquilizer (to relieve anxiety and tension). The major tranquilizer also has the effect of reducing nausea and vomiting and stopping hiccoughs. Apparently, it is assumed that many bowel conditions are associated with anxiety and can be relieved by a tranquilizer. Whether this combination is really more effective than an antispasmodic alone is not known.

Adult dosage Usually one capsule every 10 to 12 hours.

Adverse effects Side effects of both ingredients can occur. The antispasmodic can cause dry mouth, blurred vision, and difficulty in urinating, especially in older people. The major tranquilizer (infrequently) can cause drowsiness, various allergic reactions, liver or blood-cell abnormalities, and also can cause neurological reactions, such as "Parkinsonian" symptoms (symptoms resembling those of Parkinson's disease—tremor, rigid extremities) and acute spasm of the neck and jaw muscles (the latter is more common in young people).

Precautions Combid should not be taken by pregnant or potentially pregnant women or nursing mothers, particularly since the major tranquilizer can be very hazardous for unborn babies and infants. This combination should be used with caution in those with glaucoma, prostate trouble, and chronic lung disease. Those with a history of sensitivity to Thorazine or other phenothiazines should not take this drug. If drowsiness occurs, driving or operating machinery may be hazardous.

Drug interactions The antispasmodic can add to the effects of antihistamines, cough/cold medicines and tricyclic antidepressants, causing dry mouth, bladder difficulties, or constipation. The major tranquilizer can enhance the effects of alcohol and other sedating drugs and block the effect of Ismelin, a drug for high blood pressure.

See *Nausea, stomach upset, and ulcers,* page 75; *Major tranquilizers,* page 49.

Compazine

Generic name

prochlorperazine

Action and uses A member of the major tranquilizer group of drugs, used primarily to treat nausea and vomiting. Ideally, it should be used for this only if the cause is known and the symptoms are not controlled by less hazardous drugs. The same antinausea action is also used to stop hiccoughs. It is commonly used to prevent nausea after surgery. It is also frequently used with an antispasmodic drug in a combined preparation (Combid Spansules). Although it shares the antipsychotic effects of all phenothiazines (e.g.,Thorazine), it is used only infrequently to treat thought disorders such as schizophrenia.

Adult dosage 5–10 mg orally or by injection every six to eight hours for nausea. The Spansule and suppository forms are given every 12 hours as needed. Dose should be adjusted for each individual. Lower doses are usually required for older patients.

Adverse effects Compazine may cause a dry mouth, constipation, and, in younger adults,there is more likelihood of acute neurological reactions, expressed by grimacing and spasms of the neck and facial muscles (which can be relieved by drugs such as Cogentin or Benadryl). Some people may experience hypersensitivity reactions such as jaundice, rashes, or a fall in the white blood-cell count. Prolonged use can give rise to "Parkinsonian" symptoms (symptoms resembling those of Parkinson's disease)—trembling of the hands, rigidity of the arms and legs, and loss of facial expression.

Precautions Compazine should not be taken by pregnant or potentially pregnant women or nursing mothers, particularly since this drug can be very hazardous for unborn babies and infants. Persons who have had allergic reactions to Thorazine or other phenothiazines should not take this drug.

Drug interactions Oversedation may occur if Compazine is used with alcohol, tranquilizers or sleeping pills, and antihistamines. It can counteract the effect of some antihypertensive drugs such as Ismelin.

See *Nausea, stomach upset, and ulcers,* page 75; *Major tranquilizers,* page 49.

Cordran Cream, Ointment & Lotion

Generic name

flurandrenolide (available by generic name)

Action and uses A commonly used preparation of a synthetic corticosteroid (cortisone-like drug) for local (topical) application. It is used primarily for its anti-inflammatory effects in the treatment of many types of skin disorders such as psoriasis, certain types of neurodermatitis (inflammation of the skin associated with emotional factors), and a variety of other conditions where infection is not present. In many cases, the effects are dramatic. Because it retards the formation of scar tissue, it can also prevent scarring.

Adult dosage The 0.025–0.05% preparation is applied sparingly (two or three times daily). It is available in ointments, lotions, and creams in several strengths, the choice depending upon where it is to be used.

Adverse effects If the preparation is not used for long periods or on infected areas, there are virtually no important adverse effects; however, if the preparations are used for long intervals on the face, they can cause eruptions and redness. If Cordran preparations are used for long periods on a large portion of the body, the corticosteroid can be absorbed into the body through the skin. This can cause weight gain, ulcers or stomach upset, decreased resistance to infection and stress, and can be quite dangerous. If used on an infected area of the skin it can cause the infection to spread, and it can be very hazardous if used for any viral skin lesions such as those of herpes simplex ("cold sores"), shingles, or chickenpox.

Precautions Do not use without a physician's specific instructions, and use only on affected areas. Do not use on a skin area which appears to be infected without consulting a physician.

Drug interactions No significant interactions occur with Cordran, although other topical preparations placed on the same skin area may interfere with its effects.

See *Steroids, or cortisone-like drugs,* page 102; *Skin and local disorders,* page 125.

Cortisporin

Generic ingredients

> antibiotics : polymixin B, neomycin, gramicidin
> steroid : hydrocortisone

Action and uses A combination product used to treat local infections of the skin, eyes, and ears. Cortisporin combines three antibiotics and a steroid (cortisone-like drug). Each of the antibiotics acts against different types of bacteria. The steroid acts to reduce inflammation and irritation. It is available as an ointment for use in a variety of skin irritations with mild infection; eyedrops and eardrops are used for similar local problems in those areas. This type of mixture has been criticized because it represents "shotgun" therapy—using a combination of ingredients in a somewhat random, nonspecific way—when one specific ingredient may often be adequate.

Adult dosage Cortisporin is available as a cream, ointment, lotion and suspension, and also as eardrops and eyedrops; it is usually applied two to four times per day.

Adverse effects Allergy to any of the ingredients of Cortisporin may occur and skin conditions may worsen rather than improve. This is particularly true of neomycin, which has a high rate of allergic reactions. The steroid may rarely worsen infections, especially if they are caused by a virus, as in shingles. Serious adverse effects can occur from all the ingredients if the preparation is used on large areas for a long time, due to absorption. Also, resistant bacteria or fungi can appear and cause reinfection.

Precautions Cortisporin should not be used over large parts of the body at any one time. It should not be used to treat the sores of herpes simplex ("cold sores") or on smallpox vaccinations or chickenpox sores.

Drug interactions If properly used, drug interactions are not a problem.

See *Infections,* page 111; *Skin and local disorders,* page 125; *Steroids, or cortisone-like drugs,* page 102.

Coumadin

Generic name

warfarin

Action and uses An anticoagulant drug used to treat patients who have developed or are in danger of developing, a life-threatening clot (thrombosis) in an artery, a vein, or the heart itself. Although often referred to as a "blood thinner," Coumadin actually works by slowing down the time it takes the blood to clot. Coumadin is a very effective drug, but it operates within an extremely narrow safety margin: if the dose is too low, there is the danger of a blood clot forming; if the dose is too high, there is the opposite danger of uncontrolled hemorrhage.

Adult dosage Coumadin is usually taken just once a day. The exact dose necessary to prevent clotting while keeping the possibility of excessive bleeding to a minimum varies from person to person and must be carefully determined for each patient; it is established by regular laboratory tests of the "prothrombin time" (a measure of blood-clotting speed). Coumadin tablets come in six color-coded strengths: the 2 mg tablet is lavender; the 2.5 mg tablet is orange; the 5 mg tablet is peach; the 7.5 mg tablet is yellow; the 10 mg tablet is white; and the 25 mg tablet is red.

Adverse effects Excessive bleeding is the most serious and common side effect of Coumadin. Because the drug works to slow down the clotting mechanism, even a small cut or internal injury can lead to uncontrolled bleeding. Patients on Coumadin should inform their doctor right away if they notice any of the following warning signals: red or dark brown urine; red or black bowel movements; increased or prolonged menstrual bleeding; continued bleeding from minor cuts, nose or gums; prolonged stomachache, headache, or backache; or the sudden appearance of black and blue marks. Skin rash, nausea, and diarrhea are among the other, far less frequent side effects possible with the drug.

Precautions The narrow margin of safety of Coumadin can be adversely affected by a number of other drugs; it is *vital* for the patient taking Coumadin to know what they are (see below). Patients on an anticoagulant such as Coumadin must be under close medical supervision; they should also carry a card and/or wear some identification indicating that they are on this drug in case of accident. Naturally, they should inform their dentist or any other health professional they see for treatment that they are taking Coumadin, and report to their own doctor right away if pregnancy is discovered or suspected, or if any illness, infection or injury occurs.

Drug interactions Potentially serious interactions are possible when Coumadin is taken concurrently with *any* of the following: aspirin and all medications containing it (including the scores of different preparations for headache, hangover, aching muscles, and cold symptoms); many of the drugs for arthritis; tranquilizers, sleeping pills and sedatives; oral contraceptives; cortisone-like drugs; thyroid gland supplements; drugs for diabetes; drugs to lower cholesterol; antibiotics; antidepressants; antihistamines; digitalis drugs; drugs for epilepsy; alcohol; leafy green vegetables; and the vitamin K present in multivitamin tablets. All these, as well as numerous other drugs, can affect Coumadin's action in the body. Some increase its anticoagulant effect, others decrease it, but so dangerous are the results of either interaction that it is unwise to take any other medication, whether prescribed by a medical professional or just purchased over-the-counter, without first consulting the doctor.

See *Anticoagulants,* page 73.

Cyclandelate (generic name). See CYCLOSPASMOL.

Cyclospasmol

Generic name

cyclandelate (available by generic name)

Action and uses A drug promoted and used to improve the circulation in the arms, legs or brain. Known as a "vasodilator," it acts in normal people to relax the blood vessels, causing them to expand and let more blood through. However, it has not been shown that the drug has any significant dilating effect on diseased or abnormal blood vessels, for example, arteries clogged by fatty deposits (arteriosclerosis). The drug is nevertheless used in conditions caused by spastic decrease in the size of the blood vessels, including nocturnal leg cramps, in-

179

termittent cramping of leg and foot muscles on exercise, and Raynaud's phenomenon.

Adult dosage The initial dose is usually 1200–1600 mg per day in four divided doses, taken with an antacid at meals and at bedtime. If a favorable effect is noted, the dose may be reduced to 400–800 mg per day.

Adverse effects Cyclospasmol may cause stomach upset, headache, dizziness or heart palpitation, flushing of the face, and a feeling of weakness.

Precautions Cyclospasmol should be used with caution by patients with coronary heart disease or ulcers. It should be avoided if possible by pregnant or potentially pregnant women.

See *Poor circulation,* page 68

Dalmane

Generic name

flurazepam

Action and uses A minor tranquilizer which is very popular as a nighttime sedative (sleeping medication). Dalmane is closely related to a group of tranquilizers which includes Librium and Valium, and its actions are very similar. Dalmane decreases the time it takes to fall asleep, decreases the number of awakenings, and increases the total length of sleep without suppressing dreaming (REM sleep). Barbiturates and most other sleeping pills tend to suppress dreaming, and Dalmane is considered better in this respect; however, Dalmane does block other parts of the sleep cycle so that the sleep produced is still different from normal.

Adult dosage Usually 15 to 30 mg at bedtime.

Adverse effects In some people Dalmane causes a "hangover" in the morning. It can also cause depression and dizziness. When Dalmane is stopped after regular use (three weeks or more), there is usually an increase in the deep stage of sleep and often nightmares are experienced. These probably represent withdrawal symptoms.

Precautions There is a possibility that minor tranquilizers may cause birth defects and the manufacturers therefore warn against the use of Dalmane by pregnant and potentially pregnant women. In some cases, the sedation may interfere with working and driving.

Drug dependence Dalmane is not addictive in the same way as narcotics are but, like other sedatives, it can be habit-forming to a certain extent if taken for a long period of time. If it is then stopped suddenly, some withdrawal symptoms may occur. There is a tendency toward physical and psychological dependency on the drug.

Drug interactions Dalmane can increase the sedative effect of alcohol, antihistamines, other tranquilizers, and narcotics, sometimes to a dangerous extent. Unlike many sleeping pills, Dalmane does not interfere with the effect of the anticoagulant Coumadin.

See *Minor tranquilizers,* page 45; *Sleeping pills,* page 47.

Darvocet-N

Generic ingredients

pain relievers : propoxyphene, acetaminophen

Darvon

Generic name

propoxyphene

Darvon Compound 65

Generic ingredients

pain relievers : propoxyphene, aspirin, phenacetin
mild stimulant : caffeine

Action and uses Like aspirin, Darvon and its variants are used for the relief of mild to moderate pain. Unlike aspirin, however, Darvon's main ingredient, propoxyphene, cannot reduce fever and inflammation. Darvon Compound 65 has the added pain-relieving effects of the aspirin and phenacetin, and Darvocet-N has the added pain reliever acetaminophen which can reduce fever but not inflammation. In recent years, the Darvon drugs have been among the most frequently prescribed in the United States. Though tests have shown that Darvon alone is usually no more effective in relieving pain than aspirin, and in some cases no more effective than a placebo (a pill with no active ingredient), there is a widespread belief that it is "stronger than aspirin." This may well be true of Darvon Compound and Darvocet-N, which include additional pain relievers. But psychological factors probably also play a role in the Darvon drugs' potent image. For one thing, Darvon and its variants can only be obtained on prescription, a fact which automatically suggests a special power. This impression is reinforced by their colorful packaging; a bright red tablet (such as Darvocet-N) or a pink and gray capsule (such as Darvon Compound 65) simply *looks* as though it would be more effective than two plain white aspirins. As is the case with many medications, the user's expectations of the drug can be an influential factor in determining its effectiveness.

Adult dosage Usually 32–65 mg (of propoxyphene) every four hours as needed for pain.

Adverse effects Side effects with Darvon alone are minimal, though some patients do experience nausea, dizziness, headache, or allergic skin rashes. In the case of Darvon Compound 65 and Darvocet-N, their extra ingredients may cause additional side effects. The aspirin in Darvon Compound 65 can cause stomach irritation and bleeding if the drug is taken in large quantities or over an extended period. The phenacetin in Darvon Compound 65 can, if taken in large doses or over an extended period, cause kidney damage, while large doses of Darvocet-N can cause liver damage.

Precautions Darvon Compound 65 should be used with caution by patients with stomach disorders or impaired kidney function, and by pregnant or potentially pregnant women. Darvocet-N should be used with caution by patients with impaired liver function.

Drug interactions The propoxyphene in all Darvon drugs may cause increased sedation in combination with sedatives, sleeping pills, tranquilizers, alcohol, and drugs containing narcotics. Because it contains aspirin, Darvon Compound 65 can add to the effects of anticoagulants (to increase the risk of bleeding) and cortisone-like drugs (to increase the risk of ulcer).

Drug dependence The propoxyphene these drugs contain is chemically related to the narcotic analgesics and both addiction and death through overdose have occurred. For this reason, the Darvon group of drugs has been placed under scrutiny by the Food and Drug Administration for possible restriction.

See *Pain and/or inflammation,* page 37. *Non-narcotic pain relievers,* page 42.

Demerol

Generic name

> meperidine (available by generic name)

Action and uses
A common narcotic pain reliever used by injection in hospitals and occasionally taken orally. It is used in preoperative preparation for surgery, but primarily it is used to relieve severe pain—after surgery, for example, and in patients suffering from cancer. It is available outside the hospital only on restricted prescriptions.

Adult dosage
75–150 mg orally or by injection every three to six hours for pain.

Adverse effects
A number of people experience nausea and vomiting when given this drug. This is not an allergy, but an increased sensitivity to one of its effects. It can also cause constipation, and in some people, dizziness, or unusual sensations or dreams.

Precautions
Demerol should be used only when other less potent pain relievers are not effective. It should be used with caution in people with chronic lung disease or emphysema.

Drug dependence
Tolerance and addiction to Demerol can occur with continued use, and withdrawal symptoms will occur if it is discontinued suddenly.

Drug interactions
Demerol can add to the sedative and breathing depression effects of sedatives, tranquilizers, and alcohol. It can also add to the constipating effects of many antispasmodic drugs and antihistamines.

See
Narcotic pain relievers, page 41.

Demulen-21

Generic ingredients

> progestogen : ethynodiol diacetate
> estrogen : ethinyl estradiol

Action and uses
An oral contraceptive. Demulen is one of many birth control pills containing a combination of two synthetic hormones—an estrogen and a progesterone-like hormone (a progestogen). It acts, like most other oral contraceptives, to prevent conception by affecting the pituitary gland's control of the normal menstrual cycle, as well as acting locally on the lining of the uterus and the cervical mucus, and possibly in other ways.

183

When taken regularly it is a very effective contraceptive drug. It is similar to Ovulen except for a somewhat lower amount and slightly different kind of estrogen.

Adult dosage In general, one tablet is taken daily (usually at night) for the first cycle, beginning on the 5th day of menstruation and continuing for 21 days. No tablets are taken for the following 7 days, during which time menstrual bleeding occurs, and on the 8th day they are started again for another 21-day cycle, and so on.

Adverse effects As with all oral contraceptives, a variety of side effects may occur including weight gain, increased appetite, depression or fatigue, breast changes, gastrointestinal upset, headache, and increased vaginal discharge or infection. More significant but less common side effects include the risk of thrombophlebitis (blood clotting and inflammation in the veins of the legs), increased blood pressure, increased blood sugar, and gallbladder disease. The risk of certain side effects such as heart disease and gallbladder disease appear to increase with age (especially over the age of 35). If a woman has a history of true migraine headaches, she may experience a higher incidence of headaches while on the pill, and she also runs a slightly higher risk of having a stroke (though the risk remains small). A history of heavy smoking is associated with an increased risk of heart disease, particularly in the age group over 40.

Precautions A history of thrombophlebitis, blood clots, and migraine headaches is usually a contraindication to the use of oral contraceptives. For women over the age of 35, or those with other risk factors, such as a history of heavy smoking, gallbladder disease, diabetes, or high blood pressure, use should be weighed carefully against alternative birth control methods.

Drug interactions Several drug interactions have been suggested but none have been well-documented as significant in most cases.

See *Hormonal drugs,* page 87; *Oral contraceptives,* page 96.

Diabinese

Generic name

chlorpropamide

Action and uses A drug which lowers glucose levels in the blood, used to treat diabetes. Because Diabinese can be taken orally (unlike insulin), it is termed an "oral hypoglycemic" drug (hypoglycemic means "blood-sugar-lowering"). It is similar to other oral antidiabetic drugs such as Orinase and Tolinase, but not to DBI. Diabinese works by stimulating the pancreas to produce insulin and by helping the cells of the body to use glucose. It is of value only in diabetics who are able to make insulin. Such patients usually have the milder type of diabetes, which often becomes evident toward middle age (and is therefore known as maturity-onset diabetes). Oral hypoglycemic drugs should be taken only if dietary measures alone have failed to control the condition. Resistance to the effects of Diabinese often develops after a few months or years. It is recommended that withdrawal of oral antidiabetic drugs be tried every six months to one year, since their continued use may not be needed. The benefits versus risks of long-term use of this and related drugs are now widely debated.

Adverse effects The most common and hazardous adverse effect is excessive *lowering* of the blood sugar (hypoglycemia), which can cause symptoms of dizziness, weakness, cold sweats and mental dullness. Older people, those taking several other drugs (see drug interactions below), and those with liver or kidney disease are more prone to this. With proper doses, other side effects are unusual, but rashes, blood or liver abnormalities, and water retention can occur.

Adult dosage This is adjusted according to each individual patient's response. Initially 250 mg is given once daily and adjusted. Older patients may require lower doses.

Precautions The drug should be avoided by pregnant or potentially pregnant women and nursing mothers and also by those with significant kidney or liver diseases. Those allergic to sulfa drugs may develop an allergy to this drug.

Drug interactions Thiazide diuretics (e.g., hydrochlorothiazide, Diuril, Hygroton) can aggravate diabetes and may increase the dose requirement of the oral antidiabetic drug. A number of drugs can increase the risk of low blood sugar due to increased levels of drug. These include insulin, sulfa drugs, anti-inflammatory drugs such as aspirin, Butazolidin and Tandearil, and the anticonvulsant Dilantin. Inderal (propranolol) can also cause dangerous interactions and disguise the symptoms of hypoglycemia. Alcohol can cause a flushing reaction when taken with this drug.

See *Diabetes,* page 90.

Diamox

Generic name

acetazolamide (available by generic name)

Action and uses   A mild diuretic which promotes the loss of water from the body. It is used to treat glaucoma (loss of vision caused by increased pressure of the fluid within the eye) and it also has a use in the treatment of epilepsy. Rarely it is used to treat other conditions involving water retention. Diamox acts by inhibiting an enzyme, *carbonic anhydrase,* which is important for the excretion of excess acid by the kidney. When the enzyme is inhibited by the drug the kidney retains acid but excretes more sodium and potassium and, as a result, more urine is formed. The acid accumulated in the blood causes the drug to lose its effectiveness and the drug's action is only seen for a few days.

In glaucoma, Diamox exerts a local effect in the eye, and although the same enzyme is acted upon by the drug, the same loss of the drug's activity does not occur. The action of Diamox in epilepsy is not fully understood, but inhibition of the enzyme carbonic anhydrase in the brain is thought to cut down the nervous discharges which lead to convulsions.

Adult dosage   Acetazolamide is supplied as tablets of 125 mg and 250 mg (Diamox), and as a sustained-release preparation (Sequels) of 500 mg. The dosage varies with the condition being treated, but is often one Sequel twice daily or one 250 mg Diamox tablet one to four times daily.

Precautions   Diamox is chemically related to the sulfa drugs, so if there is some allergy to this group of drugs, there may be allergy to Diamox as well. Diamox should be avoided by pregnant or potentially pregnant women and nursing mothers.

Adverse effects   Tingling feelings in the fingers and toes may be experienced and if the drug is taken for longer periods, weakness, drowsiness, and dizziness may also occur.

Drug interactions   Diamox makes the urine alkaline and this can prevent the action of certain bladder antiseptics, and increase the action of certain drugs which are eliminated in the kidneys, such as quinidine and Pronestyl.

See   *Diuretics,* page 63; *Seizures (convulsions),* page 130.

Dicyclomine (generic name). See BENTYL.

Diethylpropion (generic name). See TENUATE.

Digoxin

Trade names

Lanoxin, SK-Digoxin

Action and uses A drug used in treating heart failure. It increases the force of the heart muscle's contraction, slows the heart rate, and enables the heart to pump more efficiently. Like digitalis, of which it is a purer form, digoxin is derived from the foxglove plant, whose usefulness as a heart medicine was known to folk practitioners centuries before it was first written up by a British doctor in the late 1700s.

Adult dosage Dosage must be carefully adjusted according to individual responses and requirements. Usually, however, it is 0.125 mg to 0.25 mg taken once a day. It is sometimes given in a larger dose at first, but this has to be individually determined, often with careful checking of the pulse and an electrocardiogram, plus laboratory checks on blood levels of the drug.

Adverse effects For each patient, there is a very narrow margin between the amount of digoxin necessary to benefit the heart and the amount liable to cause toxic effect. The symptoms of overdosage can include loss of appetite, nausea, vomiting, diarrhea, headache, blurred vision, and/or rapid, fluttering, irregular or skipped heartbeat.

Precautions Any of these symptoms should be reported to the doctor promptly. It cannot be overemphasized that this drug must be taken only under the strict supervision of a physician who can monitor its effect.

Drug interactions The diuretics ("water pills") often prescribed along with digoxin to treat excess fluid retention can increase the body's vulnerability to digoxin's toxic effects by causing excessive potassium loss. (Exceptions are the *potassium-retaining* diuretics Aldactazide, Aldactone, Diazide, and Dyrenium.) It may be necessary therefore to supplement the body's potassium level daily with oral potassium preparations (KCl) or potassium-rich foods, such as orange or tomato juice, bananas, or dried fruit. The possibility of toxic effects with digoxin can also be increased by drugs for high blood pressure containing reserpine, by cortisone-like drugs such as prednisone, and by thyroid preparations.

See *Heart failure,* page 65.

Dilantin

Generic name

> diphenylhydantoin or phenytoin
> (available by generic name)

Action and uses   A drug used to prevent or reduce the frequency of epileptic seizures which occur without apparent cause or are due to brain damage from accidents, surgery, or strokes. If ineffective alone, it is given in combination with other anticonvulsant drugs such as phenobarbital. It is used rarely to treat irregular heart rhythms.

Adult dosage   The usual dose is 300 mg orally once daily or in divided doses. The requirements vary widely so the need for dose adjustment is frequent when the drug is started.

Adverse effects   The most common adverse effects are related to excess dosage and include unsteadiness in walking and difficulty in coordination or speech, and bizarre behavior or confusion. These effects will decrease with lower doses. Although Dilantin is usually well tolerated at proper doses, some people may experience gastric upset, constipation, allergic skin rashes (which require stopping the drug), and swelling of the gums (often prevented by good dental hygiene and gum massage). Also, abnormalities of the blood cells and lymph glands can occur infrequently.

Precautions   Dilantin should not be used in pregnancy unless the benefits outweigh the risks, since some studies have suggested this drug may harm the fetus.

Drug interactions   Dilantin can interact with several drugs. When given with oral antidiabetic drugs, certain sulfa drugs, the anticoagulant Coumadin, the anti-inflammatory drug Butazolidin, and the anti-tuberculosis drug INH, the effects of Dilantin itself, as well as those of these drugs, may be hazardously increased. Since some tricyclic antidepressants (e.g., Elavil) and major tranquilizers (e.g., Thorazine) increase the likelihood of seizures, they may decrease the effect of Dilantin and require an increased dose. Further, Dilantin may affect the metabolism of other drugs and decrease their effectiveness.

See   *Seizures (convulsions),* page 130

Dimetane

Generic name

brompheniramine (available by generic name)

Action and uses   A commonly prescribed antihistamine which is used to treat allergic conditions, especially allergic rhinitis, sinusitis, or conjunctivitis (redness of the eye). In common with most other antihistamines it acts by blocking the effects of histamine and thus can decrease itching of the skin caused by allergies, hives or rashes. It also can sometimes have a sedating effect, although it is not customarily used for this. It is not useful for the treatment of asthma. It is usually much less expensive in generic form, as brompheniramine.

Adult dosage   Dimetane is available in oral tablets and liquids and for injections. The usual oral dose is 4 mg two to six times daily or one 8 mg or 12 mg Extentab twice daily as needed for treatment of allergic conditions.

Adverse effects   Dimetane may cause significant sedation in some people, although possibly less frequently than some other antihistamines. Other side effects are relatively rare, but can include dry mouth, blurred vision, or difficulty in urinating, especially in older people or those with glaucoma or prostate trouble.

Drug interactions   Dimetane is additive to other sedative or tranquilizing drugs and alcohol. It is also additive to other antispasmodic drugs used to treat ulcers or stomach problems, such as Pro-Banthine or Librax, causing excessive dry mouth, constipation, and difficulty in urinating.

Precautions   The sedative effects may interfere with driving or operating machinery. This drug should be used with caution by those with glaucoma or prostate trouble. It should also be avoided by pregnant or potentially pregnant women and nursing mothers.

See   *Antihistamines,* page 121.

Dimetane Expectorant

Generic ingredients

antihistamine : brompheniramine
decongestants : phenylephrine, phenylpropanolamine
expectorant : guaifenesin

Dimetane Expectorant-DC

Generic ingredients

> antihistamine : brompheniramine
> decongestants : phenylephrine, phenylpropanolamine
> expectorant : guaifenesin
> cough suppressant : codeine

Action and uses This is a compound mixture of cough/cold ingredients, aimed at several of the symptoms of a cold; it includes an antihistamine and decongestants for nasal congestion, an expectorant and, in the Dimetane Expectorant-DC, an antitussive for symptoms of cough. Whether all of these components can act effectively together is difficult to determine, but the inclusion in the "DC" preparation of codeine, which is a narcotic, makes the use of that mixture restricted to cases where coughing might be harmful. If this is not the case, then the mixture without codeine is preferable.

Adult dosage The usual dose is one teaspoon (5 ml) of the syrup three or four times per day.

Adverse effects Side effects may include drowsiness caused by the antihistamine and possibly palpitation caused by the decongestants. Although the amount of codeine is small, it may cause nausea and vomiting, and if used for several days, constipation. The expectorant may also cause nausea.

Precautions Driving or operating heavy equipment may be hazardous as sedation is an effect of this medication. Persons taking medicine for high blood pressure or heart ailments should check with their physicians before using, since the decongestants may elevate the blood pressure. Repeated use for any period of more than two to four days is undesirable in most cases. Dimetane should be avoided by pregnant or potentially pregnant women and nursing mothers.

Drug dependence The codeine in the "DC" compound can cause habituation if taken for prolonged periods.

Drug interactions The sedative effects of the antihistamine, and, to a lesser extent of the codeine, can be additive to any other sedating drugs such as tranquilizers and alcohol. The decongestants can raise the blood pressure and thus counteract the effect of any drug used to treat high blood pressure.

See *Coughs and colds,* page 117.

Dimetapp

Generic ingredients

antihistamine : brompheniramine
decongestants : phenylpropanolamine, phenylephrine

Action and uses This mixture of an antihistamine and two decongestants is used for the usual symptoms of a cold: nasal congestion and a runny nose. It is one of many similar mixtures of decongestants and antihistamines sold for this purpose. It is also relatively effective for nasal congestion related to other causes such as allergies, but it is not useful in asthma.

Adult dosage Extentab: One tablet every 8–12 hours.
Elixir: 1–2 teaspoonfuls three or four times a day (the elixir has a slightly lower dose of the separate ingredients so it can be taken more frequently).

Adverse effects Side effects may include drowsiness caused by the antihistamine, and, possibly, palpitations caused by the decongestants.

Precautions This drug should be avoided by pregnant or potentially pregnant women and nursing mothers. Driving or operating heavy equipment may be hazardous if sedation is a side effect. People taking medicines for high blood pressure or heart ailments should check with their physicians before using Dimetapp since the decongestants may elevate the blood pressure.

Drug interactions The sedative effect of the antihistamine can add to other sedating drugs such as tranquilizers and alcohol. The decongestants can also raise the blood pressure and thus counteract the effect of any drug used to treat high blood pressure, such as Aldomet and Inderal.

See *Coughs and colds,* page 117.

Diphenhydramine (generic name). See BENADRYL.

Diphenylhydantoin (generic name). See DILANTIN.

Diupres

Generic ingredients

antihypertensive : reserpine
diuretic : chlorothiazide

Action and uses   One of several popular fixed-combination drugs prescribed for the control of high blood pressure. The reserpine in Diupres lowers blood pressure by blocking the sympathetic nervous system (which constricts the blood vessels). The other component in Diupres, chlorothiazide, is a diuretic ("water pill"), which lowers blood pressure by promoting the elimination of excess salt and water from the system, thus decreasing blood volume and slightly dilating the blood vessels. Diupres is a fixed-dose combination drug—that is, it combines two ingredients in fixed amounts. This can be a drawback, because it limits the possibilities for adjusting the dose according to the requirements of each individual patient, so often necessary with drugs for high blood pressure. If the amount of one of the ingredients in Diupres suits a patient, but the amount of the other does not, it may be simpler (and less expensive) for the patient to take the two drugs separately.

Adult dosage   Usually 1–4 tablets per day if Diupres-250 has been prescribed, or 1–2 tablets per day if Diupres-500 has been prescribed. Often one daily dose only is required.

Adverse effects   The reserpine in Diupres can cause drowsiness and lethargy, nasal stuffiness, stomach upset or ulceration, and sometimes severe depression. The chlorothiazide in Diupres can cause allergic skin rash, nausea, diarrhea, and excessive loss of potassium. This last-mentioned side effect may be signaled by muscle cramping and weakness, and can be corrected by eating potassium-rich foods (tomato and orange juice, bananas and dried fruit) or by taking a supplement of potassium chloride (KCl). Less frequently, chlorothiazide can precipitate gout or diabetes, possibilities which should be checked by blood tests at intervals.

Precautions   Diupres should be used with caution by patients with gout or diabetes, a history of depression, heart failure, epilepsy, or peptic ulcers. It should be avoided if possible by pregnant or potentially pregnant women and nursing mothers. Women taking this drug for long periods of time should have regular breast checks because of a possible link between long-term use of reserpine and breast cancer, though this link remains controversial.

Drug interactions   Because of the reserpine it contains, Diupres can cause oversedation when taken concurrently with sedatives, sleeping pills, tranquilizers, antihistamines, and alcohol. Some drugs for asthma, weight loss, depression, and colds can interact with reserpine to increase blood pressure. Diupres and any of these drugs, therefore, should not be taken concurrently except under a doctor's supervision. The chlorothiazide in Diupres can interact with steroids such as prednisone to cause excessive potassium loss. The increased potassium loss due to chlorothiazide can also increase sensitivity to the toxic effects of digoxin.

See *High blood pressure,* page 58; *Diuretics,* page 63.

Diuril

Generic name

chlorothiazide (available by generic name)

Action and uses A diuretic ("water pill") used to treat high blood pressure and the excessive retention of water associated with certain heart, liver, and kidney disorders, and premenstrual tension. Its primary action is to cause a loss of excess salt and water via the kidneys, thus relieving edema (the swelling of body tissue due to retained fluid). It is also very useful in treating high blood pressure because it slightly relaxes the blood vessels and increases the effectiveness of other drugs used to lower blood pressure. This drug is one of a group of diuretic drugs called *thiazide diuretics.* The term "thiazide" refers both to a chemical structure and to a class of several similar drugs, including HydroDIURIL, Hygroton, Renese and Naturetin, which all share similar actions and side effects.

Adult dosage Usually 0.5 to 1.0 gram per day in divided doses of 250 or 500 mg. Increased urination occurs one or two hours after taking the drug and may last for three to six hours. Once the urination pattern is established the time at which the drug is taken can be determined for convenience. A nighttime dose is usually impractical.

Adverse effects If taking Diuril causes the loss of too much of the essential mineral salt potassium, side effects may occur. These include muscle cramps, weakness, tiredness, and dizziness. If potassium loss is very great it may be hazardous. Potassium supplements (KCl) are sometimes used in conjunction with Diuril. Potassium replacement can also be accomplished by dietary means (orange juice, tomato juice, bananas, or dried fruit). Other side effects include a tendency to cause high blood sugar in individuals predisposed to diabetes. In some people Diuril can cause an elevation in the levels of uric acid in the blood (the substance which can cause gout). On long-term therapy these factors are checked but seldom cause a problem. Allergies to Diuril can occur but are not common.

Precautions This drug should be used with careful supervision, if at all, by pregnant or potentially pregnant women and by people with gout or diabetes.

Drug interactions Taken in conjunction with cortisone-like drugs such as prednisone, Diuril can cause excessive potassium loss. Potentially serious interactions may also occur if Diuril is taken in conjunction with digitalis drugs for the heart, because if too much potassium is eliminated from the system through the effects of the chlorothiazide, the heart can become sensitive to the toxic effects of digitalis. Medical supervision is essential.

See *High blood pressure,* page 58; *Heart failure,* page 65.

Donnagel-PG

Generic ingredients

> antispasmodics : atropine, hyoscine, hyoscyamine
> narcotic : opium
> bulk producers : kaolin, pectin

Action and uses A mixture used to treat diarrhea. The exact cause of diarrhea is often never established. Donnagel-PG, which treats the symptoms rather than the cause, reduces diarrhea in several ways. Kaolin and pectin provide bulk which reduces the looseness of the feces, and also bind with the irritant substances so that the latter leave the body in the stools. The antispasmodic drugs atropine, hyoscine, and hyoscyamine all reduce the activity of nerves which stimulate intestinal motion. The small dose of opium (equivalent to 6 ml of paregoric) relaxes the muscle of the intestine, relieving cramp and slowing intestinal movements. Although Donnagel-PG may be effective on a short-term basis, some authorities feel that prolonged use of this type of antidiarrheal may actually prolong the illness by allowing retention of the bacteria or toxins in the bowel.

Adult dosage Two tablespoonfuls every three hours, as needed.

Adverse reactions The antispasmodics atropine, hyoscine, and hyoscyamine can cause dry mouth, blurring of vision, and difficulty in urinating. If taken in excessive doses, Donnagel-PG may cause vomiting, sedation, fever, or flushing.

Precautions Persons with glaucoma or prostate trouble should take Don-nagel-PG with caution. If diarrhea persists for more than a few days, the doctor should be consulted as the cause should be investigated.

Drug dependence Opium is a narcotic and, though present in Donnagel-PG in small amounts, it can be habit-forming—another reason why Donnagel-PG should not be taken for more than a few days at a time.

Drug interactions The effects of the antispasmodics and opium can be additive to those of other anticholinergic drugs such as antihista-mines, cough/cold medicines, and tricyclic antidepressants.

See *Diarrhea,* page 86.

Donnatal
Donnatal No. 2

Generic ingredients

antispasmodics : atropine, hyoscine, hyoscyamine
tranquilizer : phenobarbital

Action and uses A fixed-combination drug used to treat the symptoms of ul-cers and intestinal disorders. The antispasmodics relax the smooth muscle of the stomach and small and large intestine and reduce spasm by acting on the nervous system. The phenobarbital is a sedative or anti-anxiety agent, added on the (unproven) assumption that decreased anxiety will help relieve gastrointestinal symptoms. Donnatal is used to treat stomach and duodenal ulcers, irritable colon, spastic colon, and intestinal upsets. Single antispasmodic drugs are likely to be as effective.

Adult dosage Usually one or two tablets, capsules or teaspoonfuls of liquid, three or four times per day. Donnatal No. 2 contains twice as much phenobarbital as ordinary Donnatal. The dose must be adjusted to the individual needs of the patient, but is usually one or two tablets three times per day.

Adverse effects Most side effects are due to the antispasmodics. They can in-clude blurred vision, dryness of the mouth and skin, and dif-ficulty in urinating, especially in older people. They can also cause drying of bronchial secretions. Although the amount of phenobarbital present is small, it may cause sedation, and al-lergic reactions can occur.

Precautions Donnatal should be used with caution by people with glau-coma, enlargement of the prostate, and chronic lung disease. If drowsiness occurs, driving or operating machinery may be hazardous.

Drug dependence	Phenobarbital, one of the ingredients of Donnatal, is a barbiturate which may cause physical or psychological dependence if used over a long period.
Drug interactions	The effects of the antispasmodics can be additive to those of antihistamines, cough/cold medicines, and tricyclic antidepressants, causing excessive dry mouth, constipation, and occasional bladder problems. The phenobarbital can decrease the effect of the anticoagulant Coumadin, and might potentially add to the effects of other sedatives, tranquilizers or alcohol.
See	*Nausea, stomach upset, and ulcers,* page 75; *Minor tranquilizers,* page 45.

Doxycycline (generic name). See VIBRAMYCIN.

Drixoral

Generic ingredients	antihistamine : brompheniramine maleate decongestant : disoephedrine sulfate
Action and uses	A combination drug used to treat symptoms of colds and allergies. The antihistamine and decongestant help relieve nasal congestion and stop runny nose.
Adult dosage	The usual dose is one tablet once or twice a day.
Adverse effects	Side effects include drowsiness due to the antihistamine and possibly palpitation due to the decongestant.
Precautions	This drug should be avoided by pregnant or potentially pregnant women and nursing mothers. Driving or operating heavy equipment may be hazardous if sedation is an effect of this medication. Those taking medicine for high blood pressure or heart ailments should check with their physicians before using, since the decongestant may elevate the blood pressure. Repeated use for any period of more than two to four days is undesirable in most cases.
Drug interactions	The sedative effects of the antihistamine can be additive to those of any other sedating drug, e.g.,tranquilizers or alcohol. The decongestant can raise the blood pressure and thus counteract the effect of any drug used to treat high blood pressure.
See	*Coughs and colds,* page 117.

Dyazide

Generic ingredients

diuretics : triamterene, hydrochlorothiazide

Action and uses A fixed-combination diuretic ("water pill") used in the treatment of high blood pressure and heart failure. Dyazide combines the action of two diuretics, one which retains potassium (triamterene), and one which causes loss of potassium (hydrochlorothiazide). Together they produce the desired loss of excess salt and water without the undesirable effect of potassium loss. The fixed combination may present problems, however, since it does not allow dose adjustments of each of the individual ingredients. Increased urination usually occurs 1–2 hours after taking the drug.

Adult dosage Usually one or two capsules once or twice a day.

Adverse effects In some cases there may be a tendency to retain more potassium in the body than is needed or safe. When potassium levels rise too high there is a danger of heart failure and treatment to remove excess potassium is complex. This is not usually a problem in people with normal kidney function, but Dyazide can cause a decrease in kidney function, especially if there is pre-existing abnormal function. Dyazide can cause nausea or loss of appetite, which can sometimes be associated with more serious abnormalities and requires careful checking.

The hydrochlorothiazide in the drug may cause increased levels of sugar in the blood in people predisposed to diabetes. In some people it may cause an elevation in blood levels of uric acid (the substance which can cause gout). Allergies to both of the ingredients in Dyazide can occur.

Precautions Dyazide should not be used by pregnant or potentially pregnant women. Dyazide is not generally indicated for use by people with any degree of kidney disease unless the blood is monitored for potassium levels and kidney function.

Drug interactions Preparations containing potassium can raise blood levels hazardously if given with Dyazide.

See *High blood pressure,* page 58; *Diuretics,* page 63; *Heart failure,* page 65.

E.E.S. (erythomycin ethyl succinate). See
ERYTHROMYCIN.

Elavil

Generic name

amitriptyline

Action and uses
A commonly prescribed antidepressant drug. Like Tofranil and Sinequan, it belongs to a group of closely related drugs called *tricyclic antidepressants* and is used to treat certain types of moderately severe and longstanding depression. The tricyclic antidepressants are not true tranquilizers, although they can cause some sedation. Elavil's ability to improve mood and to relieve depression is often quite marked, but there is usually a significant time-lag before its beneficial effects are felt.

Adult dosage
The effective dose of Elavil varies greatly and must be carefully adjusted for each individual; dosage adjustment may take one or two months. Initially, the dose is usually 25–75 mg per day and may be increased to 150 mg per day. (The dose may be lower for elderly patients.) Because the drug is long-acting and may cause some sedation, it is usually taken just once a day, at bedtime.

Adverse effects
Initially, Elavil may cause dry mouth, blurred vision, drowsiness, confusion or dizziness, constipation, and difficulty in urinating. (These effects are especially a problem in older people.) Other significant side effects may include effects on the heart rhythm.

Precautions
Elavil should be taken with caution by people with glaucoma, prostate gland problems, liver or heart disease, epilepsy, or a hyperthyroid condition. It should not be taken by pregnant or potentially pregnant women or nursing mothers. It may interfere with driving or operating machinery.

Drug interactions
Elavil can cause oversedation when taken in combination with alcohol, sleeping pills, tranquilizers, antihistamines, and drugs containing narcotics. It can add to the side effects of antispasmodic drugs and decrease the effects of drugs to lower blood pressure such as Ismelin. It can dangerously interfere with drugs to regulate heart rhythm, thyroid drugs, and drugs of the MAO inhibitor family (e.g., Marplan, Parnate and Nardil). Taken with drugs of the latter type or with the sedative Placidyl, Elavil can cause delirium.

See *Antidepressants,* page 52.

Elixophyllin

Generic name

> theophylline (available by generic name)

Action and uses Elixophyllin is a preparation of theophylline, available in both capsule and liquid form, used to treat asthma. Theophylline is frequently the mainstay of the treatment of asthma and it can be prescribed as a less expensive generic form. It relaxes the smooth muscle constricting the small bronchi (airways) of the lungs and dilates the local arteries. The liquid form of Elixophyllin is rapidly absorbed and therefore rapidly effective. It is sometimes used for treatment of mild asthmatic attacks.

Adult dosage Capsule: One, taken three or four times daily.
   Elixir: One or two teaspoonfuls, three or four times daily. In general, the dose varies considerably from person to person and is adjusted according to clinical response, change in lung function, and/or blood level of the drug (measured by tests).

Adverse effects The most common side effect is gastric irritation from the direct effect of the drug in the stomach, as well as nausea and vomiting, which are related to indirect effects of the theophylline. The nausea and vomiting may be decreased by lowering the dose. Other dose-related effects also include headache, muscle cramps, palpitations, and, occasionally, nervousness or insomnia.

Precautions The use of Elixophyllin by people with irregular heart rhythms or other types of heart disease should be carefully supervised by the physician.

Drug interactions Elixophyllin is additive to other drugs used to treat asthma, and its side effects can also be additive. It is important for the prescribing physician to be aware of *all* prescription and over-the-counter drugs the patient is using for this condtion.

See *Asthma and lung disease,* page 109.

Empirin Compound with Codeine

Generic ingredients

> narcotic pain reliever : codeine
> pain relievers : aspirin, phenacetin
> mild stimulant : caffeine

Action and uses A combination drug used to treat moderate to severe pain. In addition to the ingredients found in Empirin Compound (the analgesics aspirin and phenacetin, plus the mild stimulant caffeine), this preparation contains the narcotic analgesic codeine, which makes the drug available on restricted prescription only.

Adult dosage Usually one or two tablets every three to six hours as needed for pain.

Adverse effects Like other combination pain relievers, the side effects of Empirin Compound with Codeine may include those of any of its ingredients, although the various components are present in smaller amounts than the normal dose when used alone. Nonetheless, the aspirin in Empirin Compound with Codeine can irritate the stomach, causing nausea, pain, and even bleeding if taken in large quantities. The phenacetin in the preparation can, over a period of months, cause kidney damage, and the codeine can cause nausea, constipation, and drowsiness.

Precautions Empirin Compound with Codeine should be avoided by patients with stomach disorders or impaired kidney function, and used with caution by pregnant or potentially pregnant women and nursing mothers.

Drug dependence Because of the codeine in this combination drug, habituation may occur if it is taken over a prolonged period of time.

Drug interactions The aspirin in this combination drug can add to the effects of the anticoagulant Coumadin to increase the risk of bleeding; taken in combination with cortisone-like drugs, it can increase the risk of stomach ulceration. The codeine in the preparation can add to the sedative effects of alcohol, tranquilizers, and antidepressants.

See *Narcotic pain relievers,* page 41.

E-Mycin (brand name for erythromycin). See
ERYTHROMYCIN.

Enduron

Generic name

methyclothiazide

Action and uses One of many diuretics ("water pills") of the thiazide type. Thus, it is very similar in its actions and side effects to hydrochlorothiazide, Esidrix, HydroDIURIL and Diuril. It is used in the therapy of hypertension (high blood pressure), heart failure, and various other ailments where edema (swelling of the feet and/or hands due to retained fluid) is a problem. It acts by causing loss of water, sodium, and potassium.

Adult dosage 2.5 to 5 mg, once or twice daily.

Adverse effects Like all thiazide diuretics, Enduron can cause excessive loss of the mineral potassium, which is seldom a problem at lower doses; at doses greater than 5 mg per day, however, the patient may need to take potassium supplements. This becomes more important if a person is taking digoxin or related drugs. Extra potassium in the diet can be obtained from orange and tomato juice and from bananas and dried fruit. Liquid potassium chloride (KCl) can also be taken. A significant lack of potassium can cause symptoms of weakness or dizziness or muscle cramp. In addition, Enduron can increase levels of sugar in the blood and also of uric acid, and predispose to gout in some people. It may also cause occasional allergic reactions.

Precautions Long-term use may require occasional checks of blood potassium, sugar, and uric acid levels, especially if digitalis or digoxin is also taken. This drug should be used with caution by pregnant or potentially pregnant women.

Drug interactions Potentially serious interactions may occur if Enduron is taken in conjunction with digitalis or digoxin; the potassium loss caused by Enduron can render the heart sensitive to the toxic effects of digitalis and related drugs. Since Enduron and other thiazide diuretics cause calcium retention, the use of calcium-containing antacids, calcium supplements, or vitamin D may cause elevated levels of calcium in the blood. The potassium loss with steroid drugs (e.g.,prednisone) can be additive to the effects of this drug.

See *High blood pressure,* page 58; *Heart failure,* page 65; *Diuretics,* page 63.

Equagesic

Generic ingredients

analgesics : aspirin, ethoheptazine
muscle relaxant : meprobamate

Action and uses A combination drug, made up of two pain relievers and a muscle relaxant, used to treat muscle pain and soreness. Interestingly enough, Equagesic's component drugs are present in lower doses than those usually thought necessary for effectiveness. For example, aspirin is usually taken in doses of 600 mg for relief of pain, but there are only 250 mg of aspirin in one Equagesic tablet. Similarly, meprobamate is usually administered in doses of 400–800 mg, when used for its muscle-relaxant effect, but there are only 150 mg of meprobamate in one Equagesic tablet. The apparent explanation for the minimal presence of the components in Equagesic is that they are additive to one another's effects. But whether they are truly additive and whether they are at all effective at these low doses is not completely clear. It is probable that an adequate dose of aspirin and the application of heat will often be as effective in treating sore muscles as this more expensive drug.

Adult dosage　Usually two tablets three or four times daily.

Adverse effects　Like other combination drugs, Equagesic has the side effects of its various components. The aspirin in Equagesic can irritate the stomach, causing nausea, vomiting, pain, and bleeding. The ethoheptazine can cause dizziness and drowsiness. The meprobamate can cause headache, blurred vision, stomach upset, and allergic skin rashes.

Precautions　Because of the meprobamate it contains, Equagesic should not be taken by pregnant or potentially pregnant women or nursing mothers. Because of its aspirin content, it should be taken with caution by patients who have stomach disorders or a sensitivity to aspirin. It should not be used by people taking Coumadin.

Drug dependence　Because of the meprobamate it contains, Equagesic can, if taken in large doses over an extended period, cause psychological and/or physical dependence.

Drug interactions　The aspirin in Equagesic can add to the effects of anticoagulants such as Coumadin and increase the risk of bleeding. The meprobamate in Equagesic can increase the sedative effects of alcohol, tranquilizers, sleeping pills, and antidepressants, and counteract the effects of the anticoagulant Coumadin.

See　*Non-narcotic pain relievers,* page 42.

Equanil

Generic name

meprobamate (available by generic name)

Action and uses　A minor tranquilizer used to relieve mild tension and anxiety. Both Equanil and Miltown (another trade name for meprobamate) are very similar to barbiturates in their sedative effects. Their use as sedatives, however, has diminished somewhat since the introduction of Librium and Valium. Equanil is also frequently used in cases of muscle strain (as in back strain) as a muscle relaxant. Whether its beneficial effect in such cases is due to sedation or to true muscle relaxation is not clear.

Adult dosage Usually 200–400 mg four times a day and sometimes double that dose.

Adverse effects The incidence of allergic reactions to Equanil is relatively high. Such reactions may include skin rashes or hives. Other common side effects may include nausea, headache, dizziness, and excessive drowsiness.

Precautions Equanil should not be taken by pregnant, potentially pregnant women or nursing mothers. It may interfere with driving or operating machinery.

Drug dependence Equanil can produce psychological and/or physical dependence. Once habituation to the drug has developed, convulsions can occur if the drug is suddenly stopped, especially if the daily dose has been more than 800 mg four times a day.

Drug interactions Equanil's sedative effects can be increased by alcohol, other sedatives and tranquilizers, sleeping pills, and antidepressants. Equanil can decrease the effects of anticoagulants, oral contraceptives, and the estrogens used in hormone replacement therapy, because it affects the way the liver metabolizes these drugs.

See *Minor tranquilizers,* page 45.

Erythrocin (erythromycin ethyl succinate). See
ERYTHROMYCIN.

Erythromycin

Trade names

E-Mycin, E.E.S., Erythrocin, Pediamycin, Ilotycin, Robimycin

Action and uses A commonly used antibiotic which comes from the mold *Streptomyces*. It acts on bacteria to inhibit production of proteins but has no effect on human cells. Erythromycin is most commonly used in mild to moderate infections where penicillin would normally be indicated but the patient is allergic to penicillin. These infections include bacterial sore throat ("strep throat"), respiratory or lung infections, and some venereal diseases. It is seldom used in very serious infections.

Adult dosage The usual adult dosage is 250 to 500 mg every six hours, preferably on an empty stomach.

Adverse effects The most frequent side effect is gastrointestinal upset, including nausea, belching, and diarrhea. Rashes and other allergic reactions can occur but are not as frequent as with other antibiotics.

Precautions This antibiotic, like all others, should be taken for the full course prescribed, and every dose should be taken. Failure to do this can result in inadequate treatment of the infection, recurrence, or development of resistant strains of bacteria. Erythromycin should be used with caution by pregnant or potentially pregnant women and nursing mothers.

Drug interactions Erythromycin may interfere with the effectiveness of penicillin and Cleocin.

See *Infections,* page 111.

Esidrex (brand name for hydrochlorothiazide). See HYDROCHLOROTHIAZIDE.

Feosol

Generic name

ferrous sulfate (available by generic name)

Action and uses A dietary supplement of iron used for treating anemia resulting from iron deficiency. Iron is an important part of the protein hemoglobin, which is responsible for transporting oxygen to all parts of the body in the red blood cells. If there is insufficient hemoglobin, not enough oxygen will reach the tissues of the body. Iron deficiency may be due to lack of iron in the diet, increased demand (as in pregnancy), failure of the body to absorb iron from the diet, or severe or chronic bleeding. Women lose iron through blood loss during menstruation. In pregnancy iron is transferred from the mother to the developing child. Women therefore need more iron than men and this can be provided by a dietary supplement, though a well-balanced diet usually provides adequate iron without the need for pills. Men almost never need iron supplements, except when prescribed by a doctor for special conditions.

Adult dosage	Usually one tablet or two teaspoonfuls three or four times per day, taken before meals.
Adverse effects	Iron preparations can cause vomiting, abdominal cramping, and diarrhea, although this is not usually severe. Long-term use may lead to constipation. Feosol and other iron preparations will tend to produce black bowel movements. Prolonged intake of unnecessary iron supplements can cause harmful iron deposits in the liver and heart.
Precautions	If iron supplements are really needed in addition to the iron in the diet, they should be prescribed by a doctor.
Drug interactions	Certain drugs can bind with iron to prevent its absorption from the intestine. These include tetracycline and antacids.
See	*Vitamins and minerals,* page 134.

Ferrous sulfate (generic name). See FEOSOL.

Fiorinal

Generic ingredients	pain relievers : aspirin, phenacetin minor tranquilizer : butalbital mild stimulant : caffeine

Fiorinal with Codeine

Generic ingredients	narcotic pain reliever : codeine pain relievers : aspirin, phenacetin minor tranquilizer : butalbital mild stimulant : caffeine

Action and uses	Both these combination drugs are prescribed for the relief of mild to moderate pain, particularly the pain of tension headaches. Both are typical of the many drugs which add a sedative, tranquilizer or anti-anxiety drug (in this case, butalbital) to a drug or drugs aimed at relieving the actual problem (in this case, the pain relievers aspirin, phenacetin, and codeine). In many cases, relief of the headache or other problem will in itself relieve the accompanying anxiety, so whether the addition of a sedative is useful, effective, or worth the extra cost is somewhat doubtful. As for the inclusion of caffeine, the combined effect of a stimulant plus a sedative on tension or anxiety is equally unclear and unproven.

Adult dosage   Usually two tablets every three to six hours as needed.

Adverse effects   As with other combination drugs, Fiorinal and Fiorinal with Codeine have all the side effects of their various components. The aspirin they contain can cause severe stomach irritation and bleeding. The phenacetin can, over extended periods, cause kidney damage. The butalbital in both preparations can cause dizziness, headache, or allergic reactions. Finally, the codeine in Fiorinal with Codeine can cause nausea and constipation.

Precautions   Fiorinal and Fiorinal with Codeine should both be used with caution by patients with stomach disorders or impaired kidney function, those taking the anticoagulant Coumadin, and they should be avoided by pregnant or potentially pregnant women and nursing mothers.

Drug dependence   The butalbital in both preparations and the codeine in Fiorinal with Codeine can both cause psychological and/or physical dependence if taken over extended periods.

Drug interactions   The aspirin in both these preparations can add to the effect of anticoagulant drugs to increase the risk of bleeding, and with cortisone-like drugs and other anti-inflammatory drugs to increase the risk of ulcer. The butalbital in both preparations and the codeine in Fiorinal with Codeine, can add to the sedative effect of other pain relievers, sleeping pills, tranquilizers, antidepressants, sedatives, alcohol, and antihistamines. The butalbital can decrease the effect of the anticoagulant Coumadin.

See   *Narcotic pain relievers,* page 41; *Non-narcotic pain relievers,* page 42.

Flagyl

Generic name

metronidazole

Action and uses   The drug of choice for the treatment of vaginal infections caused by the parasite *Trichomonas,* as well as certain other types of parasite infections, especially amebiasis. Trichomonas infections of the vagina are extremely common and usually cause a white, foamy, itching discharge. A chronic infection can sometimes cause inflammation of the cervix and changes in the appearance of cervical cells seen in a Pap smear, which is one important reason for treatment if an infection persists. Since the infection is transmitted by sexual contact, the woman's sexual partner is treated at the same time to prevent reinfection. (A man may harbor the parasite in his urethra and be able to reinfect a woman even though, in most cases, Trichomonas causes no symptoms in men.) Flagyl was once available as a local suppository, but this form of treatment was found to be generally ineffective. Until recently, the drug was used routinely on discovery of Trichomonas, but because of concern for one potential side effect, described below, local treatment, including the use of cotton underwear and acid douches, is often tried before Flagyl is prescribed.

Adult dosage For treatment of vaginal infections, the usual dose is 250 mg orally three times a day for seven days. More recently, it has been found that a single dose of 2000 mg (8 tablets) is effective in many cases, so this may also be suggested. The dose for other parasite infections is usually higher and adjusted to each individual case.

Adverse effects In general, serious side effects are unusual but certain bothersome side effects are common. Nausea, loss of appetite or gastric upset, as well as a metallic taste or furry tongue may be experienced. Less commonly, dizziness, headache, vertigo or burning on urination may occur. Flagyl may cause a temporary fall in the white blood-cell count. Flagyl has been shown to cause increased numbers of tumors in rats and mice, and this has given rise to concern that the drug may be carcinogenic in humans. As yet, however, this has not been shown to be the case.

Precautions Alcohol should be avoided while taking this drug since reactions may occur. This drug should not be taken by pregnant or potentially pregnant women or nursing mothers, nor by people with neurological disorders.

Drug interactions When Flagyl and alcohol are taken together, a certain number of people will experience marked nausea, vomiting, flushing, headaches, and faintness. Flagyl can also interact with Antabuse, a drug used to treat alcoholism, to cause unpleasant reactions, including mental changes and confusion.

See *Skin and local disorders,* page 125.

Flurandrenolide (generic name). See CORDRAN.

GANTANOL

Gantanol

Generic name

sulfamethoxazole (available by generic name)

Action and uses A sulfonamide or "sulfa" drug. Gantanol is not an antibiotic, but it prevents the growth of bacteria and is therefore used to treat some bacterial infections. It is particularly effective against infections of the kidney, bladder, and urinary tract, including cystitis. Occasionally it is used to treat meningitis.

Adult dosage The initial dose is usually 2 grams, followed by 1 gram three times a day.

Adverse effects This drug may sometimes cause nausea, vomiting, or other gastrointestinal symptoms, as well as headache or dizziness. Like all sulfa drugs, Gantanol may cause allergic reactions ranging from rashes to very serious, life-threatening reactions with fever, severe rash, and kidney failure.

Precautions It is always important to drink plenty of water while taking this drug to prevent crystal formation in the kidneys. If any fever, nausea, or rash occurs after starting the drug, it should be discontinued and the doctor notified. It should be avoided by people with severe kidney disease and those with G6PD deficiency (a congenital enzyme deficiency). As in the treatment of all infections, it is important to take the drug for the full course prescribed to prevent recurrence of the infection. Pregnant or potentially pregnant women and nursing mothers should avoid this drug.

Drug interactions Like many sulfa drugs, Gantanol may increase the effect of oral antidiabetic drugs (to cause low blood sugar) and Dilantin, Butazolidin, and phenobarbital (to increase the likelihood of toxicity of these drugs).

See *Infections,* page 111.

Gantrisin

Generic name

sulfisoxazole (available by generic name)

Action and uses A sulfonamide or "sulfa" drug. Gantrisin is not an antibiotic, but it prevents the growth of bacteria and is therefore used to treat some bacterial infections. It is particularly effective against infections of the kidney, bladder, and urinary tract, including cystitis. Occasionally it is used to treat meningitis.

Adult dosage	Usually 2 to 4 grams initially, followed by 4 to 8 grams per day divided into at least four doses.
Adverse effects	This drug may sometimes cause nausea, vomiting, or other gastrointestinal symptoms, as well as headaches or dizziness. Like all sulfa drugs, Gantrisin may cause allergic reactions ranging from rashes to very serious, life-threatening reactions with fever, severe rash, and kidney failure.
Precautions	It is always important to drink plenty of water while taking this drug to prevent crystal formation in the kidneys. If any fever, nausea, or rash occurs after starting the drug, it should be discontinued and the doctor notified. It should be avoided by people with severe kidney disease and those with G6PD deficiency (a congenital enzyme deficiency). As in the treatment of all infections, it is important to take the drug for the full course prescribed to prevent recurrence of the infection. Pregnant or potentially pregnant women and nursing mothers should avoid this drug if possible.
Drug interactions	Like many sulfa drugs, Gantrisin may increase the effect of oral antidiabetic drugs (to cause low blood sugar), and Dilantin, Butazolidin, and phenobarbital (to increase the likelihood of toxicity of these drugs).
See	*Infections,* page 111.

Haldol

Generic name	haloperidol

Action and uses	Haldol is a major tranquilizer which is chemically different but similar in action to the "antipsychotic" phenothiazine drugs such as Thorazine, Mellaril, Stelazine, and Trilafon. Though not capable of curing the underlying illness, Haldol does relieve the severe thought disorders (such as hallucinations, loss of orientation, or delusions) that characterize schizophrenia and certain other psychiatric and neurological disorders. Haldol has gained greater popularity as a first-line treatment for acute episodes because it has somewhat lower sedative effects and possibly less effects on the heart than the phenothiazines. It is also available as an alternative when allergies develop to the other group of drugs.
Adult dosage	Dosage is adjusted to suit each patient and varies widely, ranging from 1–2 mg per day, especially for older patients, to much higher doses, 20–40 mg or more per day for acutely agi-

tated people. It is usually given in pill form but occasionally it is injected.

Adverse effects Haldol can produce significant side effects and thus should be reserved for use only when necessary. The most common side effects are various types of involuntary movement, including restlessness and trembling of the arms, legs, or head—symptoms which resemble those of Parkinson's disease. These are usually controlled by an anti-Parkinsonian drug such as Cogentin or Artane. Less common but more acute is the occurrence of another disorder of movement, *acute dystonia,* which can produce grimacing, but this is also readily treated. A small proportion of patients who have taken Haldol may develop *tardive dyskinesia,* or involuntary movement of the tongue, lips, and extremities, and this is not readily treatable. Rarely, allergies may also occur.

Precautions Prolonged use of Haldol requires continued medical supervision, and driving or operation of machinery may not be possible.

Drug interactions Although Haldol has relatively minimal sedative effects in most people, these can be additive to the effects of other sedating drugs, including other major tranquilizers, minor tranquilizers (e.g.,Valium, Librium), sleeping pills, and antihistamines. Haldol has been shown to interact with Lithium to produce, in some cases, severe side effects.

See *Major tranquilizers,* page 49.

Hydergine

Generic name

dihydroergotoxine

Actions and uses This drug generally relaxes blood vessels and as a result increases blood flow. Its main use now is to treat certain mental and emotional problems of the elderly which are thought to arise from a reduced blood flow to the brain. Infrequently it is used to treat conditions where there is not enough blood flowing through peripheral vessels. It has also been used to lower high blood pressure. It has been shown to be effective in elderly confused patients only when they also had elevated blood pressure.

Adult dosage Hydergine is available as sublingual tablets containing 0.5 mg or 1.0 mg of the drug. These tablets are not to be swallowed but must be allowed to dissolve slowly under the tongue. The recommended dose is 1 mg three times a day.

Adverse effects Side effects include nausea and vomiting, blurred vision, skin rashes, and nasal stuffiness.

Precautions Excessive dosing may constrict some blood vessels and limit blood flow to the extremities. This drug should not be taken by pregnant or potentially pregnant women.

Drug interactions Hydergine may be additive to the effects of some drugs used to treat high blood pressure.

See *Poor circulation,* page 68.

Hydralazine (generic name). See APRESOLINE.

Hydrochlorothiazide

Trade names

Esidrex, HydroDIURIL, Oretic

Action and uses The prototype diuretic ("water pill") used to treat high blood pressure and the excessive retention of water associated with certain heart, liver, and kidney disorders, and premenstrual tension. Its primary action is to cause a loss of excess salt and water via the kidneys, thus relieving edema (swelling of body tissue due to retained fluid). It is also very useful in treating high blood pressure because it slightly relaxes the blood vessels and increases the effectiveness of other drugs used to lower blood pressure. This drug is a prototype of a group of drugs called *thiazide diuretics.* The term "thiazide" refers both to a chemical structure and to a class of several similar drugs, including Diuril, Hygroton, Renese and Naturetin, which all share similar actions and side effects.

Adult dosage Usually 50–100 mg per day (sometimes 200 mg per day). If the daily dose is more than 50 mg it is taken in divided doses. Hydrochlorothiazide usually takes effect within two hours and remains effective for three to six hours thereafter. During this period there may be a need to urinate frequently as the kidneys eliminate the body's excess fluid.

Adverse effects A dose of 50 mg per day of hydrochlorothiazide is rarely accompanied by side effects, but, with long-term use and at higher doses, certain side effects may occur. Chief among these is the loss of the essential mineral potassium, which is eliminated from the body along with the excess salt and water. Symptoms of a significant drop in the body's natural potassium level may include dizziness, unusual tiredness, muscle cramps, and/or tingling in the extremities. Fortunately, it is easy to replace lost potassium—by adding potassium-rich foods to the diet (orange and tomato juice, dried fruits and bananas), by using salt substitutes (Co-Salt or Lite-salt), or by taking a supplement of potassium chloride (KCl). The amount of loss and the need for potassium replacement is usually evaluated at an early stage in therapy by checking blood levels of potassium at intervals. Other side effects of hydrochlorothiazide may include an elevation of the blood sugar level in people predisposed to diabetes and a rise in the body's uric acid level, which can precipitate gout. Both of these effects can be watched for and rarely produce problems. Finally, some people are allergic to hydrochlorothiazide, developing reactive skin rashes or nausea; this is slightly more likely in people who are allergic to sulfa drugs or oral antidiabetic drugs.

Precautions This drug should be used with caution by pregnant or potentially pregnant women and nursing mothers, and by patients with gout or diabetes.

Drug interactions Taken in conjunction with cortisone-like drugs such as prednisone, hydrochlorothiazide can cause excessive potassium loss. Potentially serious interactions may also occur if hydrochlorothiazide is taken in conjunction with digitalis drugs for the heart, because, if too much potassium is eliminated from the system by the action of hydrochlorothiazide, the heart can become sensitive to the toxic effects of digitalis. Medical supervision is essential.

See *High blood pressure,* page 58; *Diuretics,* page 63.

HydroDIURIL (brand name for hydrochlorothiazide).
See HYDROCHLOROTHIAZIDE.

Hydropres

Generic ingredients

antihypertensive drug : reserpine
diuretic : hydrochlorothiazide

Action and uses One of several popular fixed-combination drugs prescribed for the control of high blood pressure. The reserpine in Hydropres lowers blood pressure by blocking the sympathetic nervous system (which causes the blood vessels to constrict); as a result, the blood vessels relax and dilate (widen). Hydropres' other component, hydrochlorothiazide, is a diuretic ("water pill"). It lowers blood pressure by promoting the elimination of excess salt and water from the system, thus decreasing blood volume, and by slightly dilating the blood vessels. Hydropres is a fixed-dose combination drug—that is, it combines two ingredients in fixed amounts. This can be a drawback because it is not possible to adjust the dose of each drug individually to suit the patient—a process that is often necessary with drugs for high blood pressure. If the amount of one of the ingredients in Hydropres suits a patient, but the amount of the other does not, it may be simpler (and less expensive) for the patient to take the two drugs separately.

Adult dosage Usually 1–4 tablets per day if Hydropres-25 has been prescribed, or 1–2 tablets per day if Hydropres-50 has been prescribed. Often it can be taken only once daily.

Adverse effects The reserpine in Hydropres can cause drowsiness and lethargy, nasal stuffiness, and stomach upset or ulceration, and sometimes severe depression. The hydrochlorothiazide in Hydropres can cause allergic skin rash, nausea, diarrhea, and excessive loss of the mineral potassium. This last-mentioned side effect may be signaled by muscle cramping and weakness and can be corrected by eating potassium-rich foods (tomato and orange juice, bananas and dried fruit) or by taking a supplement of potassium chloride (KCl). Less frequently, hydrochlorothiazide can precipitate gout or diabetes, possibilities which should be checked with blood tests at intervals.

Precautions Hydropres should be used with caution by patients with gout or diabetes, a history of depression, heart failure, epilepsy, or peptic ulcers. It should be avoided if possible by pregnant or potentially pregnant women and nursing mothers. Women taking this drug for long periods should have regular breast examinations because of a possible link between long-term use of reserpine and breast cancer (though this finding is still controversial).

Drug interactions Because of the reserpine it contains, Hydropres can cause oversedation when taken concurrently with sedatives, sleeping pills, tranquilizers, antihistamines, and alcohol. Some drugs for asthma, weight loss, depression, and colds can interact with reserpine to increase blood pressure. Hydropres,

213

therefore, should not be used concurrently with any of the drugs except under a doctor's supervision. The hydro chlorothiazide in Diupres can interact with steroids such a prednisone to cause excessive potassium loss. Hydrochlor thiazide can also cause a potentially serious interaction wit digitalis or digoxin, as the increased potassium loss can re der the heart sensitive to the toxic effects of these drugs.

See *High blood pressure,* page 58; *Diuretics,* page 63.

Hygroton

Generic name

chlorthalidone

Action and uses A diuretic ("water pill") used to treat high blood pressur and the excessive retention of water associated with certai heart, liver, and kidney disorders, and premenstrual tensior Its primary action is to cause a loss of excess salt and wate via the kidneys, thus relieving edema (the swelling of bod tissue due to retained fluid). It is also very useful in treatin high blood pressure because it slightly relaxes the blood ves sels and increases the effectiveness of other drugs used t lower blood pressure. This drug is one of a group of diureti drugs called *thiazide diuretics.* The term "thiazide" refer both to a chemical structure and to a class of several simila drugs, including Diuril, HydroDIURIL, Renese, and Nature tin, which all share similar actions and side effects.

Adult dosage Usually 50–100 mg per day, although in some cases it can b taken on alternate days or less frequently, since it has slightly greater effect than the same dose of hydrochlorothia zide. Increased urination occurs for 3–12 hours or longer afte taking the drug and once this pattern is determined, a con venient time for dosing can be decided.

Adverse effects Hygroton can cause excessive loss of potassium, especiall when taken daily. If this occurs potassium can be replaced ei ther in the diet (with extra orange juice, tomato juice, ba nanas or dried fruit) or with liquid potassium chloride (KCl) Hygroton also tends to cause an increased blood sugar leve in those predisposed to diabetes and may increase levels o uric acid in the blood (the substance which can cause gout). If used to excess, Hygroton or any diuretic can cause dehy dration and may affect kidney function and the amount o waste products in the blood. The effects of the initial use o Hygroton are therefore usually followed carefully.

Precautions	This drug should be used with caution by pregnant or potentially pregnant women and by patients with gout or diabetes.
Drug interactions	Taken in conjunction with cortisone-like drugs, such as prednisone, it can cause excessive potassium loss. Potentially serious interactions may also occur if Hygroton is taken in conjunction with digitalis and related drugs (e.g.,digoxin) for the heart, because if too much potassium is eliminated from the system by the action of Hygroton, the heart can become sensitive to the toxic effects of digitalis. Medical supervision is essential.
See	*Diuretics,* page 63; *High blood pressure,* page 58.

Ilosone

Generic name	erythromycin estolate (available by generic name)

Action and uses	A commonly used antibiotic which comes from the mold *Streptomyces.* It acts on bacteria to inhibit production of proteins but has no effect on human cells. Erythromycin is most commonly used in mild to moderate infections where penicillin would normally be indicated but the patient is allergic to penicillin. These infections include bacterial sore throat ("strep throat"), respiratory or lung infections, and some venereal diseases. It is seldom used in very serious infections. Ilosone, unlike other erythromycins, is not easily destroyed by stomach acid; this gives more flexibility in time of dosing, but may not be worth the extra cost or risk of this special form.
Adult dosage	The usual adult dosage is 250 to 500 mg every six hours.
Adverse effects	The most frequent side effect is gastrointestinal upset, including nausea, belching, and diarrhea. Rashes and other allergic reactions can occur but are not as frequent as with another antibiotics. However, unlike other erythromycin preparations, Ilosone can have an allergic effect on the liver producing a yellowing of the skin and eyes (jaundice). This effect is rare and usually only appears if Ilosone is taken for more than ten days. It is preceded by nausea, vomiting, pain in the abdomen, and loss of energy. These symptoms disappear when the drug is discontinued.
Precautions	This antibiotic, like all others, should be taken for the full course prescribed, and every dose should be taken. Failure to do this can result in inadequate treatment of the infection,

recurrence, or development of resistant strains of bacteria. If symptoms of adverse effects occur, for example abdominal pain, the doctor should be consulted promptly. Ilosone should be used with caution by pregnant or potentially pregnant women and nursing mothers.

Drug interactions Erythromycin may interfere with the effectiveness of penicillin and Cleocin.

See *Infections,* page 111.

Imipramine (generic name). See TOFRANIL.

Inderal

Generic name

propranolol

Action and uses A drug used to treat high blood pressure, angina pectoris, and certain types of irregular heart rhythm. The exact mechanism by which it lowers blood pressure is not known, although it does block part of the sympathetic nervous system (which is responsible for constricting the blood vessels), and it does decrease both heart rate and the force of heart contraction, thus saving work for the heart. In the treatment of high blood pressure, Inderal is often used in conjunction with a diuretic ("water pill") such as hydrochlorothiazide, and/or a drug to dilate blood vessels such as Apresoline.

Adult dosage Initially, usually 10–20 mg, three or four times per day, with a gradual increase until the desired blood pressure response is achieved. The usual effective dosage range is 120–320 mg daily in divided doses, usually taken before meals and at bedtime. It is normally recommended that if Inderal is to be discontinued, the drug should be stopped gradually, over a period of days or weeks.

Adverse effects The major side effects of Inderal tend to occur early in therapy and include dizziness, slow heart rate, tiredness and depression, increased dreaming, gastrointestinal upset, skin rashes, cold hands and feet, and increased wheezing in patients who have asthma or chronic lung disease.

Precautions Inderal should be used with caution by pregnant or potentially pregnant women. It should be avoided by those with asthma, diabetes, and in most cases by those with definite heart failure, except when the heart failure is caused by high blood pressure or certain irregular heart rhythms.

Drug interactions Inderal may interact harmfully with insulin and antidiabetic drugs, with MAO inhibitor drugs (e.g. the antidepressants Marplan, Nardil and Parnate), the antibiotic Furoxine, and the drug Tegretol. Inderal can usefully add to the effects of drugs for high blood pressure but can interact harmfully, to increase the blood pressure, with nasal decongestants like Neosynephrine and cough/cold preparations. Inderal may cause oversedation if taken in conjunction with reserpine, barbiturates, and narcotics.

See *High blood pressure,* page 58; *Diuretics,* page 63; *Angina pectoris,* page 71; *Abnormal heart rhythms,* page 67.

Indocin

Generic name

indomethacin

Action and uses Indocin is one of several drugs used as alternatives to aspirin in the treatment of various types of arthritis. It has the ability to relieve pain and decrease inflammation associated with arthritis, but it has no effect on the progress of the disease. Indocin was released over 10 years ago as a potential alternative to aspirin and received wide use. However, the occurrence of its various side effects has resulted in reduced and more selective use. It is one of several anti-inflammatory drugs which serve as alternatives in arthritis therapy when after an adequate trial aspirin has proved unsuccessful or has not been tolerated (others include Motrin, Naprosyn, Nalfon, and Tolectin).

Adult dosage 25 mg two or three times a day with gradual increases of dose, according to response, up to a daily dose of 150 to 200 mg.

Adverse effects The most common side effects are due to irritation of the gastrointestinal tract and can include ulceration and bleeding. In addition, visual changes, hearing changes, headache, edema, and dizziness may occur. Rarely, abnormalities of the blood and liver have been observed.

Precautions Indocin should not be used by pregnant or potentially pregnant women or nursing mothers. It is not advised for people with known ulcer disease or allergy to aspirin. If taken for long periods, periodic eye examinations are indicated. Occasionally Indocin may cause sufficient drowsiness to interfere with driving or operating machinery. The prescribing physician should be notified if any symptoms of headache, visual or hearing changes, or personality changes occur.

Drug interactions Indocin may interact with oral anticoagulants such as Coumadin to increase the risk of bleeding. The likelihood of peptic ulcer is also increased when used with other drugs predisposing to ulcer such as prednisone or aspirin.

See *Pain with inflammation,* page 43.

Insulin-NPH

Action and uses Insulin-NPH, or Isophane insulin suspension, is the most commonly used "intermediate-acting" insulin in the long-term treatment of diabetes. The N in NPH is for a neutral solution; P is for Protamine-zinc insulin (the suspension which allows for its longer action); and H is for Hagedorn, the laboratory where the process originated. Like all insulins, it is made by extracting and purifying the insulin from the pancreas glands of cows or pigs. More highly purified forms of insulin are now being developed, but it is unclear how great their advantage will be. Insulin-NPH acts to lower blood sugar; its effects begin within two hours of injection and can last 18–24 hours. Accordingly, it is most frequently used once daily, in the morning, to cover the times of food intake (when blood sugar is at its highest).

Adult dosage The dosage varies greatly and is carefully adjusted to suit each individual patient. Adjustment is made on the basis of periodic measurements of the levels of sugar in the blood and in the urine. Dose may range from 5 units per day to 100 units or more per day—common dosages are in the 20–40 units per day range, usually given in an early morning subcutaneous injection.

Side effects The most common side effect occurs when the insulin dose is slightly excessive for the actual meal intake (for example, when a meal is skipped) and the person's blood sugar level falls too low (hypoglycemia), most frequently at the time of peak action, or in the late afternoon. The hypoglycemia, usually manifested by shakiness or dizziness, can be curtailed by a high-sugar snack such as a candy bar or orange juice. Such episodes usually signal the need for reevaluation of the dose and dietary intake. Other side effects, also usually avoidable, include shrinkage of the skin in areas of repeated injection (avoided by a plan of continually alternating injection sites), and, relatively infrequently, insulin resistance.

Precautions   A person requiring insulin injections should be know-ledgeable about his illness, his diet, and how to care for and use his needles and syringes. If both the short-acting "regular" insulin and Insulin-NPH are required, they should not be mixed in the same syringe.

Drug interactions   Persons also taking beta-blocking drugs such as Inderal (propranolol) or Lopressor may have more difficulty with control of their diabetes. Dosage requirements may also be increased if a person also takes certain diuretics such as HydroDIURIL, hydrochlorothiazide, Esidrex, or cortisone-like drugs such as prednisone.

See   *Diabetes,* page 90.

Ionamin

Generic name

phentermine (available by generic name)

Action and uses   An appetite suppressant used as an aid to weight reduction. Its effect in decreasing the appetite tends to diminish after 7–14 days. Its true effectiveness in causing weight loss can be questioned. Like amphetamine sulfate, to which it is related, it also stimulates the nervous system, producing an increase in energy and mental alertness and a lift in mood. Though Ionamin is less effective in suppressing appetite than amphetamine sulfate, it is probably preferable because it may have a smaller tendency to cause dependence.

Adult dosage   Usually 25 mg before meals, three times daily.

Adverse effects   Like amphetamine sulfate, Ionamin can cause dry mouth; nervousness; headache; anxiety; nausea; vomiting; rapid, irregular heartbeat; and elevation of the blood pressure. (In most patients, however, the side effects of Ionamin on the nervous system and cardiovascular system are less marked than those of amphetamine sulfate.) Withdrawal symptoms of fatigue and depression are likely when the drug is stopped, particularly if it has been taken in doses exceeding those prescribed.

Precautions   Ionamin should only be used for short periods under careful supervision. It should not be used by anyone with any type of heart disease, irregular heart rhythm, or high blood pressure.

Drug dependence   Like amphetamine sulfate, Ionamin can cause severe psychological and/or physical dependence, and tolerance to its effects develops quickly.

Drug interactions Ionamin can counteract the effect of drugs for high blood pressure and of some drugs used to regulate heart rhythms. When used with decongestants or nasal sprays and drugs for asthma, Ionamin can add to their effects and increase the likelihood of side effects.

See *Weight loss,* page 106.

Ismelin

Generic name

guanethidine

Action and uses A potent drug for the treatment of moderate to severe high blood pressure. It acts to block the nerves which cause the arterial blood vessels to constrict. It is usually reserved for use when less potent drugs (e.g.,Inderal or Aldomet) are not effective. It is customarily used in conjunction with some type of diuretic. It is long acting, and its effects may continue for days to weeks after discontinuation.

Adult dosage The dose varies widely, from 5 mg to 100 mg daily. It is usually started at a low dose which is gradually increased every three to seven days until the desired effect is obtained.

Adverse effects Ismelin has a higher incidence of side effects than many antihypertensive drugs. It can cause a rapid fall in blood pressure, and therefore dizziness, when the patient suddenly changes position. This is most noticeable early in the morning. Diarrhea may occur, and changes in sexual function are frequent. Other less common side effects include nausea, nasal stuffiness, depression, or unusual dreams.

Precautions This drug should be avoided by pregnant or potentially pregnant women and nursing mothers, and by people who have ulcers.

Drug interactions Tricyclic antidepressants (Elavil, Tofranil) counteract the effect of Ismelin, as do the decongestants in some nasal sprays and in medicines for allergy or coughs and colds. Stimulants and weight-control drugs also have this effect. Ismelin can also increase the effects of alcohol.

See *High blood pressure,* page 58.

Isopto Carpine

Generic name	
	pilocarpine

Action and uses   An eyedrop preparation used for the treatment of glaucoma. Glaucoma is a disease of the eye in which the normal flow of fluid through the chambers of the eye is obstructed and pressure within the eye increases. It often runs in families. The increased pressure can gradually (or suddenly, in acute glaucoma) cause blindness. When applied to the eye, pilocarpine causes the pupil to constrict and this subsequently causes a fall in pressure inside the eye. This effect takes place within 15–30 minutes and lasts four to eight hours.

Adult dosage   Initially, one drop of a 0.25–1% solution is placed in the eye every six to eight hours, and the concentration and dose are adjusted individually.

Adverse effects   Occasionally aching over the eye, decreased vision in the dark, local irritation, or allergic reactions may occur. If an excessive dose is used, other effects such as sweating, slowed heart rate or gastrointestinal disturbance may occur.

Precautions   It is important to avoid contaminating the eyedrop container by not touching the eye on application and by keeping the lid tightly closed. If more than one eye medicine is being used, they should be carefully marked.

Drug interactions   Since pilocarpine is a cholinergic drug (one that stimulates the parasympathetic nervous system), its action can be counteracted by excessive doses of the many anticholinergic antispasmodic drugs such as Pro-Banthine, by antihistamines, or by tricyclic antidepressants such as Elavil.

Isordil

Generic name	
	isosorbide dinitrate (available by generic name)

Action and uses   A drug used to relieve pain in the treatment of angina pectoris—the characteristic pain felt in the chest (or sometimes in the arm) which results from inadequate supply of oxygen to the heart muscle. Angina pectoris is often brought on by exercise, exertion, or emotion. The deficiency of oxygen (which is carried to the heart by the blood) most often results from narrowing of the blood vessels supplying the heart, the *coronary arteries,* which become "furred up" with fatty deposits and are unable to conduct enough oxygen-rich blood to the heart. Isordil acts in two ways: to open up the often partly blocked blood vessels to the heart, and to dilate peripheral blood vessels, which reduces the amount of work the heart must do to pump blood around the body. Isordil is also sometimes used to treat conditions where blood circulation is poor, e.g.,Raynaud's disease and certain other heart failure conditions.

Adult dosage For acute attacks the usual dosage is 2.5 to 10 mg; the tablets are placed under the tongue and allowed to dissolve. The tablets each contain either 2.5 mg or 5 mg. For regular use tablets containing 5 mg, 10 mg, or 20 mg are *swallowed* to reduce the frequency of angina attacks. For this purpose the usual dosage is 5–30 mg taken four times per day by swallowing. Long-acting tablets and long-acting capsules, containing 40 mg isosorbide dinitrate, are also available. These should be taken every six to twelve hours.

Adverse effects Flushing is a very common side effect and is due to increased blood flow to the skin. Throbbing headache often occurs and is also the result of changes in blood flow. A feeling of faintness or dizziness can occur (particularly in hot weather) more commonly in people with high blood pressure.

Precautions If more than two or three tablets do not relieve the pain, the doctor should be notified at once.

Drug interactions Excessive alcohol intake tends to dilate blood vessels, thereby increasing the effects of Isordil, as do certain antihypertensive drugs, e.g.,Apresoline.

See *Poor circulation,* page 68; *Angina pectoris,* page 71.

Isosorbide dinitrate (generic name). See ISORDIL, SORBITRATE.

Isoxsuprine (generic name). See VASODILAN.

Keflex

Generic name

cephalexin

Action and uses An antibiotic which is similar chemically and in its actions to penicillin. It is one of a group of drugs widely used in hospitals (and now thought to be overused) called *cephalosporins.* The proper primary use of Keflex is as a substitute for ampicillin where allergy to the penicillin group of antibiotics is present or where a bacterium especially sensitive to it is involved, for example, *Klebsiella.* It is used more widely, however, in a variety of infections of the urinary tract, chest, and elsewhere, although in many cases less costly drugs are equally effective.

Adult dosage Usually 250 mg–500 mg every six hours on an empty stomach. The maximum dose is 4 grams per day. Keflex should be taken regularly for the number of days recommended (usually 7–10 days) to be fully effective and to prevent recurrence of the infection and the development of resistant strains of bacteria.

Adverse effects Some people are allergic to Keflex and may develop skin rashes, itching, or difficulty in breathing. People who have had severe allergies to penicillin are more likely to be allergic to Keflex. Keflex may also cause nausea, other stomach problems, or diarrhea since it also can effect the bacteria in the lower gastrointestinal tract. More rarely, it can cause headaches, dizziness, changes in the blood, and abnormalities in the kidney.

Precautions A person who has had a severe (anaphylactoid) reaction to penicillin should probably not take Keflex. Pregnant or potentially pregnant women and nursing mothers should use caution in taking this drug.

Drug interactions The likelihood of damage to the kidneys is increased if Keflex is taken at the same time as the diuretic Lasix or with certain other antibiotics, e.g., gentamycin (Garamycin). Keflex can increase the effects of the anticoagulant Coumadin to increase the risk of bleeding.

See *Infections,* page 111.

Kenalog Cream & Ointment

Generic name
triamcinolone (available by generic name)

Action and uses A commonly used preparation of a synthetic corticosteroid (cortisone-like drug) for local (topical) application. Its main use is in the treatment of many types of skin disorder where its anti-inflammatory effects are helpful—examples are pso-

223

riasis, certain types of neurodermatitis (inflammation of the skin associated with emotional factors) and a variety of other conditions where there is no infection. In many cases, the effects are dramatic. Because it retards formation of scar tissue, it can also prevent scarring.

Adult dosage The 0.025–0.1% preparation is applied sparingly two or three times daily. It is available as an ointment or a cream in several strengths, the choice depending on where it is to be used.

Adverse effects If Kenalog is not used for long periods or on infected areas, there are virtually no important adverse effects; however, if the preparations are used for long periods on the face, they can cause eruptions and redness. If Kenalog preparations are used for long periods on a large area of the body, the corticosteroid can be absorbed through the skin into the body. This can cause weight gain, ulcers or stomach upset, decreased resistance to infection and stress, and can be quite dangerous. If used on an infected area of the skin it can cause the infection to spread, and it can be very hazardous if used for any viral skin lesions such as those of herpes simplex ("cold sores"), shingles, or chickenpox.

Precautions Do not use without a physician's specific instructions, and use only on affected areas. Do not use on a skin area which appears to be infected without consulting a physician.

Drug interactions No significant interactions will occur although other topical preparations placed on the same skin area may interfere with the effects of Kenalog.

See *Steroids, or cortisone-like drugs,* page 102; *Skin and local disorders,* page 125.

K-Lyte

Generic name

potassium bicarbonate

K-Lyte DS

Generic name

potassium citrate

Action and uses K-Lyte is a preparation used to treat potassium deficiency. It is added to water to make an effervescent solution. Potassium deficiency most commonly occurs as a result of the use of diuretic drugs. (Diuretics, or "water pills," are drugs which cause increased excretion of water and salts. Most of them cause increased loss of salts of potassium, which is an essential mineral, but there are exceptions—the *potassium-retaining diuretics,* e.g.,Aldactazide, Aldactone, Diazide, and Triamterene.) Potassium deficiency may also occur with the use of many cortisone-like drugs (e.g.,prednisone) and with severe vomiting and diarrhea. However, the K-Lyte preparations are less effective means of correcting potassium deficiency than potassium chloride (see POTASSIUM CHLORIDE, p.275) since the chloride allows more of the potassium to be retained in the body than the more pleasant-tasting citrate or bicarbonate salts in K-Lyte.

Adult dosage Dose is adjusted according to the needs of each patient, but is customarily one or two tablets in water, one to four times per day.

Adverse effects Nausea, vomiting, or gastric distress may occasionally occur.

Precautions K-Lyte should not be used if there is an excessive amount of potassium in the blood, as may occur in kidney failure or Addison's disease. Prolonged use of K-Lyte usually requires occasional monitoring of the blood potassium level.

Drug interactions If given in conjunction with potassium-retaining diuretics, K-Lyte can cause dangerously high levels of potassium in the blood, which can lead to severe effects on the heart.

See *Vitamins and minerals,* page 134.

Kwell

Generic name

gamma benzene hexachloride

Action and uses A liquid medication used to treat scabies and lice. Kwell kills both the microscopic-sized scabies parasites, which get into the skin, and lice, which live and multiply in areas of the body covered by hair. It is only effective when combined with other measures to eliminate the parasites and their eggs, including careful laundering of clothes, bedding, and other personal items.

Adult dosage Kwell comes as a lotion, a cream, and a shampoo. It is either shampooed into the affected area or applied for a brief period. It should not be left on the skin for long periods.

Adverse effects Kwell can produce a red eruption on the skin where it is applied due to local irritation or allergic reactions. If left on large body areas for a long time, or ingested, it can be absorbed and may produce hazardous effects on the liver and blood cells.

Precautions Kwell is a poison if taken by mouth and must be kept out of the reach of small children. It should not be applied repeatedly or left on the skin for long periods.

Drug interactions None have been reported.

See *Skin and local disorders,* page 125.

Lanoxin (brand name for digoxin). See DIGOXIN.

Larotid

Generic name

amoxicillin (available by generic name)

Action and uses An antibiotic used to treat many infections including those of the urinary tract, ear, nose, and throat. It is one of several so-called "semi-synthetic" penicillins, which are made by both chemical and biological manipulation of penicillin produced by the mold *penicillium*.

Amoxicillin, like penicillin, acts by preventing bacteria from forming their cell walls. They therefore break up. It has no effect on human cells since they have a different structure. Though basic penicillin (penicillin G) is still one of the most important of all the antibiotics, it has several disadvantages. One is the somewhat limited effectiveness against certain types of bacteria—the "gram-negative" organisms. Another disadvantage is that it is not totally effective when taken by mouth because penicillin G is broken down by stomach acid. Amoxicillin, however, is highly effective when taken by mouth because it is not broken down by stomach acids. It differs from ampicillin only in that it may be taken in the presence or absence of food (whereas ampicillin must be taken on an empty stomach), and it is more costly.

Because it is active against many kinds of bacteria, it is called a "broad-spectrum" antibiotic. It is less effective than penicillin G against "gram-positive" cocci (found in abscesses and ear infections), but more effective against gram-negative bacteria (which cause urinary tract infections). It is not effective against fungal or viral diseases. Antibiotics should not be used for trivial infections or to treat nonsensitive bacteria (those against which they are not effective); such use only produces resistant bacteria which are difficult to eliminate.

Adult dosage The average adult dose is 250 mg or 500 mg every six hours. The dose should always be established by a physician and will vary with the type and severity of infection.

Adverse effects Many people develop allergic reactions to the penicillin group of drugs. Once sensitization develops, *all* forms of penicillin, including amoxicillin, can produce a reaction. An allergic reaction may be manifested by any of the following symptoms: skin rashes, hives, itching, fever, difficulty in breathing, and swelling of the lips and tongue. Persons who have infectious mononucleosis often develop rashes in response to amoxicillin and should not take it while they are ill with the disease. Amoxicillin can also produce stomach upset due to the killing of certain bacteria in the intestine and may cause diarrhea. It may also cause mild fungal infections of the anorectal area or the vagina.

Precautions This antibiotic should not be used if there is a history of allergy to any type of penicillin. It should not be taken by people with infectious mononucleosis because it is accompanied by a high incidence of rashes. Once treatment with amoxicillin is begun, the prescribed course of not less than five to seven days should be completed (unless, of course, side effects occur). It should *not* be stopped when the infection seems to be gone, since despite the disappearance of symptoms the bacteria may not be entirely eliminated and the infection could recur. The frequent starting and stopping of any antibiotic only leads to the development of resistant bacteria which are much more difficult to treat. Pregnant or potentially pregnant women and nursing mothers should use with caution.

Drug interactions The effectiveness of amoxicillin may be hindered by the antibiotics erythromycin and chloramphenicol, if they are used together.

See *Infections,* page 111.

Lasix

Generic name

furosemide

Action and uses A potent diuretic ("water pill") used to treat excessive retention of water in, for example, congestive heart failure and some forms of kidney disease. Lasix is also sometimes used for high blood pressure, but it offers no particular advantage over the less potent diuretics such as hydrochlorothiazide, which work on a different part of the kidney. Its primary action is to promote the excretion of excess salt and water by the kidneys, thus relieving edema (the swelling of body tissue due to retained fluid).

Adult dosage Usually 20–80 mg per day taken as a single morning dose, or in divided doses. Higher doses are sometimes needed. The diuretic response is usually seen within one or two hours.

Adverse effects Lasix can cause excessive loss of potassium, especially when taken daily. If this occurs extra potassium can be obtained either in the diet (orange juice, tomato juice, bananas or dried fruit) or by taking liquid potassium chloride (KCl). Lasix also tends to cause an increased level of sugar in the blood in those predisposed to diabetes and may increase the levels of uric acid in the blood (the subtance which can cause gout). If used to excess, Lasix or any diuretic can cause dehydration and may affect kidney function and the amount of waste products in the blood. Therefore, the initial use of Lasix is usually carefully supervised to avoid these effects.

Precautions This drug should be used with caution by pregnant or potentially pregnant women and by patients with gout or diabetes.

Drug interactions Taken in conjunction with cortisone-like drugs such as prednisone, Lasix can cause excessive potassium loss. Potentially serious interactions may also occur if Lasix is taken in conjunction with digitalis drugs for the heart (e.g.,Lanoxin, digoxin), because if too much potassium is eliminated from the system by the Lasix, the heart can become sensitive to the toxic effects of digitalis. Medical supervision is essential.

See *High blood pressure,* page 58; *Diuretics, page 63.*

Librax

Generic ingredients

tranquilizer : chlordiazepoxide
antispasmodic : clidinium

Action and uses Librax is a popular combination drug used in the treatment of peptic ulcer and other types of gastrointestinal spasm. Like many other similar preparations, it combines an anticholinergic-antispasmodic compound, which decreases the contractions of the bowel and stomach, with a commonly used tranquilizer, in this case Librium. Apparently it is assumed that the bowel symptoms are associated with anxiety and thus can be relieved by a tranquilizer. Whether in fact the combination is more effective than an antispasmodic alone is not known.

Adult dosage The usual dose is one or two capsules three or four times per day, adjusted according to clinical response of the patient.

Adverse effects Both components of this preparation have side effects. The Librium can cause drowsiness, dizziness, or confusion, especially in older people. If taken for long periods and then discontinued, withdrawal symptoms of anxiety, insomnia, and nightmares can occur. The antispasmodic clidinium can cause dry mouth, bladder dysfunction (usually in people with prostate problems), or blurring of vision.

Precautions Lower doses may be necessary for older people, for those sensitive to tranquilizing drugs, and for those with prostate trouble or glaucoma. If drowsiness occurs, driving or operating machinery may be hazardous. Librax should be avoided by pregnant and potentially pregnant women.

Drug dependence Prolonged use of Librax has the potential to cause dependence, and there may be withdrawal symptoms if it is discontinued suddenly.

Drug interactions The Librium in this combination can add to the effects of alcohol, tranquilizers, and sedatives. The effects of the clidinium can be additive to those of other antispasmodic drugs, antihistamines, some cough/cold medicines, and some tricyclic antidepressants such as Elavil, causing excessive dry mouth or constipation.

See *Nausea, stomach upset, and ulcers,* page 75; *Minor tranquilizers,* page 45.

Librium

Generic name

chlordiazepoxide (available by generic name)

Action and uses A minor tranquilizer widely used to treat anxiety and nervousness. The primary effect of Librium is to produce calm and decrease feelings of anxiety. Librium is one of a group of related drugs which includes Valium, Serax, Dalmane, and Tranxene; they are the most frequently prescribed medications in the United States. Librium is usually prescribed to

229

relieve the symptoms of a condition in the same way that narcotics are used to relieve pain. In general it has no effect on
the cause of the symptoms. Librium is also often used in the
treatment of withdrawal from certain drugs, especially alcohol. It can also be used as a sleeping medication in a similar
way to the related drug, Dalmane. Exactly how these drugs
work is not known.

Adult dosage The usual dose of Librium ranges from 10 mg per day to 10–
25 mg three or four times per day, depending on individual
requirements. Some people are strongly sedated by 10–20
mg, while others are not especially affected by that dose.

Adverse effects The most common side effect of Librium is sedation (tiredness) and depression, and sometimes dizziness, but this can
usually be relieved by lowering the dose. Other side effects
are relatively uncommon. A few individuals may suffer from
increased anxiety when taking Librium, but this is rare.
When Librium is taken in combination with alcohol the two
drugs act together and marked sedation may occur. In some
cases the sedation may interfere with working and driving.

Precautions There is a possibility that minor tranquilizers may cause
birth defects and the manufacturers therefore warn against
the use of Librium by pregnant or potentially pregnant
women.

Drug dependence Librium is not addictive in the same way as narcotics but,
like other sedatives, it can be habit-forming to a certain extent if taken for a long period of time. If it is then stopped
suddenly some withdrawal symptoms may occur, especially
after large doses. These can include anxiety, insomnia, and
nightmares.

Drug interactions Librium can enhance the sedative effect of alcohol, antihistamines, sleeping pills, and narcotics, sometimes to a dangerous extent. Unlike many sedatives, Librium does not interfere with the actions of the anticoagulant Coumadin.

See *Minor tranquilizers,* page 45.

Lidex

Generic name
fluocinonide (available by generic name)

Action and uses A commonly used preparation of a synthetic corticosteroid
(cortisone-like drug) for local (topical) application. Its main

use is in the treatment of many types of skin disorder where its anti-inflammatory effects are helpful—examples are psoriasis, certain types of neurodermatitis (inflammation of the skin associated with emotional factors), and a variety of other conditions which are not infected. In many cases, the effects are dramatic. Because it retards formation of scar tissue, it can also prevent scarring.

Adult dosage The 0.05% preparation is applied sparingly three or four times daily. It is available both as an ointment and as a cream in several strengths, the choice depending on where it is to be used.

Adverse effects If the preparation is not used for long periods or on infected areas, there are virtually no important adverse effects; however, if the preparations are used for long periods on the face, they can cause eruptions and redness. If Lidex preparations are used for long periods on a large area of the body, the corticosteroid can be absorbed into the body through the skin. This can cause weight gain, ulcers or stomach upset, decreased resistance to infection and stress, and can be quite dangerous. If used on an infected area of the skin it can help the infection to spread, and it can be very hazardous if used for any viral skin lesions such as those of herpes simplex ("cold sores"), shingles, or chickenpox.

Precautions Do not use without a physician's specific instructions and use only on affected areas. Do not use on a skin area which appears to be infected without consulting a physician.

Drug interactions No significant interactions will occur, although other topical preparations placed on the same skin area may interfere with the effects of Lidex.

See *Steroids, or cortisone-like drugs,* page 102; *Skin and local disorders,* page 125.

Lomotil

Generic ingredients

antidiarrheal : diphenoxylate
antispasmodic : atropine

Action and uses A drug used to treat diarrhea. Since its introduction in 1961, it has become increasingly popular with overseas travelers as a medication for the common hazard "traveler's diarrhea." One of its two components, diphenoxylate, is a synthetic narcotic similar to Demerol. At normal doses of Lomotil, this ingredient does not produce the euphoria, pain relief, or dependence associated with Demerol. It does, however, act like morphine to reduce the movement of the bowel and thus decrease diarrhea. The other ingredient, atropine, is added because it too has a constipating effect, and because its presence is supposed to discourage any possible drug abuse with Lomotil. However, the actual amount of atropine in Lomotil is probably too small to have any significant effect except when the medication is taken in overdose. Interestingly enough, many authorities have expressed the opinion that, although Lomotil can be effective on a short-term basis, continued use when traveler's diarrhea occurs can prolong certain diarrheal illnesses by allowing retention of the toxins or bacteria in the bowel.

Adult dosage	Initially, one or two 2.5 mg tablets, followed by a single 2.5 mg tablet every four to six hours until diarrhea stops.
Adverse effects	Lomotil can cause dry mouth, nausea, and dizziness. In excessive amounts, it can cause vomiting, sedation, depression, along with signs of atropine poisoning (flushed skin, fever). Allergic reactions may rarely occur.
Precautions	Lomotil should be used with caution by people with glaucoma or prostate trouble. If diarrhea persists for more than a few days, the cause should be investigated.
Drug dependence	Because of the presence of diphenoxylate, Lomotil may be capable of causing psychological and/or physical dependence, but only when taken daily over an extended period.
Drug interactions	Oversedation may rarely result from concurrent use of Lomotil and sedatives, sleeping pills, tranquilizers, or alcohol. Certain antihistamines and antidepressants can be additive to the antispasmodic effects of Lomotil.
See	*Diarrhea,* page 86.

Lo Ovral

Generic ingredients

progestogen : norgestrel
estrogen : ethinyl estradiol

Action and uses An oral contraceptive. Like many other birth-control pills, Lo Ovral is made up of a combination of two synthetic hormones—an estrogen compound and a progesterone-like compound (a progestogen). This newer pill differs from any other birth control pills in that it contains a lower dose of estrogen, which tends to alter its effects somewhat. (It is similar to Ovral [see p. 261] but has only 60% of Ovral's hormone content.) Recent studies have suggested that lower doses of estrogen in birth control pills such as Lo Ovral may be associated with fewer side effects. However, the lower dose of estrogen also results in a greater incidence of "breakthrough" or mid-cycle bleeding, which may in turn cause a greater dropout rate and therefore lessen Lo Ovral's effectiveness as a contraceptive. The tendency to breakthrough bleeding often decreases with more prolonged use. At present, its effectiveness in contraception appears to be similar to the higher-dose birth-control pills.

Adult dosage In general, one tablet is taken daily (usually at night) for 21 consecutive days, beginning on the 5th day of menstruation. No tablets are taken for the following 7 days, during which time menstrual bleeding occurs, and on the 8th day they are started again for another 21-day cycle, and so on.

Adverse effects Use of oral contraceptive pills has been associated with a variety of side effects. Lo Ovral may be associated with a higher incidence of intermenstrual bleeding "breakthrough bleeding," or "spotting," but it appears to produce a slightly lower incidence than some other pills with a higher estrogen content of the effects of estrogen excess, such as nausea, edema, and leg cramps. Other possible minor side effects include acne, breast discomfort, depression, gastrointestinal upset, headaches, and vaginal infections. More significant but less common side effects include the risk of thrombophlebitis (blood clotting associated with inflammation of the veins of the legs), increased blood pressure, increased blood sugar, and gallbladder disease. The risk of certain side effects such as heart disease and gallbladder disease appear to increase with age (especially over the age of 35). If a woman has a history of true migraine headaches she may experience increased headaches while on the pill, and she may also run a slightly higher risk of having a stroke (though the risk remains small). A history of heavy smoking is associated with increased risk of heart disease, particularly in the age group over 40.

Precautions A history of thrombophlebitis, blood clots, or migraine headaches is usually a contraindication to the use of oral contraceptives. For women over the age of 35, or those with other risk factors, such as a history of heavy smoking, gallbladder

233

disease, diabetes or high blood pressure, use should be weighed carefully against alternative birth-control methods.

Drug interactions Several drug interactions have been suggested but none have been well-documented as significant in most cases.

See *Hormonal drugs,* page 96; *Oral contraceptives,* page 96.

Lotrimin

Generic name

clotrimazole

Action and uses A "broad-spectrum" antifungal drug used topically to treat skin infections such as athletes' foot (*tinea pedis*), "jock itch" (*tinea cruris*), and Candida (Monilia) infections due to the fungus *Candida albicans.* It is available both as a cream and as a liquid and, because fungal skin infections are often very persistent, it must be used regularly for at least 10–14 days to prevent recurrence; the primary action of the drug is to inhibit growth of the fungi and to allow tissues to heal.

Adult dosage The cream or solution is massaged into the skin twice daily.

Adverse effects Some people may experience local irritation, burning, and itching with the drug, and this may be difficult to differentiate from symptoms of the disorder. If they persist, the prescribing doctor should be notified.

Precautions Its effects on pregnancy and during nursing are unknown, but it should generally be avoided by pregnant women or nursing mothers.

Drug interactions No drug interactions are known.

See *Infections,* page 111; *Skin and local disorders,* page 125.

Macrodantin

Generic name

nitrofurantoin (available by generic name)

Action and uses An antibacterial drug used to treat infections of the kidneys, bladder, and urinary system; it is specifically designed to treat urinary infections and is not customarily used against any other infections. Macrodantin is active against many of the bacteria which commonly affect the urinary tract, but there are a few varieties of bacteria which are resistant to it. It is the same chemical as Furadantin but is made in larger crystals and is therefore absorbed more slowly into the system. This form was developed to reduce the likelihood of the gastrointestinal distress often associated with Furadantin.

Adult dosage Usually 50–100 mg, four times a day. Macrodantin can be given with food or milk. It should be taken for the full period of time directed, unless adverse effects occur.

Adverse effects The most common side effects are nausea, vomiting, and diarrhea. These are reduced if the drug is taken with milk or other food. Some people may develop allergies to Macrodantin and may suffer from rashes, hives, fever, chills, cough, or other symptoms. This drug can cause serious effects on nerve function, especially in people with diabetes, kidney disease, or serious chronic disease. It can also cause lung scarring and effects on red blood cells.

Precautions Macrodantin should not be used by pregnant or potentially pregnant women, by patients with kidney disease, severe diabetes, or G6PD deficiency (a congenital enzyme deficiency). Because of the potential for serious reactions, its use should be carefully supervised.

Drug interactions Macrodantin blocks the effect of nalidixic acid (Neg-Gram), which is also used to treat urinary infections, and therefore the two drugs should not be taken together.

See *Infections,* page 111.

Marax

Generic ingredients

bronchodilators : theophylline; ephedrine
antihistamine/sedative : hydroxyzine

Action and uses A combination preparation used to treat asthma. It contains two drugs which relax the bronchi, theophylline and ephedrine, plus hydroxyzine, an antihistamine with sedative properties. Theophylline and ephedrine act on the muscles of the bronchi, relax them, and open up the airways. Hydroxyzine theoretically provides a mild sedative for anxious asthmatic patients and counteracts any stimulant effect of the ephedrine. However, neither effect is proven, or even likely at the small dose of hydroxyzine used. It is contended by some that the hydroxyzine has a beneficial antihistamine effect, but this again is unproven. Most often, theophylline alone in proper doses is equally effective, less costly, and has fewer side effects. Further, this fixed combination does not allow adjustment of the dose of the ingredients relative to each other.

Adult dosage   One or two tablets every four to six hours (to treat attacks or to prevent them).

Adverse effects   Adverse effects from the ephedrine component can include nervousness, high blood pressure, fast heart rate, or palpitations. The theophylline can cause nausea, headaches or muscle cramps, and also palpitations.

Precautions   This drug should be avoided by pregnant and potentially pregnant women. Marax should be used cautiously by people who have heart disease or high blood pressure. It can be additive to certain over-the-counter drugs for asthma, so the prescribing physician should be informed of *all* drugs being used, including aerosols or inhalers.

Drug interactions   The ephedrine can be additive to drugs for coughs and colds (and thus increase side effects), but can counteract antihypertensive drugs. The theophylline can interact with anticoagulant drugs such as Coumadin.

See   *Asthma and lung disease,* page 109.

Meclizine (generic name). See ANTIVERT.

Medrol

Generic name

methylprednisolone

Action and uses   Medrol is one of several drugs referred to as "steroids" or "corticosteroids." Corticosteroids are hormones produced by the cortex (outer part) of the adrenal glands. Drugs with very similar properties to these hormones can also be made by chemical synthesis. Medrol is one of these "synthetic" steroid hormones, and is used in a wide variety of disorders usually associated with severe inflammation and/or destruction of tissue, such as acute arthritis or serious allergic reactions, as in severe asthma. Medrol is very similar to prednisone, although it is much more costly, but it may have slightly fewer side effects.

Medrol and related corticosteroids act on may cells in the body to change the production of proteins and the way cells handle carbohydrates, fats, and certain minerals. This produces several desirable effects when the drug is given in higher doses.

First, it acts to suppress inflammation, which can be use-

236

ful in certain types of arthritis (although it is used as a last resort in this situation); in inflammatory disease of the bowel, such as ulcerative colitis; and in a large variety of skin diseases where there is inflammation of the skin, for example psoriasis or eczema.

Second, it acts to suppress certain types of white blood cell and lowers the body's immunity (defenses against infection), which can be useful in the treatment of certain types of "auto-immune" diseases (where the body reacts to its own tissues), for example lupus erythematosus and certain types of leukemia where there is overproduction of white blood cells; it is also useful in preventing the "rejection" of transplanted organs.

Third, it acts to inhibit allergic reactions in severe allergic conditions (e.g. asthma) and serious skin allergies (e.g. poison ivy and poison oak). Medrol has a variety of other actions which are sometimes made use of in treatment, but which more often represent undesirable side effects as noted below.

Adult dosage The dose is carefully adjusted to suit each case and varies widely: it may be as high as 100 mg or more per day, or as little as 5 mg per day. When first started, it is often taken in high doses, sometimes several times a day, but when taken over long periods it is usually taken once daily in the morning or once every other day, depending on the circumstances.

Adverse effects The adverse effects of Medrol are related to both the dose and the length of time the drug is taken. A single dose of any amount may usually be taken without significant adverse effects. However, the incidence of serious adverse effects increases considerably with time at any dose greater than the physiological equivalent (approximately 7.5 mg per day). The most common adverse reaction observed in a large series of hospitalized patients on the similar drug prednisone included disturbances of water and salt balance to produce edema (or water retention) and loss of potassium (which can cause weakness); however, because it has less effect on salt and water, Medrol is believed to cause fewer problems of this type than prednisone.

Other common side effects include the development of abnormal fat deposits around the face ("moon face"), neck ("buffalo hump"), or abdomen, weight gain, increased bruising, gastrointestinal bleeding and/or upset, mental confusion, and diabetes. Antacids are frequently given to prevent the gastrointestinal problems. A continuing effect is the increased susceptibility to infections and often the masking of the symptoms of these infections. For this reason, those with a history of (or those who are exposed to) chronic infections such as tuberculosis are observed carefully. With longer-term use, there is often gradual degeneration of bone and muscle, which can cause fractures and muscle weakness, and cataracts may develop. Obviously, the use of this drug for long periods requires very careful analysis of benefits versus risks. It has been found that certain, but not all, chronic ailments which require this drug for very long periods can be controlled by giving Medrol every other day. This is desirable whenever possible since it tends to eliminate most of the severe side effects.

Another practical effect of using Medrol relates to the fact that it tends to suppress the normal function of the adrenal gland. In stress, the adrenal gland releases increased amounts of steroid hormones to help the body deal with the stressful or threatening situation. The absence of this extra reserve can be life threatening. A person taking corticosteroid drugs does not have this reserve, so that if an accident occurs, or if surgery is required, higher doses may be needed for a few days.

Precautions Use of Medrol, especially for more than seven days, should be under the careful supervision of a physician. The doctor should be notified of any changes which occur, especially after altering the dose or adding any other drug. People taking this drug for long periods should carry a card or wear a bracelet giving this information in case of emergency.

Drug interactions Medrol can interact additively with many diuretics such as hydrochlorothiazide or Lasix, to cause excessive loss of potassium, which can cause weakness. Diuretics are often used to treat the edema caused by corticosteroids, so this interaction can be anticipated and prevented by supplementing the potassium intake. Since aspirin and several other anti-inflammatory drugs used to treat arthritis, e.g., Motrin, also cause gastric upset and ulcer, they may be additive to this effect of Medrol.

See *Steroids, or cortisone-like drugs,* page 102.

Medroxyprogesterone (generic name). See PROVERA.

Mellaril

Generic name

thioridazine

Action and uses A major tranquilizer used to treat disorders of thinking and anxiety. Mellaril is one of a group of tranquilizers (which includes Thorazine and Stelazine) that have been widely used to treat conditions in which a person's perception of reality is disturbed. This disturbance may cause a person to think, for example, that he is in a different time or place (disorientation), or that he can fly (a delusion), or that he hears voices or sees visions (hallucinations). Mellaril is used to treat these disturbances in conditions such as schizophrenia, manic-depression, severe alcohol withdrawal and some neurological disorders such as multiple sclerosis. It is also used to treat patients who have taken LSD and amphetamines. Mellaril has the effect of "returning to reality" a person with disordered thinking, but it has little effect on normal thinking. Mellaril also has sedative effects, but is not used primarily for these. It is sometimes used in preference to other similar drugs because it causes fewer neurological side effects.

Adult dosage For the treatment of thought disorders, the initial dose of Mellaril may be 25–200 mg per day, eventually rising to 800 mg per day in some cases. The dose is adjusted to suit each patient, and is likely to vary greatly, because sensitivity to the drug varies widely from person to person. Generally speaking, however, the dose tends to be lower for older people, and, whatever the patient's age, it may usually be taken just once a day (often at bedtime, to take advantage of its sedative effect) when used over a long period of time.

Adverse effects Mellaril may produce a number of significant side effects, and can occasionally cause serious drug reactions. Its use, therefore, must be carefully supervised. When first taken, it is likely to produce heavy sedation, a sensation of mental dullness, and, in some cases, blurred vision, dry mouth, and constipation. These effects usually diminish if the drug is continued for two to three weeks or more. Mellaril also lowers the blood pressure, an effect which may manifest itself in a sensation of dizziness when a person stands up suddenly. In some people, Mellaril can cause restlessness, a fixed facial expression, and trembling in the hands, arms or legs. These side effects, which resemble the symptoms of Parkinson's disease, can usually be controlled with an anti-Parkinson drug, e.g., Cogentin. A few people who have taken Mellaril for a long time experience an involuntary movement of the tongue and lips. Occasionally, Mellaril can cause a skin rash, jaundice, or a fall in the white blood cell count, which increases the patient's vulnerability to infection; under these circumstances the drug must be discontinued.

Precautions Prolonged use requires regular medical evaluation at intervals. There may be some interference with driving or operating machinery.

Drug interactions Oversedation is possible when Mellaril is taken in combination with alcohol, other sedatives and tranquilizers, sleeping pills, antidepressants, antihistamines, and drugs containing narcotics. If taken with the antihypertensive drugs Ismelin and Aldomet it can counteract their blood pressure-lowering effect. It can also cause constipation or bladder dysfunction in some people if combined with antispasmodic drugs, anti-Parkinson drugs such as Cogentin, and tricyclic antidepressants such as Elavil.

See *Major tranquilizers,* page 49.

Meprobamate

Trade names

Equanil, Miltown

Action and uses A minor tranquilizer used to relieve mild tension and anxiety. Both Equanil and Miltown (trade names for meprobamate) are very similar to barbiturates in their sedative effects. Their use as sedatives has, however, diminished somewhat since the introduction of Librium and Valium. Meprobamate is frequently used in cases of muscle strain (as in back strain) as a muscle relaxant. Whether its beneficial effect in such cases is due to sedation or to true muscle relaxation is not clear.

Adult dosage Usually 200–400 mg four times a day and sometimes double that dose.

Adverse effects The incidence of allergic reactions to meprobamate is significant. Such reactions may include skin rashes or hives. Other common side effects may include nausea, headache, dizziness, and excessive drowsiness.

Precautions Meprobamate should not be taken by pregnant or potentially pregnant women or nursing mothers. Its sedative effects may make driving or operating machinery dangerous.

Drug dependence Meprobamate can produce psychological and/or physical dependence. Once habituation to the drug has developed, convulsions can occur if the drug is suddenly stopped, especially if the daily dose has been more than 800 mg four times a day.

Drug interactions The sedative effects of meprobamate can be increased by alcohol, other sedatives and tranquilizers, sleeping pills, and antidepressants. It can decrease the effects of anticoagulants, oral contraceptives, and the estrogens used in hormone replacement therapy because it affects the way the liver metabolizes these drugs.

See *Minor tranquilizers,* page 45.

Minocin

Generic name

minocycline

Action and uses A newer and slightly different member of one of the most commonly used oral antibiotic groups, the tetracyclines. There are a number of tetracycline drugs available, and most are comparable in their actions and side effects; Minocin, however, differs in some respects, as does Vibramycin. In general, the tetracyclines are known as "broad-spectrum" antibiotics because they can be used in a wide variety of different infections, although they are first choice drugs in very few common infections. They act by stopping the production of proteins in sensitive bacterial cells and have little effect on human cells. Minocin is currently very commonly used in low doses to inhibit the bacteria on the face which are believed to contribute to acne. It is also frequently used by those with chronic bronchitis or other lung disease. It has no effect on viral illnesses, including colds or fungal infections. Minocin is distinguished from other tetracyclines by its longer action, requiring less frequent dosing, its somewhat greater safety in people with kidney disease, and a higher incidence of vertigo as well as a higher cost.

Adult dosage *The dosing of Minocin is not the same as for other tetracyclines.* The usual adult dose is 200 mg initially, then 100 mg every 12 hours for a prescribed number of days as specified by the physician. It is very important to take this on an empty stomach. The dose may vary in some conditions, for example, in acne, where it may be lower.

Adverse effects   Minocin can cause various gastrointestinal symptoms, including nausea and vomiting, burning stomach or belching, cramps, and diarrhea. The latter symptom is often due to the fact that tetracyclines inhibit some bacteria in the lower intestine and elsewhere and allow overgrowth of other bacteria and minor fungi. These symptoms may, however, occur less frequently with Minocin.

Normally the symptoms tend to disappear when the drug is discontinued. Less commonly, Minocin can cause rashes or other allergic reactions and sensitivity of the skin to sunlight (photosensitivity), which may lead to rashes. It can also tend to worsen certain types of kidney disease, and rarely can cause liver damage or blood-cell abnormalities.

Precautions   Minocin should not be taken by pregnant or potentially pregnant women or nursing mothers and should be used with caution when significant liver disease is present. This antibiotic, like all others, should be taken for the full course prescribed, and every dose should be taken. Failure to do this can result in inadequate treatment of the infection, recurrence or the development of resistant strains of bacteria.

Drug interactions   The most common interaction occurs with antacids or milk products, since Minocin binds to these in the stomach and fails to be absorbed into the body. Minocin can potentially increase the effect of the anticoagulant Coumadin and increase the hazard of bleeding.

See   *Infections,* page 111.

Monistat

Generic name

miconazole

Action and uses   An antifungal cream used to treat fungus or yeast infections of the vagina. Monistat is effective in killing several fungi, including the one called *Candida* which most commonly infects the vagina. This kind of infection causes a thin, itchy discharge and often occurs after broad-spectrum antibiotic therapy or in diabetes.

Adult dosage   The cream is usually applied at bedtime for 10–14 days with a measured-dose applicator. It is important to use the drug for the full period of time, since otherwise the microorganisms will not be completely eradicated and infection will recur.

Adverse effects	The most common side effects are occasional local irritation or burning. Sometimes allergic reactions may occur.
Precautions	It is currently believed that Monistat is safe for use during the last six months of pregnancy but earlier use should be avoided.
Drug interactions	None are currently known.
See	*Skin and local disorders,* page 125.

Motrin

Generic name	
	ibuprofen

Action and uses	One of the several recently introduced drugs, called "non-steroidal anti-inflammatory drugs," used to treat the symptoms of various types of arthritis. It has some ability to relieve pain and also acts to decrease inflammation. Motrin, like the other recently introduced drugs with similar actions (e.g., Tolectin, Naprosyn, and Nalfon), is often used as an alternative to aspirin in the therapy of osteoarthritis and rheumatoid and other types of arthritis. In some cases, its effect is seen in a few days; and in other cases, chronic osteoarthritis for example, its effects may be seen only after a longer period of use. Because of its considerably greater cost, it is usually reserved for those people on whom aspirin is not effective or is not tolerated.
Adult dosage	The currently recommended dose is 300–400 mg three or four times daily, usually adjusted according to response.
Adverse effects	The most common side effects are gastrointestinal irritation, occurring in between 4% and 16% of patients, some of whom experience bleeding. Other side effects include dizziness, headaches, rash, decreased appetite, and fluid retention. It can also cause visual changes.
Precautions	Motrin should be avoided by pregnant or potentially pregnant women and nursing mothers. Motrin should be used with caution by people with heart failure or a history of peptic ulcer. If bleeding or visual changes occur, the prescribing physician should be notified at once.
Drug interactions	Motrin may possibly interact with anticoagulant drugs such as Coumadin and predispose to bleeding. The use of aspirin with Motrin may decrease the effectiveness of Motrin, and their stomach-irritant effects can be additive.

See *Pain with inflammation,* page 43.

Mycolog

Generic ingredients

> antibiotics : nystatin, neomycin sulfate, gramicidin
> steroid : triamcinolone acetonide

Action and uses A combination product used to treat local infections of the skin. Mycolog combines three antibiotics and a steroid (cortisone-like drug). Each of the antibiotics acts against different types of bacteria or fungi. The steroid acts to reduce inflammation and irritation. The ointment is used in a variety of skin irritations where mild infection is present. This type of mixture has been criticized because it represents "shotgun" therapy—using a mixture of ingredients in a somewhat random, nonspecific fashion when often one specific ingredient may be adequate.

Adult dosage Mycolog is available as a cream, ointment, lotion, and suspension; it is usually applied two to four times per day.

Adverse effects Allergy to any of the ingredients of Mycolog may occur and skin conditions may worsen rather than improve. This is particularly true of neomycin which has a high rate of allergic reactions. The steroid may rarely worsen an infection, especially if it is caused by a virus, as in shingles. Serious adverse effects can occur from all the ingredients if the preparation is used on large areas for a long time, due to absorption through the skin. Also, resistant bacteria or fungi can appear and cause reinfection.

Precautions Mycolog is for topical (local) application and should not be used over large parts of the body at any one time. It should not be used to treat the sores of herpes simplex ("cold sores") or those of shingles, chickenpox, or of smallpox vaccinations.

Drug interactions If used properly, drug interactions are not a problem.

See *Infections,* page 111; *Skin and local disorders,* page 125; *Steroids, or cortisone-like drugs,* page 102.

Mycostatin

Generic name

> nystatin (available by generic name)

Action and uses An antibiotic used to treat fungal infections. Mycostatin is not active against infections caused by bacteria, but is effective in treating many fungal infections, particularly those caused by a family of fungi known as *Candida* (or *Monilia*). This causes candidiasis (moniliasis), an infection which can affect the vagina to produce a clear discharge, itching, or burning. The mouth and anus can also be affected. This often occurs after treatment with broad-spectrum antibiotics or in diabetes.

Adult dosage Usually one or two tablets inserted into the vagina daily for two weeks. The tablets are supplied with an applicator and should be used regardless of an intervening menstrual period. Creams, ointments, and suspensions are usable for other infections. It is very important to use them nightly for the full time period since infections may otherwise recur.

Adverse effects There are no serious side effects except for occasional minor irritations.

Precautions No special precautions are necessary with Mycostatin and it can be used during pregnancy.

Drug interactions None are known.

See *Infections,* page 111; *Skin and local disorders,* page 125.

Naldecon

Generic ingredients

decongestants : phenylpropanolamine, phenylephrine antihistamines : chlorpheniramine, phenyltoloxamine

Action and uses Naldecon is a combination of two decongestant drugs, phenylpropanolamine and phenylephrine (which are related to epinephrine), and two antihistamine drugs, chlorpheniramine and phenyltoloxamine. It is used to treat nasal congestion associated with allergy, sinusitis, and the common cold. The two decongestants cut down blood flow to inflamed nasal areas and help to dry up a runny nose. The antihistamines act to prevent the action of histamine, a substance released by cells damaged by allergy or infection, which is responsible for causing the redness and inflammation experienced in allergy.

Adult dosage Naldecon is available as sustained-action tablets and as syrup. One dose (5 ml) of syrup should be taken every four hours; not more than four doses should be taken in any 24-hour period. The sustained-action tablets are formulated to be taken three times daily, at eight-hourly intervals.

Adverse effects Prolonged use of Naldecon may lead to a chronic runny nose condition and can be followed by a rebound congestion when the drug is discontinued. Because of its two epinephrine-like components, Naldecon can cause palpitations and raise the blood pressure. The antihistamines in Naldecon can cause drowsiness, occasional blurring of vision, and difficulty in passing urine.

Precautions This drug should be avoided by pregnant or potentially pregnant women and nursing mothers. Naldecon may interfere with driving or using machinery. People with heart disease or high blood pressure should use this drug only after checking with their physician.

Drug interactions The antihistamines can add to the sedative effects of alcohol, tranquilizers, and sleeping pills. They can also add to the antispasmodic effects of drugs for gastric distress (e.g.,Pro-Banthine, Librax), causing mouth dryness and difficulty in urinating.

   The decongestants can counteract the effects of drugs for high blood pressure and cause a dangerous interaction with MAO inhibitor drugs such as Nardil, Parnate, Eutonyl, and Eutron.

See *Coughs and colds,* page 117.

Nalfon

Generic name
fenoprofen

Action and uses One of several recently introduced drugs, called "non-steroidal anti-inflammatory drugs," used to treat the symptoms of various types of arthritis. It has some ability to relieve pain and also acts to decrease inflammation. Nalfon, like the other new drugs with similar actions (e.g.,Motrin, Naprosyn, Tolectin, and Clinoril), is often used as an alternative to aspirin for rheumatoid and other types of arthritis. In some cases, its effect is seen in a few days, but in others it may take longer.

Adult dosage Usually 300 –600 mg orally on an empty stomach, four times a day, with some dose adjustment as needed. Doses higher than 750 mg per day are not recommended.

Adverse effects Gastrointestinal side effects, including heartburn, nausea, stomach upset, and gastrointestinal bleeding may occur in one out of seven patients taking Nalfon. Less frequently, peptic ulcer, skin rashes, ringing in the ears, fluid retention, visual and hearing disturbances have been reported in those taking the drug.

Precautions Nalfon should be avoided by pregnant or potentially pregnant women and nursing mothers. It should be used with caution by people with a history of allergy to aspirin or other non-steroidal anti-inflammatory drugs, heart failure, peptic ulcer, and kidney failure as well as those taking anticoagulants, antiepileptic drugs, and oral drugs for diabetes. If bleeding, rash, or unusual changes occur, the prescribing physician should be notified at once.

Drug interactions Nalfon may interact with the anticoagulant drug Coumadin to increase the risk of bleeding and with Dilantin and oral drugs for diabetes to increase their toxic effects. Aspirin and phenobarbital may reduce the effectiveness of Nalfon.

See *Pain with inflammation,* page 43.

Naprosyn

Generic name

naproxen

Action and uses One of several recently introduced drugs, called "non-steroidal anti-inflammatory drugs," used to treat the symptoms of various types of arthritis. It has some ability to relieve pain and also acts to decrease inflammation. Naprosyn, like the other new drugs with similar actions (e.g.,Motrin, Nalfon, Tolectin and Clinoril), is often used as an alternative to aspirin for rheumatoid and other types of arthritis. In some cases, its effect is seen in a few days, but, in others, it may take longer. Naprosyn's major advantage over the similar drugs is that it need be taken only twice daily; however, because of its considerably greater cost, it is usually reserved for those people on whom aspirin therapy is not effective or not tolerated.

Adult dosage Usually 250 mg orally twice daily on an empty stomach with some individual dose adjustment. Doses higher than 750 mg per day are not recommended.

Adverse effects Gastrointestinal side effects, including heartburn, nausea, stomach upset, and gastrointestinal bleeding may occur in one out of seven patients taking Naprosyn. Less frequently, peptic ulcer, skin rashes, ringing in the ears, fluid retention, visual and hearing disturbances have been reported in those taking the drug.

Precautions Naprosyn should be avoided by pregnant or potentially pregnant women and nursing mothers. It should be used with caution by people with a history of allergy to aspirin or other non-steroidal anti-inflammatory drugs, heart failure, peptic ulcer, and kidney failure as well as those taking anticoagulants, antiepileptic drugs, and oral drugs for diabetes. If bleeding, rash, or unusual changes occur, the prescribing physician should be notified at once.

Drug interactions Naprosyn may interact with the anticoagulant drug Coumadin to increase the risk of bleeding, and with Dilantin and oral drugs for diabetes to increase their toxic effects. Aspirin and phenobarbital may reduce the effectiveness of Naprosyn.

See *Pain with inflammation,* page 43.

Nembutal

Generic name

pentobarbital (available by generic name)

Action and uses A barbiturate similar to Seconal and Butisol. Nembutal is chiefly used as a sleeping pill, although is occasionally used as a daytime sedative to relieve anxiety and tension. It takes effect 15–30 minutes after being taken and its effect lasts 5–6 hours. When used as a sleeping medication, Nembutal decreases the time it takes to go to sleep but suppresses dreaming. After a few days tolerance can develop and it is necessary to increase the dose to produce the same sleep-inducing effect. Some of the effects of Nembutal may last longer than 5–6 hours, such as a "hangover" which may occur the morning after taking the drug.

Adult dosage For sleep the usual dose is 100 mg at bedtime. If used in the daytime for relief of anxiety and tension, the usual dose is 30 mg, two to four times per day.

Adverse effects When used as a sleeping pill Nembutal may cause a "hangover" effect the following morning. It may also cause a feeling of depression and tiredness, together with nausea, vomiting, and diarrhea. In older people it may cause excitement rather than sedation. If it is discontinued after several weeks of use withdrawal symptoms may appear: there is often a tendency for increased dreaming and even nightmares; there may be insomnia (difficulty in sleeping) and nervousness; if the dose has been high (over 400 mg per day) seizures may occur. All these effects are due to the withdrawal of the drug. Other mild side effects of the drug include allergic skin reactions, upset stomach, and muscular aches. Nembutal can suppress breathing in people with severe lung disease.

Precautions Nembutal and other barbiturates have long been a major cause of self-poisoning and death through overdose, both accidental and deliberate. If taken in high doses they can be very dangerous and sometimes fatal. They are particularly dangerous if taken with alcohol or other tranquilizers.

Drug dependence If used for longer than seven to ten days, "tolerance" to Nembutal may build up. If this occurs, dependence on the drug may develop, and if it is suddenly discontinued withdrawal symptoms may occur. Therefore, it must be stopped slowly if it has been used for a long time. Because of this problem, as well as its potential for abuse, the prescribing of Nembutal is restricted.

Drug interactions Nembutal can interact with many other drugs, particularly the anticoagulant Coumadin, whose effect it decreases. Its effect is additive to the effects of other tranquilizers, sleeping pills, and alcohol. The combination of Nembutal with any such drugs can be very hazardous, causing suppression of breathing and even death.

See *Sleeping pills,* page 47; *Minor tranquilizers,* page 45.

Neosporin Ophthalmic

Generic ingredients

antibiotics : neomycin; polymyxin B; bacitracin

Action and uses A sterile preparation for use in the eye. Neosporin is a combination of three antibiotics which between them kill a large range of bacteria. It is used for short-term treatment of infected eye conditions, including conjunctivitis.

Adult dosage Supplied as ointment and drops. The ointment should be applied every three or four hours. If the drops are used, one or two drops should be instilled into the affected eye two to four times daily; it is often necessary to commence therapy by using the drops every 30 minutes.

Adverse effects As with all antibiotics, "overgrowth" of bacteria which are not sensitive to the drug can occur with prolonged use of Neosporin. Allergic reactions are not uncommon, and can be confused with the disorder being treated.

Precautions If the condition shows no improvement after a few days, or if it worsens, the treatment should be re-evaluated by the physician.

See *Infections,* page 111; *Skin and local disorders,* page 125.

Nicotinic Acid (Niacin)

Trade names

Nicobid, Nico-400, Nicotinex

Action and uses One of the B group of vitamins, which is used to lower cholesterol levels in the blood. Its effectiveness in preventing diseases associated with high blood cholesterol, such as coronary heart disease, is limited by its side effects. The cholesterol-lowering action is due to an effect on metabolism and transport of particles containing cholesterol (this is not related to the action of niacin in treating pellagra). In high doses, it is used to dilate blood vessels in circulation disorders, but it does not usually act on the diseased vessels, only the tiny ones such as those in the face. It is also used to treat the symptoms of pellagra (a skin condition due to niacin deficiency and characterized by sensitivity to light, red blotches, diarrhea, and swollen tongue). Niacin is essential for normal body function, but deficiency seldom arises as it is a normal dietary constituent, found mainly in proteins. It does not come from nicotine and does not have any effects associated with tobacco.

Adult dosage The dose recommended for the treatment of pellagra is up to 500 mg daily in divided doses.

Much higher doses are used if the drug is employed for lowering cholesterol levels in the blood: 2–6 grams daily, taken regularly over a long period of time.

Adverse effects In the doses given for pellagra and, particularly, for high cholesterol levels, niacin frequently produces an intense flushing of the skin, often accompanied by itching. Although this reaction decreases in intensity after several weeks' therapy, it is very unpleasant. Vomiting and diarrhea and indigestion may also occur with niacin, as well as ulcers, diabetes, liver damage, and allergic reactions.

Precautions Niacin may affect the levels of uric acid and sugar in the blood; it should therefore be taken with caution by people suffering from gout, having a predisposition to diabetes, or with ulcer disease.

Drug interactions   There are no significant interactions in normal doses.

See   *Poor circulation,* page 68; *Vitamins and minerals,* page 134.

Nitro-Bid (trade name). See NITROGLYCERIN.

Nitrofurantoin (generic name). See MACRODANTIN.

Nitroglycerin

Trade names

> Nitro-Bid, Nitrobon, Nitroglyn, Nitrol,
> Nitrong, Nitrospan, Nitrostat

Action and uses   A drug used to relieve pain in the treatment of angina pectoris, the characteristic pain felt in the chest (or sometimes in the arm) which is due to inadequate supply of oxygen to the heart muscle. Angina pectoris is often brought on by exercise, exertion, or emotion. The deficiency of oxygen (which the heart receives from the blood) most often results from narrowing of the blood vessels which supply the heart, the *coronary arteries,* which become "furred up" with fatty deposits and are unable to conduct enough oxygen-rich blood to the heart. Nitroglycerin acts in two ways: to open up the blood vessels to the heart, which are often partially blocked, and to dilate peripheral blood vessels in order to reduce the work the heart must do.

Nitroglycerin is sometimes also used to treat conditions where blood circulation is poor, such as Raynaud's disease, and in certain other heart-failure conditions.

Adult dosage   The tablets of nitroglycerin should be placed under the tongue and allowed to dissolve. The drug is quickly absorbed from the lining of the mouth. Up to three 0.2 mg tablets may be taken when an attack of angina pectoris occurs. The tablets may be chewed and retained in the mouth, but they should never be swallowed (if they are, absorption will be too slow to have any effect). Nitroglycerin is also available as a paste and applied in measured amounts to a skin area, usually the back. This has a more prolonged action.

Adverse effects   Flushing is very common and is due to increased blood flow to the skin. Throbbing headache often occurs and is also associated with changes in blood flow. A feeling of faintness or dizziness can occur (particularly in hot weather), more commonly in people with high blood pressure.

Precautions If more than two or three tablets do not relieve the pain, the doctor should be notified at once. Nitroglycerin tends to deteriorate in 2–6 months, so that fresh tablets should always be used (old tablets are not dangerous, just ineffective).

Drug interactions Excessive alcohol intake tends to dilate blood vessels and add to the action of nitroglycerin, as do certain antihypertensive drugs, such as Apresoline.

See *Poor circulation,* page 68; *Angina pectoris,* page 71.

Nitrostat (trade name). See NITROGLYCERIN.

Norgesic
Norgesic Forte

Generic ingredients

> antihistamine : orphenadrine citrate
> pain relievers : aspirin, phenacetin
> mild stimulant : caffeine

Action and uses An analgesic drug used for the relief of muscular pain. Orphenadrine citrate is an antihistamine drug which acts in the brain to reduce muscle rigidity (it is also used to treat the symptoms of Parkinson's disease). Aspirin and phenacetin are pain relievers which reduce the production of substances in the body responsible for causing the sensation of pain. The function of the caffeine present is not clear. Norgesic Forte is twice the strength of Norgesic.

Adult dosage One or two tablets of Norgesic or one-half or one tablet of Norgesic Forte are taken three or four times daily.

Adverse effects Aspirin may cause stomach upset and irritation and also affects the blood clotting system. Phenacetin can cause kidney damage, particularly if taken over a long period of time. Orphenadrine has some of the side effects of other antihistamine drugs, including dry mouth, blurring of vision, and drowsiness.

Precautions Norgesic should not be taken if you have any form of kidney disease. Because of the effects of Orphenadrine, Norgesic should be used carefully if asthma, glaucoma, or prostate trouble is present. Any sedative effect will be additive to that of alcohol or sedative drugs, including sleeping tablets and some antidepressants. When taking Norgesic, driving or operating heavy machinery may be hazardous. Norgesic should not be taken by pregnant or potentially pregnant women and nursing mothers.

Drug interactions When taken together with propoxyphene (Darvon preparations), Norgesic has been shown to cause confusion and tremors. Norgesic can add to the sedative effects of antispasmodics, antihistamines, and tricyclic antidepressants.

See *Non-narcotic pain relievers,* page 42.

Norinyl 1/50-21

Generic ingredients

progestogen : norethindrone estrogen : mestranol

Action and uses An oral contraceptive. Like many other birth-control pills, Norinyl 1/50-21 is made up of a combination of two synthetic hormones—an estrogen and a progesterone-like hormone (a progestogen). It is essentially identical to Ortho-Novum 1/50 and is one of the lower-dose preparations, containing 50 micrograms only of estrogen. Recent studies have suggested that lowering the dose of estrogen may be associated with a lower incidence of side effects, although the incidence of intermenstrual bleeding ("breakthrough bleeding," or "spotting") tends to be increased, especially during the first few cycles. It acts, like most birth-control pills, to prevent conception by affecting the pituitary gland's control of the reproductive cycle, as well as by acting locally on the lining of the uterus and the cervical mucus, and possibly in other ways. When taken regularly, it is a very effective contraceptive drug.

Adult dosage In general, one tablet is taken daily (usually at night) for 21 consecutive days, beginning on the 5th day of menstruation. No tablets are taken on the following 7 days, during which time menstrual bleeding occurs, and on the 8th day they are restarted for another 21-day cycle.

Adverse effects Use of oral contraceptive pills has been associated with a variety of side effects. Norinyl 1/50-21 may be associated with a higher incidence of breakthrough bleeding, or spotting, but there appears to be a slightly decreased incidence (as compared with some other higher-dose estrogen pills) of the effects of estrogen excess, such as nausea, edema, and leg cramps. Other minor side effects include acne, breast discomfort, depression, gastrointestinal upsets, headaches, and vaginal infections. More significant but less common side effects include the risks of thrombophlebitis (blood clotting associated with inflammation of the veins of the legs), increased blood pressure, increased blood sugar levels, and gallbladder disease. It is possible that these last-mentioned side effects also are less likely to occur with a low-dose of estrogen, as in Norinyl 1/50-21. The risk of certain side effects such as heart disease and gallbladder disease appear to increase with age (especially over the age of 35). A woman who has a history of true migraine headache may find that headaches increase while she is taking oral contraceptives, and she may also run a higher risk (though the risk is still small) of suffering a stroke.

Precautions A history of thrombophlebitis, blood clots, and migraine headaches is usually a contraindication to the use of oral contraceptives. For women over the age of 35, or for those who have other risk factors (a history of heavy smoking, gallbladder disease, diabetes or high blood pressure), use should be weighed carefully against alternative birth-control methods.

Drug interactions Several drug interactions have been suggested but none have been well documented as clinically significant in most cases.

See *Hormonal drugs,* page 87; *Oral contraceptives,* page 96.

Norlestrin 21 1/50
Norlestrin 21 2.5/50

Generic ingredients

progestogen : norethindrone
estrogen : ethinyl estradiol

Action and uses Norlestrin is an oral contraceptive available in two different doses. Like many birth-control pills, it is made up of a combination of two synthetic hormones, an estrogen and a progesterone-like hormone (a progestogen). The Norlestrin pills contain somewhat greater amounts of both types of hormones than the similar product Loestrin. Norlestrin 2.5/50, like Ovral and Ortho-Novum 10 mg, is a "progestogen-dominant" oral contraceptive, which may affect the side effects seen (see below). Norlestrin 1/50 has a lower dose of progestogen and resembles many other commonly used oral contraceptives. Like most other oral contraceptives, it acts to prevent conception by affecting the pituitary gland's control of the reproductive cycle as well as by acting locally on the lining of the uterus and the cervical mucus, and possibly in other ways. When taken regularly, it is a very effective contraceptive drug.

Adult dosage In general, one tablet is taken daily (usually at night) for 21 consecutive days, beginning on the 5th day of menstruation. No tablets are taken on the following 7 days, during which time menstrual bleeding occurs, and on the 8th day they are restarted for another 21-day cycle.

Adverse effects Compared with some other oral contraceptives, Norlestrin 2.5/50 may show a slightly higher incidence of certain side effects—increased appetite and weight gain, acne or hair loss, depression, fatigue, and decreased menstrual flow.

With both Norlestrin 2.5/50 and 1/50 the other common side effects of oral contraceptives may also be seen, including breast changes, gastrointestinal upset, and inflammation of the vagina. Less common but more significant side effects include the risk of thrombophlebitis (blood clotting associated with inflammation of the veins of the legs), increased blood pressure, increased blood sugar levels, and gallbladder disease. The risk of certain side effects such as heart disease and gallbladder disease appear to increase with age (especially over the age of 35). A woman with a history of true migraine headache may find that her headaches increase while she is taking oral contraceptives, and she may also run a slightly higher risk (though the risk is still small) of suffering a stroke. A woman with a history of heavy smoking runs an increased risk of heart attack, particularly at ages greater than 40.

Precautions A history of thrombophlebitis, blood clots, or migraine headaches is usually a contraindication to the use of oral contraceptives. For women over the age of 35, or for women with other risk factors (a history of heavy smoking, gallbladder disease, diabetes, or high blood pressure) use should be weighed carefully against alternative birth-control methods.

Drug interactions Several drug interactions have been suggested but have not been well documented as significant in the majority of cases.

See *Hormonal drugs,* page 87; *Oral contraceptives,* page 96.

Novahistine-DH

Generic ingredients

```
decongestant : phenylpropanolamine
cough suppressant : codeine
```

255

Action and uses   This is a mixture of a decongestant and codeine; it acts to reduce nasal and upper respiratory congestion and also to reduce coughing. This particular cough/cold mixture does not include an antihistamine and is not likely to cause sedation, which may be a useful attribute. Ideally it should be used only when it is necessary to reduce coughing, and this is not often the case since coughing is a useful protective reflex to get rid of secretions.

Adult dosage   Two teaspoons every four to six hours, not to exceed four doses in 24 hours.

Adverse effects   The decongestant ingredient may occasionally cause palpitations or pounding of the heart. Several days' use of any compound with codeine can cause constipation. Other side effects are relatively uncommon.

Precautions   Elderly people, or those with diabetes, heart trouble, or high blood pressure, should always check with their physician before using this drug, since they may require a lower dose. This drug should be used only for a limited time (two to four days) in most cases.

Drug dependence   The small quantities of codeine present can cause habituation if the drug is taken for prolonged periods.

Drug interactions   The decongestant ingredient can raise the blood pressure and counteract the effects of several antihypertensive drugs, e.g.,Aldomet and Inderal. Codeine can add to the effects of any other sedating drugs.

See   *Coughs and colds,* page 117.

Nystatin (generic name). See MYCOSTATIN.

Omnipen (brand name). See AMPICILLIN.

Orinase

Generic name

tolbutamide (available by generic name)

Action and uses   A drug which lowers the level of glucose (sugar) in the blood, used to treat diabetes. Because Orinase can be taken orally (unlike insulin) it is termed an "oral hypoglycemic" drug (hypoglycemic means "blood-sugar-lowering"). It is similar to other oral antidiabetic drugs such as Diabinese and Tolinase, but not to DBI. Orinase works by stimulating the pancreas to produce insulin and by helping the cells of the body to use glucose. It is only of value in diabetics who are able to make insulin. Such patients usually have the mild type of diabetes that often becomes evident toward middle age (and is therefore known as maturity-onset diabetes). Oral hypoglycemic drugs should be taken only if dietary measures alone have failed to control the condition. Resistance to the effects of Orinase often develops after a few months or years. It is recommended that a withdrawal of oral antidiabetic drugs be tried every six months to one year since their continued use may not be needed. The long-term benefits versus risks of this and related drugs are now widely debated.

Adult dosage   The dosage is adjusted according to the needs of each patient; usually 500 mg are taken twice daily initially, with subsequent adjustment according to response.

Adverse effects   The most common and hazardous adverse effect is excessive lowering of the blood sugar (hypoglycemia), which can cause symptoms of dizziness, weakness, cold sweats and mental dullness. Older people, people taking several other drugs (see drug interactions below), or those with liver or kidney disease are more prone to this effect. With proper dosage, other side effects are unusual, but rashes, blood or liver abnormalities and water retention can occur.

Precautions   This drug should be avoided by pregnant or potentially pregnant women and nursing mothers as well as by those with significant kidney or liver disease. People who are allergic to sulfa drugs may develop an allergy to this drug.

Drug interactions   Thiazide diuretics (e.g., hydrochlorothiazide, Diuril, Hygroton) can aggravate diabetes and may increase the necessary dose of the oral antidiabetic drug. A number of drugs can increase the risk of low blood sugar if taken in combination with Orinase. These include insulin, sulfa drugs, anti-inflammatory drugs such as aspirin, Butazolidin, and Tandearil, and the anticonvulsant Dilantin. Inderal (propranolol) can also cause dangerous interactions and disguise the symptoms of hypoglycemia. Alcohol can cause a flushing reaction when taken with this drug.

See   *Diabetes,* page 90.

Ornade Spansule Capsules

Generic ingredients

antihistamine : chlorpheniramine
decongestant : phenylpropanolamine
anticholinergic : isopropamide iodide

Action and uses This mixture of ingredients includes a decongestant, an antihistamine, and an anticholinergic (which causes drying of nasal secretions) for the relief of symptoms of allergic sinusitis and for severe symptoms of a cold. It is not indicated for asthma.

Adult dosage One Spansule every 12 hours as needed for symptoms.

Adverse effects The most common side effect is drowsiness, due to the antihistamine component. Less commonly, there may be excessive dryness of the mouth and nose, palpitations, or nervousness. Other side effects are infrequent but are more likely to occur in people with heart disease, high blood pressure, or prostate trouble.

Precautions This drug should be avoided by pregnant or potentially pregnant women and nursing mothers. People who are allergic to iodide should not take this drug; also because of the presence of iodide, prolonged use is not advisable. Caution in driving and operating machinery is necessary if a sedative effect is noticed. People taking medicines for high blood pressure or heart ailments should check with their physicians before using Ornade since the decongestant may elevate the blood pressure.

Drug interactions The sedative effect of the antihistamine can be additive to alcohol and to other sedatives and tranquilizers. The decongestant can raise the blood pressure and thus counteract the effects of some antihypertensive drugs. The effects of the anticholinergic component can also be additive to those of certain antispasmodic drugs used for treatment of ulcer or bladder dysfunctions (e.g.,Pro-Banthine) or can interact with tricyclic antidepressant drugs (e.g.,Elavil). The iodide in the compound can interfere with certain tests of thyroid function.

See *Coughs and colds,* page 117.

Ortho-Novum 1/50-21
Ortho-Novum 1/50-28

Generic ingredients

> progestogen : norethindrone
> estrogen : mestranol

Action and uses An oral contraceptive. Ortho-Novum 1/50, which is essentially identical to Norinyl 1/50, is a combination of two synthetic hormones, an estrogen and progesterone-like hormone (a progestogen). Like Norinyl 1/50, Ortho-Novum 1/50 contains a lower dose of estrogen (50 micrograms) than many combination oral contraceptives. Recent studies have suggested that lower doses of estrogen may be associated with a lower incidence of estrogen-related side effects, although the incidence of intermenstrual bleeding ("breakthrough bleeding" or "spotting") tends to increase, especially in the first few cycles. Like most birth-control pills, it acts to prevent conception by affecting the pituitary gland's control of reproduction, as well as by acting locally on the lining of the uterus and the cervical mucus, and possibly in other ways. When taken regularly it is a very effective contraceptive drug.

Adult dosage For Ortho-Novum 1/50-21, one tablet is taken daily (usually at night) for 21 consecutive days, beginning on the 5th day of menstruation. No tablets are taken on the following 7 days, during which time menstrual bleeding occurs, and on the 8th day, they are restarted for another 21-day cycle. With the Ortho-Novum 1/50-28 pack, one tablet is taken each day after starting.

Adverse effects Use of oral contraceptive pills has been associated with a variety of side effects. Ortho-Novum 1/50 may be associated with a higher incidence of intermenstrual bleeding ("breakthrough bleeding," or "spotting") but there appears to be a slightly decreased incidence (as compared with some other higher estrogen pills) of the effects of estrogen excess, such as nausea, edema, and leg cramps. Other minor side effects include acne, breast discomfort, depression, gastrointestinal upsets, headaches, and vaginal infections. More significant but less common side effects include the risks of thrombophlebitis (blood clotting associated with inflammation of the veins of the legs), increased blood pressure and other metabolic effects, gallbladder disease and rarely, liver tumors. It is possible that these are slightly decreased in this lower dose. The risk of certain side effects, for example heart disease and gallbladder disease, appears to increase with age (especially over the age of 35). A woman with a history of true migraine headache may find that her headaches increase while she is taking oral contraceptives; she may also run a higher risk (though the risk is still small) of suffering a stroke.

Precautions A history of thrombophlebitis, blood clots, and migraine headaches is usually a contraindication to the use of oral contraceptives. For women over the age of 35, or for those with other risk factors, such as a history of heavy smoking, gallbladder disease, diabetes, or high blood pressure, use should be weighed carefully against alternative birth-control methods. The "patient package insert" now required by law should be read carefully by every patient.

Drug interactions Reduced efficacy has been reported when barbiturates, anticonvulsants, and ampicillin are also taken.

See *Hormonal drugs,* page 87; *Oral contraceptives,* page 96.

Ortho-Novum 1/80-21

Generic ingredients

progestogen : norethindrone
estrogen : mestranol

Action and uses Ortho-Novum 1/80 is one of the four Ortho-Novum oral contraceptives combining a progesterone-like synthetic hormone (a progestogen) with an estrogen. It has a lower dose of both the progestogen and the estrogen than plain Ortho-Novum but a higher dose of estrogen than Ortho-Novum 1/50. It is sometimes used when intermenstrual bleeding ("breakthrough bleeding") occurs with a lower dose of estrogen, as in Ortho-Novum 1/50. The product is essentially identical to Norinyl 1/80. Like most other oral contraceptives, it acts to prevent conception by affecting the pituitary gland's control of the reproductive cycle, as well as by acting locally on the lining of the uterus and the cervical mucus, and possibly in other ways. When taken regularly, it is a very effective contraceptive drug.

Adult dosage In general, one tablet is taken daily (usually at night) for 21 consecutive days, beginning on the 5th day of menstruation. No tablets are taken on the following 7 days, during which time menstrual bleeding occurs, and on the 8th day they are restarted for another 21-day cycle.

Adverse effects As with all oral contraceptives, a variety of side effects may occur, including weight gain, increased appetite, depression or fatigue, breast changes, gastrointestinal upset, headache, and increased vaginal discharge or infection. More significant, but less common, side effects include the risk of thrombophlebitis (blood clotting associated with inflammation of the veins of the legs), increased blood pressure, increased blood sugar levels, and gallbladder disease. The risk of certain side effects, for example, heart disease and gallbladder disease, appears to increase with age (especially over the age of 35). A woman with a history of true migraine headache may find that her headaches increase while she is taking oral contraceptives; she may also run a slightly higher risk (though the risk is still small) of suffering a stroke.

Precautions A history of thrombophlebitis, blood clots, and migraine headaches is usually a contraindication to the use of oral contraceptives. For women over the age of 35, or for those with other risk factors, such as a history of heavy smoking, gallbladder disease, diabetes, or high blood pressure, use should be weighed carefully against alternative birth-control methods.

Drug interactions Several drug interactions have been suggested but none has been well documented as clinically significant in most cases.

See *Hormonal drugs,* page 87; *Oral contraceptives,* page 96.

Ovral

Generic ingredients

| progestogen : norgestrel |
| estrogen : ethinyl estradiol |

Action and uses An oral contraceptive. Like many birth control pills, Ovral is made up of a combination of two synthetic hormones, an estrogen and a progesterone-like hormone (a progestogen). Ovral contains somewhat greater amounts of hormones than the similar product, Lo Ovral. Norgestrel is believed to be a somewhat more potent progestogen so that Ovral, like Norlestrin 2.5 mg and Ortho-Novum 2 mg, is a "progestogen-dominant" oral contraceptive, which may affect the type of side effects seen (see below). Like most other oral contraceptives, it acts to prevent conception by affecting the pituitary gland's control of the reproductive cycle, as well as by acting locally on the lining of the uterus and the cervical mucus, and possibly in other ways. Like all oral contraceptives, when taken regularly it is a very effective contraceptive drug.

Adult dosage In general, one tablet is taken daily (usually at night) for 21 consecutive days, beginning on the 5th day of menstruation. No tablets are taken on the following 7 days during which time menstrual bleeding occurs, and on the 8th day the tablets are restarted for another 21-day cycle.

Adverse effects Compared with some other oral contraceptives, Ovral may produce a slightly higher incidence of increased appetite and weight gain, acne or hair loss, depression, fatigue and decreased menstrual flow.

The other more common side effects of oral contraceptives may also be seen, including breast changes, gastrointestinal upset, and vaginal inflammation. Less common but more significant side effects include the risk of thrombophlebitis (blood clotting associated with inflammation of the veins of the legs), increased blood pressure, increased blood sugar levels, and gallbladder disease. The risk of certain side effects, for example heart disease and gallbladder disease, appears to increase with age (especially over the age of 35). A woman with a history of true migraine headache may find that her headaches increase while she is taking oral contraceptives; she may also run a higher risk (though the risk is still small) of suffering a stroke. A history of heavy smoking is associated with an increased risk of heart attack, particularly in women of 40 and over.

Precautions A history of thrombophlebitis, blood clots, or migraine headaches is usually a contraindication to the use of oral contraceptives. For women over the age of 35, or for those with other risk factors, such as a history of heavy smoking, gallbladder disease, diabetes, or high blood pressure, use should be weighed carefully against alternative birth-control methods.

Drug interactions Several drug interactions have been suggested but have not been well documented as significant in the majority of cases.

See *Hormonal drugs,* page 87; *Oral contraceptives,* page 96.

Ovral-28

Generic ingredients

> progestogen : norgestrel
> estrogen : ethinyl estradiol

Action and uses An oral contraceptive. Like many birth control pills, Ovral-28 is made up of a combination of two synthetic hormones, an estrogen and a progesterone-like hormone (a progestogen). It is essentially identical to Ovral except that it is packaged with 21 combination pills and seven "dummy" pills, so that a pill is taken every day of the month, but the 21-day cycle and the intervening menstrual bleeding is maintained. This form is sometimes useful for those who tend to get confused. In every other respect it is identical to Ovral, and the description given under that heading applies.

Ovulen-21

Generic ingredients

> progestogen : ethynodiol diacetate
> estrogen : menstranol

Action and uses An oral contraceptive. Like many birth control pills, Ovulen contains a combination of two synthetic sex hormones, an estrogen and a progesterone-like hormone (a progestogen). Like most other oral contraceptives, it acts to prevent conception by affecting the pituitary gland's control of the reproductive cycle, as well as by acting locally on the lining of the uterus and the cervical mucus, and possibly in other ways. When taken regularly it is like all oral contraceptives, a very effective contraceptive drug.

Adult dosage In general, one tablet is taken daily (usually at night) for 21 consecutive days, beginning on the 5th day of menstruation. No tablets are taken on the following 7 days, during which time menstrual bleeding occurs, and on the 8th day they are restarted for another 21-day cycle.

Adverse effects A "patient package insert" is now included with every prescription. This should be read carefully and discussed with the prescribing physician. The information given here represents only a brief summary. As with all oral contraceptives, a variety of side effects may occur, including weight gain, increased appetite, depression or fatigue, breast changes, gas-

263

trointestinal upset, headache, and increased vaginal discharge or infection. More significant but less common side effects include the risk of thrombophlebitis (blood clotting associated with inflammation of the veins of the leg), increased blood pressure, increased blood sugar levels, and gallbladder disease. The risk of certain side effects, for example heart disease and gallbladder disease, appears to increase with age (especially over the age of 35). A woman with a history of true migraine headache may find that her headaches increase while taking oral contraceptives, and she may also run a higher risk (though the risk is still small) of suffering a stroke.

Precautions Before a doctor prescribes oral contraceptives for any woman he should take a careful medical history and perform a thorough physical exam, and discuss alternative methods of contraception with her. A history of thrombophlebitis, blood clots, and migraine headaches is usually a contraindication to the use of oral contraceptives. For women over the age of 35, or for those with other risk factors, such as a history of heavy smoking, gallbladder disease, diabetes, or high blood pressure, use should be weighed carefully against alternative birth-control methods.

Drug interactions Several drug interactions have been suggested but none have been well documented as significant in most cases.

See *Hormonal drugs,* page 87; *Oral contraceptives,* page 96.

Papaverine (generic name). See PAVABID.

Parafon Forte

Generic ingredients

muscle relaxant : chlorzoxazone
pain reliever : acetaminophen

Action and uses Parafon Forte is a combination drug used to treat various types of muscle spasm, most commonly those experienced in back or neck strain. It is a combination of the mild pain reliever acetaminophen (Tylenol, Nebs) with a drug which is believed to act on the spinal cord to inhibit local muscle spasm and thus to relieve discomfort. This "muscle-relaxing" drug, chlorzoxazone, is also used alone as the drug Paraflex.

Adult dosage One or two tablets, three or four times per day, adjusted according to need.

Adverse effects   Occasional gastrointestinal upset or drowsiness and dizziness may occur. Rarely, liver abnormalities have been reported to occur with chlorzoxazone. Some people may also have reddish-purple urine which is not thought to represent a problem.

Precautions   Parafon Forte may cause drowsiness and therefore present a hazard when driving or operating machinery. The drug should be avoided by pregnant or potentially pregnant women and nursing mothers.

Drug interactions   Both ingredients in this combination have been reported to cause liver damage in excessive doses, and it is therefore possible that they could interact to increase this risk.

See   *Non-narcotic pain relievers,* page 42.

Paregoric (camphorated tincture of opium)

Action and uses   A preparation used to treat diarrhea. It contains only a minute amount of morphine (0.04%) but, because of morphine's pronounced constipating effect on the intestinal tract, even this small quantity is enough to make paregoric an effective remedy for simple diarrhea. Paregoric is often combined with kaolin and pectin to enhance its antidiarrheal action. Among the products containing this combination are Parepectolin, Ka-Pek with paregoric, Kaoparin with paregoric, and Dia-Quel. Although paregoric is effective, some authorities feel that prolonged use may lengthen the illness by allowing retention of bacteria or toxins in the bowel.

Adult dosage   Usually one or two teaspoons one to four times per day for no more than two days.

Adverse effects   Side effects of paregoric are few, although people who are allergic to morphine may also be allergic to this drug. One minor side effect, ironically, is constipation, which may result if the paregoric is continued too long after the diarrhea stops.

Precautions   If diarrhea persists for more than two or three days, its cause should be investigated by a doctor. Paregoric should be kept in an amber bottle away from extreme heat and should be thrown away after five years.

Drug dependence   Psychological and/or physical dependence can potentially result if this drug is taken in large doses over an extended period.

Drug interactions   Oversedation might result from mixing paregoric with sedatives, sleeping pills, tranquilizers, or alcohol.

See *Diarrhea,* page 86.

Pavabid

Generic name

papaverine (available by generic name)

Action and uses   This drug is promoted and used for disorders causing decreased circulation to the brain, feet, or hands. Although it relaxes blood vessels (and therefore increases the flow of blood) when injected directly into the vessels in normal persons, there is no clear evidence that when taken orally it can increase blood flow in abnormal states, such as when there is arteriosclerosis (fatty obstruction of the blood vessels), or when a person experiences coldness of the extremities or pain with exercise (intermittent claudication). It is also used in conditions where there is temporary spasm of the arteries, such as Raynaud's phenomenon, but here again its effectiveness is questionable.

Adult dosage   100–150 mg two or three times a day.

Adverse effects   Pavabid is usually well tolerated, but it may cause various gastrointestinal reactions, as well as dizziness (especially when the patient rapidly changes position) and rapid heart rate. Allergic rashes may also occur, and, rarely, liver abnormalities.

Precautions   This drug should not be used immediately after minor or major surgery or childbirth. It should be avoided by pregnant or potentially pregnant women and nursing mothers and also by people with ulcers.

Drug interactions   Pavabid may add to effects of other more effective blood-vessel relaxing drugs, such as nitroglycerin or Apresoline, causing blood pressure to fall.

See *Poor circulation,* page 68.

Penicillin G

Trade names

Pentids, Pfizerpen

Action and uses   One of the most important of all the antibiotics and the prototype for the group of penicillin drugs. It is produced by the bread mold *penicillium* and purified for use in tablets and for injection. Penicillin G acts to prevent formation of the cell walls of bacteria. This prevents them from growing and multiplying. There is no effect on human cells, which have a very different structure. Penicillin G is most effective against the group of bacteria which commonly cause sore throats (*Streptococci,* hence the name "strep throat") and certain abscesses, although some bacteria in abscesses (*Staphylococci,* or "staph") can become resistant to penicillin G, especially in hospitals. Penicillin G is also effective against syphilis and gonorrhea in most cases; these venereal diseases are often treated with long-acting injections of penicillin G (Bicillin). Penicillin G is not so effective for treatment of serious infections caused by the group of bacteria called "Gram-negative bacilli," which cause infections in the urinary tract, bowel, and elsewhere. Penicillin G has no effect on viral or fungal infections.

Adult dosage The dose varies according to the infection. When given by injection, the dose may range from 0.6 or 1.2 million units to 4.8 million units every 4 to 6 hours, depending on the need. If taken orally, penicillin G tends to be destroyed by stomach acid, and food tends to interfere with its entry into the body. Therefore, although it is available for taking orally, penicillin V is more often used.

Adverse effects If taken orally, the most common adverse effect is gastrointestinal upset, cramps, or diarrhea. The primary concern, both when it is given by injection and when it is taken orally, is the occurrence of allergic reactions, which can include skin rashes or hives, swelling of the face or throat, difficulty in breathing, or some time later, joint pains and fever.

Precautions Penicillin G should not be taken when there is known allergy to any of the penicillin drugs. Nursing mothers should check with the physician. Penicillin G, like all antibiotics, should be taken for the full course prescribed (usually 5–10 days) and every dose should be taken even though symptoms may have disappeared. Despite the disappearance of symptoms, not all the bacteria may have been eliminated, and the infection may recur, or resistant strains of bacteria may develop.

Drug interactions In some cases, the effect of penicillin may be decreased if erythromycin or chloramphenicol is also taken.

See *Infections,* page 111.

Penicillin V (generic name). See V-CILLIN K.

Penicillin VK

Generic name

> phenoxymethyl penicillin
> (available by generic name)

Action and uses

A semisynthetic penicillin antibiotic which is almost identical to penicillin G in its action and adverse effects except that, due to a small difference in its chemical structure, it is more effective when taken orally. This is because it is not easily destroyed by stomach acid. See the discussion of PENICILLIN G.

Adult dosage

The usual oral dose is 250–500 mg (equivalent to 0.4–0.8 million units) every six hours on an empty stomach, but this is adjusted for each patient according to the infection.

Pentids (brand name for penicillin G). See PENICILLIN G.

Pentobarbital (generic name). See NEMBUTAL.

Pen-Vee-K

Generic name

> phenoxymethyl penicillin
> (available by generic name)

Action and uses

A semisynthetic penicillin antibiotic which is almost identical to penicillin G in its action and adverse effects except that, due to a small difference in its chemical structure, it is more effective orally. This is because it is not easily destroyed by stomach acid. See the discussion of PENICILLIN G.

Adult dosage

The usual oral dose is 250–500 mg (equivalent to 0.4–0.8 million units) every six hours on an empty stomach, but this is adjusted for each patient according to the infection.

Percodan

Generic ingredients

> narcotic pain reliever : oxycodone
> pain relievers : aspirin, phenacetin
> mild stimulant : caffeine

Action and uses

A strong pain reliever used in the treatment of severe pain. It combines the narcotic analgesic oxycodone, a chemical relative of codeine, with the non-narcotic analgesics aspirin and phenacetin and the mild stimulant caffeine. Oxycodone is slightly stronger than codeine and by itself would be a useful alternative narcotic for moderate to severe pain. Prescriptions for this drug are specially controlled because of the hazard of abuse.

Adult dosage Usually one or two tablets every four to six hours as needed for pain.

Adverse effects The oxycodone in Percodan can, like codeine, cause nausea and constipation and occasional allergic reactions. The aspirin in the preparation can cause stomach irritation and bleeding. The phenacetin can cause kidney damage.

Precautions Percodan should be taken with caution by patients with stomach disorders or impaired kidney function if prolonged use is necessary. Pregnant or potentially pregnant women and nursing mothers should avoid this drug if possible.

Drug dependence Percodan can cause psychological and/or physical dependence or addiction if used for extended periods of time.

Drug interactions Oversedation may result when Percodan is taken concurrently with alcohol, tranquilizers, sedatives, sleeping pills, antidepressants, and antihistamines. The aspirin adds to the effects of oral anticoagulants, increasing the risk of bleeding, and to the effects of cortisone-like drugs, increasing the risk of peptic ulcer.

See *Narcotic pain relievers,* page 41.

Periactin

Generic name

cyproheptadine

Action and uses An antihistamine drug which differs somewhat from other antihistamines in that as well as blocking the effects of histamine, it also blocks another substance in the body called serotonin. It is most commonly used as an antihistamine for treatment of allergic dermatitis and other allergy problems. However, because of its antiserotonin effect it can also be used to treat the diarrhea which occurs in patients who have had their stomachs removed (called the "dumping syndrome") and in patients with a special kind of tumor called carcinoid (a tumor which produces serotonin and causes severe diarrhea and flushing).

Adult dosage The usual dose for treatment of allergic conditions is 4 mg three or four times per day. Somewhat higher doses are sometimes used for treatment of the special kinds of diarrhea mentioned above.

Adverse effects Periactin shares the ability of antihistamines to cause drowsiness in some people, and sometimes other effects such as dry mouth and stomach distress. Unlike other antihistamines, it has been shown to cause weight gain with long-term use in some patients.

Precautions This drug may interfere with driving or operating machinery. It should be avoided by pregnant or potentially pregnant women and nursing mothers.

Drug interactions Periactin is additive to other sedative and tranquilizing drugs, e.g., sleeping pills and alcohol. It is also additive to strong antispasmodic drugs of the kind used to treat stomach problems, e.g., Pro-Banthine and Librax, as well as tricyclic antidepressants, e.g., Elavil

See *Antihistamines,* page 121.

Persantine

Generic name

dipyridamide

Action and uses A drug prescribed for people with coronary artery disease and angina pectoris; its action is to dilate the arteries to increase blood flow to the heart. Although chemically different, it is believed to act in a similar way to nitroglycerin. It is taken orally on a regular basis rather than in response to attacks of pain. Whether it is any more effective than other drugs for angina has long been debated, and this is further complicated by the fact that its effects may not be seen until it has been taken for two to three months.

Adult dosage The usual dose is one or two 25 mg tablets three times daily on an empty stomach.

Adverse effects Certain effects related to the blood vessel-dilating effects may occur elsewhere in the body, e.g., headache, dizziness, flushing and fainting; these effects may be due to excessive dosage. Skin rash and stomach upset have also been reported to occur.

Precautions The drug should be used with caution by people with low blood pressure.

See *Poor circulation,* page 68.

Phenaphen with Codeine

Generic ingredients

> narcotic : codeine
> pain reliever : acetaminophen

Action and uses A popular mild analgesic drug available with or without the additon of codeine, a narcotic analgesic. With codeine it is used to treat more severe pain than can be relieved by simple analgesics such as aspirin or acetaminophen.

Adult dosage One or two tablets every four to six hours as needed for pain.

Adverse effects The major side effects which can occur are due to the codeine, which can cause constipation, occasional nausea and vomiting, and occasionally dizziness. Large doses of acetaminophen can cause serious liver disease.

Precautions Because habitual use is a hazard, the forms containing codeine should be used only when non-narcotic analgesics are not effective.

Drug dependence Prolonged use of codeine may cause dependence.

Drug interactions The effects of codeine can be additive to those of other narcotic drugs as well as to those of other sedating drugs such as tranquilizers or alcohol.

See *Narcotic pain relievers,* page 41.

Phenazopyridine (generic name). See PYRIDIUM.

Phenergan Expectorant

Generic ingredients

> antihistamine : promethazine
> expectorant : potassium guaiacol-sulfonate, sodium citrate,
>   citric acid
> miscellaneous : ipecac, alcohol

Phenergan Expectorant with Codeine

Generic ingredients The same as for Phenergan Expectorant, but with the addition of the narcotic cough-suppressant, codeine.

Phenergan VC Expectorant

Generic ingredients The same as for Phenergan Expectorant, but with the addition of the decongestant, phenylephrine.

Phenergan VC Expectorant with Codeine

Generic ingredients The same as for Phenergan Expectorant, but with the addition of the decongestant, phenylephrine and the narcotic cough-suppressant, codeine.

Action and uses These are mixtures for the relief of upper respiratory symptoms: nasal congestion is relieved by the antihistamine, and in the VC preparations, the decongestant; dried secretions are liquefied and eliminated by the expectorants. They are used for relief of symptoms of colds and some allergies, but not for asthma. Whether these compounds actually have a useful expectorant effect is not known, since it has been difficult to test the expectorant components for their effectiveness. Phenergan VC Expectorant differs from Phenergan Expectorant only in the addition of the decongestant, phenylephrine. Both are available with or without the narcotic cough-suppressant, codeine, which should be used only when cough suppression is really needed.

Adult dosage One or two teaspoons every four to six hours as needed for the relief of symptoms.

Adverse effects Phenergan may occasionally cause drowsiness, and the expectorant may cause nausea in some cases. The codeine preparations may cause constipation and also nausea. The decongestant in the VC preparations may cause palpitations or nervousness, and a lower dose may be required for those with heart disease, high blood pressure, or diabetes. This drug should be avoided by pregnant or potentially pregnant women and nursing mothers.

Precautions If sedation is an effect, then driving or operating machinery can be hazardous. People with high blood pressure should not take Phenergan VC Expectorant.

Drug dependence Although the dose is small, prolonged use of large doses of the codeine-containing compounds can cause habituation.

Drug interactions The sedative effect of Phenergan and codeine can be additive to the effects of alcohol or tranquilizing drugs. The alcohol in the mixture can cause reactions in people taking Antabuse or Flagyl. The decongestant can counteract the effect of drugs used to treat high blood pressure.

See *Coughs and colds,* page 117; *Antihistamines,* page 121.

Phenobarbital

Trade name

Luminal

Action and uses A widely used drug for the treatment of anxiety, seizures (such as epileptic seizures), and insomnia. Phenobarbital is one of the group of drugs known as *barbiturates*. It has been used for many years both as a tranquilizer and to treat seizures. In the last 15 years, with the introduction of newer tranquilizers such as diazepam (Valium) and meprobamate (Miltown, Equanil), its use as a tranquilizer has decreased, but it is still a major anticonvulsant or antiepileptic drug. Sometimes it is used in combination with other anticonvulsant drugs, e.g. Dilantin. Phenobarbital is also incorporated into more than 50 combination products which are used for treating illness ranging from stomach ulcers to asthma, on the questionable assumption that many of these conditions are associated with anxiety.

Adult dosage For treatment of anxiety, usually 15–30 mg, two or three times per day. For sleep, usually 60–100 mg at bedtime. For prevention of seizures, 30–90 mg may be given once daily (since it stays in the body for more than a day).

Adverse effects When phenobarbital is used as a sleeping pill it may cause a "hangover" effect the following morning. It may also cause a feeling of depression and tiredness, or infrequently nausea, vomiting, and diarrhea. Allergic reactions, such as skin rashes, may also occur.

Drug dependence If used for longer than seven to ten days, "tolerance" to phenobarbital may develop, which means that a larger dose will be needed to produce the same tranquilizing effect. If this occurs, dependence on the drug may develop and if it is suddenly discontinued there may be withdrawal symptoms such as anxiety, insomnia, or even seizures (if the dose is large or if a seizure disorder is present). Therefore, it must be stopped gradually if it has been used for a long time.

Precautions Phenobarbital and other barbiturates can, if taken in high doses, be very dangerous, and sometimes fatal. They can be hazardous if taken with alcohol or other tranquilizers. They have long been a major cause of accidental overdose, sometimes resulting in death, and equally they have been used in suicide attempts, again often with fatal results.

Drug interactions Phenobarbital can interact with many other drugs, particu-

273

larly the anticoagulant Coumadin, to decrease its effectiveness and increase the risk of clotting.

Its effect is additive to the effects of other tranquilizers, sleeping pills, and alcohol. The combination with any of these drugs can be very hazardous, causing suppression of breathing and even death.

See   *Sleeping pills,* page 47; *Minor tranquilzers,* page 45; *Seizures (convulsions),* page 130.

Phenoxymethylpencillin (generic name). See
PENICILLIN VK, V-CILLIN K, PEN-VEE-K.

Phentermine resin (generic name). See IONAMIN.

Phenylbutazone (generic name). See BUTAZOLIDIN.

Pilocarpine (generic name). See ISOPTO-CARPINE.

Polaramine

Generic name	dexchlorpheniramine (available by generic name)

Action and uses   A commonly prescribed antihistamine which is frequently used to treat allergic conditions, especially allergic rhinitis, sinusitis, or conjunctivitis (redness of the eye). In common with most other antihistamines it has the effect of blocking the effects of the substance histamine, which is released by the body in response to certain noxious stimuli and causes many of the symptoms of inflammation and allergic reaction. Polaramine can thus reduce itching of the skin caused by allergies, hives, or rashes. Sometimes it can also have a sedating effect, although it is not customarily used for this. It is not useful for the treatment of asthma. It is usually much less expensive when sold under its generic name, or as chlorpheniramine.

Adult dosage   Polaramine is available in oral tablets and liquid forms. The usual oral dose is 2 mg two to four times daily or one 6 mg Repetab, twice daily as needed for treatment of allergic conditions.

Adverse effects   Polaramine may cause significant sedation in some people, although it may be less likely to cause this effect than some other antihistamines. Other side effects are relatively rare, but can include dry mouth, blurred vision, or difficulty in urinating, especially in older people or those with glaucoma or prostate trouble.

Precautions The sedative effects may interfere with driving or operating machinery. This drug should be used with caution by those with glaucoma or prostate trouble. It should also be avoided by pregnant or potentially pregnant women and nursing mothers.

Drug interactions Polaramine is additive to other sedative or tranquilizing drugs and to alcohol. It is also additive to other antispasmodic drugs used to treat ulcers or stomach problems, e.g., Pro-Banthine or Librax, and can cause excessive dry mouth, constipation, and difficulty in urinating if taken in conjunction with these drugs.

See *Antihistamines,* page 121.

Polycillin (brand name for ampicillin). See AMPICILLIN.

Poly-Vi-Flor

Generic ingredients

vitamins : A,D,C,E,B complex, folic acid
mineral : fluoride

Action and uses A fixed-combination vitamin mineral supplement for children. The vitamins are intended to supplement the regular food of infants and children. The fluoride is intended to help prevent dental cavities, but should be taken only where there is no fluoride in the water supply.

Adult dosage One chewable tablet per day.

Adverse effects Both vitamins A and D can cause serious adverse effects if taken in excess. Vitamin A can cause liver and skin abnormalities, and vitamin D, bone abnormalites.

Precautions Poly-Vi-Flor should not be used if the local water supply already contains fluoride. Only the recommended dose should be taken, preferably with a doctor's advice.

Drug interactions No significant interactions occur at the recommended dose.

See *Vitamins and minerals,* page 134.

Potassium Chloride

Trade names

Kaochlor, Kaon-Cl, Kato, Kayciel, KEFF,
K-Lor, Klorvess, K-Lyte/Cl, Kolyum, Pfiklor,
Rum-K, Slow-K

Action and uses   This is a mineral salt that is essential to the body's function and is usually given to replace the body potassium lost from the kidneys. The loss is most often caused by diuretics ("water pills") or cortisone-like drugs, but can also occur in some diseases. Thus a potassium supplement forms a common part of a regimen for high blood pressure or heart failure. Potassium is vital to the body's function, and excessive loss can cause muscle weakness, tiredness, and dizziness, and when severe, can be life-threatening.

  Potassium is present in many foods, especially fruits such as oranges, melons, dried fruits, and vegetables such as tomatoes and potatoes. If the amounts needed are small, they may be replaced by dietary means, or by use of salt substitutes which also contain this mineral, e.g., Lite-Salt. If larger amounts are required, as determined by checking the blood level of potassium, it is necessary to give potassium orally. This has been a major problem since many people find potassium chloride, the only form of potassium which is really effective, very distasteful. It commonly comes, in the much less expensive generic form, as a liquid with or without various flavorings. It also comes in a variety of trade-name preparations, both powders and liquids. Many of these are more palatable, but they are also much more costly, and many contain other forms of potassium, such as potassium citrate, which are not so effective. It is the amount of potassium *chloride* taken which is important. The pill form of potassium chloride, SLOW-K, is discussed under that name.

Adult dosage   This varies with need but is most often 40–80 milli-equivalents per day. It can be taken with juice or food to disguise the taste.

Adverse effects   The most common unwanted effect of potassium is its metallic bitter taste on the tongue. Also common is stomach irritation or nausea, which can be avoided by diluting the mineral (in concentrated form, it is very irritating). Rarely, ulceration of the stomach or bowel can occur if the potassium is concentrated in one area. If excess potassium is used in the presence of kidney failure, serious effects on the heart can occur.

Precautions   Potassium should be used only with special instructions, and if it must be given to people who have severe kidney disease or who are taking potassium-retaining diruretics (see *Diuretics,* p. 63), occasional blood tests should be performed to monitor blood levels of potassium.

Drug interactions If taken in conjunction with potassium-retaining diuretics such as Dyazide, Dyrenium, Aldactone, or Aldactazide, potassium preparations can cause dangerously high levels of potassium in the blood.

See *Vitamins and minerals,* page 134.

Prednisone

Trade names

Deltasone, Meticorten, Orasone

Action and uses Prednisone is one of several drugs referred to as "steroids" or "corticosteroids." Corticosteroids are hormones produced by the cortex (outer part) of the adrenal glands. Drugs with very similar properties to these hormones can also be made by chemical synthesis. Prednisone is one of these "synthetic" steroid hormones and is the one most commonly used. Prednisone is used in a wide variety of disorders in two major ways:

1. It is used to make up for a lack of the normally present corticosteroid hormones (replacement therapy) in cases where, for example, the adrenal glands have been removed or are not functioning due to disease (Addison's disease); in such cases the doses of prednisone are very small.

2. It is used, in much larger doses, to prevent or treat a variety of disorders usually associated with severe inflammation and/or destruction of tissue, such as acute arthritis or serious allergic reactions, as in severe asthma.

Prednisone and related corticosteroids act on many cells in the body to change the production of proteins and the ways in which the cells handle carbohydrates and fats and certain minerals. This promotes several desirable effects when the drug is given in higher doses. First, it acts to suppress inflammation, which can be useful in certain types of arthritis (although it is used as a last resort in this situation); in inflammatory disease of the bowel, such as ulcerative colitis; and in a large variety of skin diseases where there is inflammation of the skin, such as psoriasis or eczema. Second, it acts to suppress certain types of white blood cells and lowers the body's immunity (defenses against infection), which can be useful in the treatment of certain types of "auto-immune" diseases (where the body reacts to its own tissues) such as lupus erythematosus, and certain types of leukemia where there is an overproduction of the white blood cells; it

277

is also useful in preventing the rejection of donor organs after transplant operations. Third, it acts to inhibit allergic reactions in severe allergic conditions, such as asthma, and serious skin allergies, such as poison oak and poison ivy. Prednisone has a variety of other actions for which it is sometimes prescribed, but which, more often, represent undesirable side effects.

Adult dosage The dose is adjusted for each patient according to the condition for which it is prescribed, and can vary greatly; it may be as high as 100 mg or more a day, or as little as 5 mg per day. When first started, it is often taken in high doses, sometimes several times a day but when taken over long periods it is usually taken once daily in the morning or once every other day, depending on the circumstances.

Adverse effects The adverse effects of prednisone are related to both the dose and the length of time the drug is taken. A single dose of any amount of prednisone may usually be taken without significant adverse effects. However, the incidence of serious adverse effects increases considerably with time at any dose greater than the physiological equivalent (approximately 7.5 mg per day). The most common adverse reaction observed in a large series of hospitalized patients on prednisone included disturbances of water and salt balance to produce edema (or water retention) and loss of potassium (which can cause weakness).

Other common side effects include the development of abnormal fat deposits around the face ("moon face"), neck ("buffalo hump"), or abdomen, weight gain, increased bruising, gastrointestinal bleeding and/or upset, mental confusion, and diabetes. Antacids are frequently given to prevent the gastrointestinal problems. A continuing effect is an increased susceptibility to infections and often the masking of the symptoms of these infections. For this reason, people who have a history of (or those who are exposed to) chronic infections such as tuberculosis are observed carefully. With longer use, there is often gradual degeneration of bone and muscle which can cause fractures and muscle weakness, and cataracts may develop. Obviously the use of this drug for long periods requires very careful analysis of benefits versus risks. It has been found that certain, but not all, chronic ailments which require this drug for very long periods can be controlled by giving prednisone every other day. This is desirable whenever possible since it tends to eliminate most of the severe side effects.

Another practical effect of using prednisone relates to the fact that it tends to suppress the normal functioning of the adrenal gland. In stress, the adrenal gland puts out greatly increased amounts of corticosteroid hormones to help the body handle the stress. The absence of this extra reserve can be life threatening. A person on prednisone does not have this reserve, so that if an accident occurs, or surgery is required, higher doses may be needed for a few days.

Precautions Use of prednisone, especially for more than seven days, requires the careful supervision of a physician; the doctor should be notified of any changes which occur, especially after altering the dose or adding any other drug. Persons taking prednisone for long periods should carry a card or wear a bracelet giving this information in case of an emergency.

Drug interactions Prednisone interacts with many diuretics, e.g., hydrochlorothiazide or Lasix, adding to their effects to cause excessive loss of potassium, which can cause weakness. However, since diuretics are often used to treat the edema caused by corticosteroids, this interaction can be anticipated and prevented by supplementing the potassium intake. Since aspirin and several other anti-inflammatory drugs used to treat arthritis, e.g., Motrin, also cause gastric upset and ulcer, they may be additive to this effect of prednisone.

See *Steroids, or cortisone-like drugs,* page 102.

Premarin

Generic name

conjugated estrogen

Action and uses Premarin (the name is a contraction of "pregnant mare's urine") is a mixture of estrogen female hormone compounds similar to those found in the horse's urine. In 1976 it was the second most frequently prescribed drug in the United States. It is usually prescribed to replace deficient estrogen following surgical removal of the ovaries (a natural source of estrogens) or the decreased function of the ovaries which occurs at the menopause. Premarin is also used in some other types of menstrual dysfunction, in the treatment of breast swelling after childbirth, and in the treatment of certain cases of cancer of the prostate in men and cancer of the breast in women.

In the normal woman before the menopause the levels of

estrogens produced by the ovaries fluctuate during the menstrual cycle; along with the other female hormone, progesterone, they control the menstrual cycle. Estrogens also act on and partly maintain the so-called secondary sexual characteristics, including the development of the breasts and the reproductive organs, and to a certain extent, the distribution of body hair and fat. They also are believed to affect the skin, bone metabolism and brain function to some extent, as well as other metabolic functions.

At the onset of the menopause, the amount of estrogen produced by the ovaries decreases—rapidly in some women, more slowly in others. A certain proportion of women experience various symptoms during this time, including hot flashes, menstrual irregularity, irritability or anxiety, and sleep disorders. Similar symptoms may be experienced by those who have had their ovaries surgically removed.

Although the cause of these symptoms is not known to be directly due to a lack of estrogen, it has been shown that estrogens can partly relieve these symptoms.

Premarin and other similar estrogen-mixture compounds such as Formatrix, Conestron, Evex, Follestrol, Menotabs, and SK-Estrogens, are primarily prescribed to replace the deficient estrogens. There is some controversy over whether these mixtures or single estrogen compounds such as ethinyl estradiol are more likely to simulate the body's normal estrogens, but at present this has not been resolved.

The most widely publicized controversy over Premarin and the other estrogens given for menopausal symptoms relates to a possible link with an increased incidence of cancer of the uterus. This has been hotly argued but at the present the information does seem to suggest a somewhat greater risk. The arguments in favor of the use of estrogens include an improved quality of life (i.e., relief of menopausal symptoms) and prevention of fractures (which occur due to bone degeneration or osteoporosis in a certain proportion of women after the menopause).

At present, the controversy continues, but there is now a general tendency to use Premarin and related drugs more selectively—for treatment of specific symptoms when required—and with general withdrawal except when needed to prevent osteoporosis. One of the more distressing symptoms of the menopause is a reduction of glandular secretions in the vaginal area, which can result in painful intercourse due to drying of the mucous membranes in the vagina. The isolated problem is often treated locally with Premarin vaginal cream or another estrogen cream.

Adult dosage The dose varies considerably according to use. For menopausal symptoms, 0.3 to 1.25 mg per day is usually given on a cyclic basis, with 20–23 days on and 7–10 days off the drug each month. The vaginal cream is applied nightly or several times per week.

Adverse effects A variety of side effects may occur, including nausea or upper gastrointestinal distress, vaginal bleeding or "spotting," breast enlargement, weight changes, edema or swelling, headaches and mood changes.

Precautions The indications, benefits, and risks of the use of this and related drugs should be discussed thoroughly with the prescribing physician. People with a history of thrombophlebitis (blood clotting associated with inflammation of the veins of the legs), blood clots in the legs or lungs, breast or uterine cancer, or liver disease may be unable to use estrogens.

Drug interactions At present, although several theoretical interactions with other drugs have been suggested, clearcut instances have not been established.

See *Estrogen and progestogen therapy,* page 99.

Principen (brand name for ampicillin). See AMPICILLIN.

Pro-Banthine

Generic name

propantheline bromide (available by generic name)

Action and uses A drug used to treat ulcers of the stomach and symptoms of gastrointestinal spasm. Pro-Banthine reduces the movement of the muscles of the stomach and intestines and also helps reduce the secretion of stomach acid. It is often used in combination with other drugs, particularly antacids, to treat ulcers. It is sometimes used in the treatment of urinary dysfunction.

Adult dosage Usually 15 mg just before meals and two 15 mg tablets at bedtime. Pro-Banthine is available in 7.5 mg and 15 mg tablets.

Adverse effects Pro-Banthine reduces the secretion of acid in the stomach, but also affects secretions elsewhere in the body, as in the salivary glands and bronchial tubes. Consequently it may cause dryness of the mouth and drying of bronchial secretions. Other side effects include blurred vision, drowsiness, and difficulty in urinating.

Precautions Pro-Banthine should be used with caution by people with prostate trouble, hiatus hernia, glaucoma, or chronic lung disease.

Drug interactions When used with antacids, Pro-Banthine may cause constipation, and its side effects are additive to the similar side effects of antihistamines, cough/cold medicines, and tricyclic antidepressants.

See *Nausea, stomach upset, and ulcers,* page 75.

Procainamide (generic name). See PRONESTYL.

Proloid

Generic name

thyroglobulin (available by generic name)

Action and uses A purified extract of animal thyroid given as "replacement therapy" to people with a deficiency of thyroid hormone. Thyroid hormones help to regulate many of the body's functions, especially the metabolism, including the rate at which cells use oxygen. In certain diseases of the thyroid such as myxedema (hypothyroidism) and simple goiter, the hormone levels may be reduced and hormones obtained from animals, such as Proloid, can be used to make up for the lack. In most cases today, however, the pure hormones, e.g.,Synthroid, are used in preference to animal extracts. Proloid, like other thyroid preparations, has no place in weight control therapy.

Adult dosage The dosage must be adjusted according to the individual patient's requirements. Proloid is produced in seven different strengths: 16 mg, 32 mg, 65 mg, 100 mg, 130 mg, 200 mg, and 325 mg. Laboratory tests are usually necessary to determine the correct dose.

Adverse effects If too high a dose of Proloid is given, symptoms of overdose will occur. These include nervousness, sweating, irregular and rapid heartbeat, chest pains (angina), and irregular menstruation.

Precautions The required dose of Proloid may vary, so regular checks of thyroid function may be needed. Careful regulation of the dose is also important if high blood pressure or heart disease is also present.

Drug interactions	When taken with thyroid drugs, certain tricyclic anti-depressant drugs (e.g.,Elavil) and decongestants or drugs for asthma can increase the likelihood of palpitations, rapid heart rate, and elevation of the blood pressure.
See	*Thyroid disorders,* page 89.

Promethazine (generic name). See PHENERGAN.

Pronestyl

Generic name	procainamide (available by generic name)
Action and uses	A drug used to regulate abnormal heart rhythm and secondarily to increase the heart's efficiency. Pronestyl can decrease the number of extra heartbeats, and is sometimes also able to convert an irregular heart rhythm to a regular one and maintain it. It is usually administered orally, except in emergencies, when it may be injected.
Adult dosage	Usually carefully adjusted to suit each individual according to body weight, the specific type of abnormal heart rhythm, and the patient's response to therapy. Per day, the suggested dosage is in the range of 50 mg per kilogram of body weight, given in divided doses at 3–4 hour intervals (usually 300–400 mg every 3–4 hours).
Adverse effects	Large doses may cause loss of appetite, nausea, vomiting, diarrhea, mental confusion, or hallucinations. These effects can sometimes be prevented by measuring blood levels of the drug and adjusting the dose accordingly. Use may result in a disorder called *lupus erythematosus* which is characterized by chills and fever, by pains in the joints, chest, or abdomen, and by facial rash; if it develops, the drug must be stopped. Any of these symptoms should be reported to the doctor promptly.
Precautions	People allergic to Novocain (procaine), the local anesthetic frequently used by dentists, are often allergic to this drug. Pronestyl should be monitored carefully in patients with impaired kidney function and myasthenia gravis.
Drug interactions	Pronestyl can be additive to the blood-pressure-lowering effects of antihypertensive drugs. The diuretic Diamox, used for glaucoma, can increase the amount of Pronestyl in the blood and the dose may have to be reduced.
See	*Abnormal heart rhythm,* page 67.

Propantheline (generic name). See PRO-BANTHINE.

Propoxyphene (generic name). See DARVON.

Provera

Generic name

> medroxyprogesterone acetate

Action and uses A female hormone used to treat irregular menstrual cycles and so called "functional" uterine bleeding. It is also used to relieve painful menstruation and occasionally to relieve the tension which frequently occurs before menstruation (premenstrual tension). Provera is a progestogen—a synthetic version of progesterone, which is normally produced by the female ovary and by the placenta during pregnancy. Provera and other related progesterone drugs are also used in the treatment of certain types of severe chronic lung disease.

Adult dosage The dose varies according to the condition it is used to treat. Usually 5–10 mg per day for five to ten days beginning between the 16th to the 21st days of the menstrual cycle. Provera should never be taken without the advice and supervision of a physician.

Adverse effects The progesterone hormones are believed to have fewer serious side effects than the estrogens. They can, however, cause various menstrual abnormalities (e.g.,"breakthrough bleeding," or "spotting"), fluid retention, weight changes, skin changes, and depression. Liver damage has also occurred in some rare cases.

Precautions Provera should not be used by pregnant or potentially pregnant women and nursing mothers, and should not be taken by women with serious liver disease or who have (or have had) cancer of the breast, cervix, uterus, or ovary. It should be taken with caution by those who have had blood clots in the legs or elsewhere.

Drug interactions Since progestogens such as Provera are seldom used alone or for long periods, drug interactions have not been identified as yet.

See *Estrogens and progestogen therapy,* page 99.

Pseudoephedrine (generic name). See SUDAFED.

Pyridium

Generic name

> phenazopyridine hydrochloride
> (available by generic name)

Action and uses A drug used to relieve bladder pain caused by infection, injury, or surgery of the bladder. It acts to anesthetize the bladder. Although at one time it was thought that Pyridium killed the bacteria which caused bladder infections, it is now known that it only relieves pain. When taken by mouth it is absorbed into the blood and goes through the kidneys and into the bladder, where it has its effect. It is then excreted in the urine.

Adult dosage Usually 200 mg three times per day after meals, only when bladder pain is present.

Adverse effects The most noticeable side effect of Pyridium is that it turns the urine a reddish-orange color. This may stain the underwear, but is otherwise harmless; the urine returns to normal when the drug is stopped. In patients with kidney disease the drug may collect in the blood and give a yellowish tinge to the eyes and skin. Pyridium can occasionally upset the stomach, or cause allergic reactions.

Precautions Pyridium should not be taken by patients with severe kidney disease. Pregnant or potentially pregnant women and nursing mothers should ask the physician's advice.

Drug interactions Pyridium can interfere with many urine and blood tests. These should not be done while the drug is being taken.

See *Infections,* page 111.

Quibron

Generic ingredients

> bronchodilator : theophylline
> expectorant : glyceryl guaiacolate

Action and uses A combination drug used for the treatment of asthma. It contains the bronchodilator theophylline in combination with the expectorant glyceryl guaiacolate. Theophylline is one of the most effective and useful bronchodilator drugs available, if taken in appropriate doses. It is often prescribed generically by itself and is generally less expensive in this form. The expectorant's usefulness in this preparation is not known, since although theoretically it would be useful to liquefy and mobilize secretions in the asthmatic, tests to demonstrate that expectorants have this effect have not been conclusive.

Adult dosage One or two capsules every six to eight hours. Since the amount of theophylline needed to produce a bronchodilator effect varies considerably from person to person, the dose is usually adjusted according to clinical relief of symptoms, testing of lung function and/or blood levels of theophylline.

Adverse effects If theophylline levels become high, nausea or stomach upset may occur. Less commonly, headaches, palpitations, muscle cramps, or jitteriness can be seen, but almost all of these will disappear with lower doses.

Precautions Quibron may be additive to the effects of certain over-the-counter drugs used to treat asthma, as well as other drugs given for asthma, so that the prescribing physician should be made aware of all drugs being used.

Drug interactions Both components may affect the clotting system and interact with blood-thinning drugs such as Coumadin or heparin. As noted above, Quibron can be additive to other drugs used for treatment of asthma.

See *Asthma and lung disease,* page 109.

Quinidine Sulfate

Trade names

Quinidex, Quinora

Action and uses A drug commonly used to control abnormal or irregular heart rhythms which result in ineffective pumping of the heart and inadequate circulation of blood. The major use of quinidine sulfate, which comes from cinchona bark, is to suppress abnormal and irregular heart rhythms. It is a dangerous drug which should be used only under strict medical supervision. It may eventually be replaced by other drugs since it is not always effective, and it is relatively costly since it must be obtained from tropical countries.

Adult dosage Usually 100–400 mg every two or three hours with careful monitoring. After a normal heart rhythm is restored the usual dosage is 100–200 mg, three or four times per day. It is given by mouth or, rarely, by injection.

Adverse effects Side effects to this drug are unpredictable and they appear in some individuals but not in others. They may include dizziness, nausea, vomiting, diarrhea and breathing problems.

Some common allergies can occur. (If so, a person will also be sensitive to quinine.) Taken in excess amounts, quinidine sulfate may accumulate in the body and cause a condition known as *cinchonism*, symptoms of which include disturbances in hearing (ringing in the ears), changes in vision, stomach upset, skin rashes, local swelling, headache, fever and confusion.

Precautions Quinidine should be used with caution by people with a history of heart block and should be avoided by pregnant or potentially pregnant women.

Drug interactions When sodium bicarbonate or certain antacids are used on a regular basis, the dose of quinidine required may be lower; the same is true of the drug Diamox. Quinidine may add to the effects of the anticlotting drug Coumadin and increase the risk of bleeding.

See *Abnormal heart rhythm,* page 67.

Regroton

Generic ingredients

antihypertensive : reserpine
diuretic : chlorthalidone

Action and uses A fixed-combination drug used to treat high blood pressure. Regroton incorporates two different drugs, each of which has a lowering effect on the blood pressure. Reserpine acts on the nervous system to block nerves causing constriction of blood vessels, and chlorthalidone causes loss of salt and water and also dilates the blood vessels. The actions of the drugs together are additive. Although this combination allows the use of smaller doses of each drug, thereby reducing the possibility of adverse side effects which occur with higher doses, it does not allow an individual drug regimen to be established by adjusting the dose of each ingredient, nor does it allow the doctor to identify which ingredient is causing any side effects that occur.

Adult dosage Usually one tablet daily.

Adverse effects Regroton can cause adverse effects related to either of its components. Reserpine can cause depression, nasal stuffiness, stomach upset, and a drop in blood pressure on changing posture (for example, standing up too quickly). Chlorthalidone can cause excessive loss of potassium, especially when taken daily. If this occurs potassium can be replaced either in the diet (extra orange juice, tomato juice, dried fruit, or bananas) or with liquid potassium chloride (KCl). Regroton also tends to cause increased levels of sugar in the blood in those predisposed to diabetes and may increase blood levels of uric acid (the substance which can cause gout). If used to excess, the diuretic can cause dehydration and may effect kidney function and the amount of waste products in the blood. Chlorthalidone may also cause allergic rashes.

Precautions Regroton should be used with caution by patients with gout, diabetes, depression, or peptic ulcers. It should be avoided if possible by pregnant or potentially pregnant women. Women taking this drug for long periods should have regular breast examinations; this is because of a possible link between long-term use of reserpine and breast cancer, though this finding is controversial.

Drug interactions Drugs for weight loss, asthma, colds, depression, and heart conditions may counteract the effect of Regroton to increase the blood pressure, and they should be taken together only under the supervision of the physician who prescribed the Regroton. Alcohol and other sedative drugs may also have enhanced effects when taken with Regroton. The chlorthalidone in Regroton can cause excess potassium loss, which can increase sensitivity to toxic effects of digoxin, and also add to the similar effects of steroids such as prednisone.

See *High blood pressure,* page 58; *Diuretics,* page 63.

Reserpine

Trade names

Sandril, Serpasil

Action and uses A commonly used antihypertensive drug which blocks the nerves causing constriction of arterial blood vessels. Formerly used in mental patients, its effectiveness in relieving high blood pressure has made it one of the more widely used drugs. Very often, it is given in various combinations such as Ser-Ap-Es, Regroton, or Diupres. Because of the controversial finding of a possible association between long-term use of reserpine and the development of breast cancer, plus the availability of new drugs such as Inderal, its use has declined. However, since it must be taken only once daily, this fact has tended to maintain it as a popular preparation.

Adult dosage 0.125–0.25 mg daily.

Adverse effects A significant number of people do experience side effects, some dose-related. The drug may have a sedating effect. A stuffy nose, gastric upset (or even ulcer) and other gastrointestinal symptoms may occur. Depression or unusual feelings or dreams can be a problem, especially in people who have a history of such symptoms. Sexual function may be altered.

Precautions This drug should be used with caution by people with a history of peptic ulcer, severe allergic sinusitis, or depression. Women taking this drug for long periods should have regular breast examinations.

Drug interactions The decongestants in nasal sprays, cough/cold medicines and drugs for asthma can counteract the blood-pressure-lowering effect. The sedating effects, if present, can be additive to those of tranquilizers and alcohol.

See *High blood pressure,* page 58.

Ritalin

Generic name

> methylphenidate

Action and uses A stimulant drug which is, at present, most commonly used in the treatment of hyperkinetic children, and although it is effective, its use is quite controversial. It is also used on occasion in the treatment of mild depression although its effectiveness for this has not been clearly established. It has also been used, though rarely, as a drug to help reduce appetite and promote weight loss. It is quite similar in its effects to the amphetamine drugs, and since it has been used as a substitute for them by drug abusers, it requires special prescriptions similar to those for narcotic drugs.

Adult dosage For adults, 10 mg are taken one to three times daily. Dosage in children differs and varies. Other sources should be consulted.

Adverse effects Nervousness, decreased appetite, and difficulty in sleeping are the most common side effects, although dizziness, palpitations, increased blood pressure, headache, and stomach upset may also occur. Prolonged use can cause weight loss and habituation, so that discontinuing the drug can cause withdrawal symptoms such as depression.

Precautions This drug should not be used by people with anxiety or nervousness, high blood pressure or any type of heart disease, epilepsy, or problems with drug or alcohol abuse.

Drug dependence   Prolonged use of Ritalin may result in dependence.

Drug interactions   Ritalin can counteract the effects of antihypertensive drugs to increase the likelihood of side effects. When used with decongestants and nasal sprays, it can add to their effects. It also counteracts the effect of anticonvulsant drugs such as Dilantin.

See   *Antidepressants and lithium,* page 52.

Salutensin

Generic ingredients

> diuretic : hydroflumethiazide
> antihypertensive : reserpine

Action and uses   Salutensin is a combination product used to treat mild to moderate high blood pressure. It combines a thiazide-type diuretic, hydroflumethiazide, which causes a dilation of blood vessels and the loss of excess salt and water, with reserpine, a drug which helps block the sympathetic nerves (which cause constriction of the arterial walls). Hydroflumethiazide is similar to many other thiazide diuretics, e.g., hydrochlorothiazide, Esidrix, and Diuril. Ideally, this combination should be prescribed for a particular patient only after it is determined that both ingredients are really needed to control blood pressure.

Adult dosage   One tablet once or twice daily.

Adverse effects   Side effects due to either ingredient may develop, and this makes use of the combination more problematic. The hydroflumethiazide can cause excess potassium loss in some people, resulting in weakness, lethargy, or dizziness. It can also elevate the level of sugar in the blood in people predisposed to diabetes and elevate the blood levels of uric acid and predispose to gout. In some, reserpine can cause depression or anxiety, peptic ulcer and nasal stuffiness, and occasionally dizziness associated with rapid postural changes.

Precautions   Use of this drug by people with a history of depression or peptic ulcer should be under careful medical supervision. Many cough/cold medicines or nasal sprays should be avoided. It should be avoided if possible by pregnant or potentially pregnant women. Women taking this drug for long periods should have regular breast examinations; this is because of a possible link between long-term use of reserpine and breast cancer, though this finding is controversial.

Drug interactions The potassium loss caused by the diuretic may increase sensitivity to the toxic effects of digoxin if the two drugs are used together. Further, since the diuretic component causes high calcium retention, the taking of calcium supplements, vitamin D and antacids containing calcium together with Salutensin can cause excessively high levels of calcium in the blood. Use of many anti-allergy, asthma, or cough/cold medicines, or of nasal sprays containing phenylephrine, ephedrine, or phenylpropanolamine may raise the blood pressure and counteract the effect of this drug. The blood-pressure-lowering effect of Salutensin can be additive to the effects of other antihypertensive drugs (e.g., Inderal) and also to general anesthetics, to cause excessively low blood pressure.

See *High blood pressure,* page 58; *Diuretics,* page 63.

Septra
Septra-DS

Generic ingredients

antibacterials : sulfamethoxazole, trimethoprim

Action and uses A fixed-combination drug used to treat infections of the urinary tract. It is the same drug as Bactrim, another trade name. Septra combines a sulfa drug, which is particularly effective against the bacteria that commonly affect the bladder and kidney, with a chemical antibacterial drug that acts against the same bacteria. Together the two drugs are more effective than either one alone, since each inhibits a separate enzyme in the bacteria; this also decreases the likelihood of resistance developing. This combination is also finding use in certain other diseases, such as typhoid fever.

Adult dosage Usually one double-strength (DS) tablet, or two ordinary tablets, or four teaspoonfuls of liquid, every 12 hours, for 10 to 14 days. It may be used for longer periods in chronic urinary tract infections.

Adverse effects This drug may sometimes cause nausea, vomiting or other gastrointestinal symptoms, and also headaches or dizziness. Like all sulfa drugs, Septra may cause allergic reactions ranging from rashes to very serious, life-threatening reactions with fever, severe rash, and kidney failure. Abnormalities of the blood cells may also occur.

Precautions It is important always to drink plenty of water while taking this drug to prevent the formation of crystals in the kidneys.

291

If any fever, nausea, or rash occurs after starting the drug, it should be discontinued and the doctor notified. It should be avoided by people with a history of allergy to sulfa drugs and by those with severe kidney disease or G6PD deficiency (a congenital enzyme deficiency). As in the treatment of all infections, it is important to take the drug for the full time recommended to prevent recurrence of the infection.

Drug interactions As with many sulfa drugs, Septra may increase the effect of oral antidiabetic drugs (to cause low blood sugar), and of Dilantin, Butazolidin, and phenobarbital to increase the likelihood of toxicity of these drugs.

See *Infections,* page 111.

Ser-Ap-Es

Generic ingredients

antihypertensive : reserpine
diuretic : hydrochlorothiazide
vasodilator : hydralazine

Action and uses A fixed-combination drug used to treat high blood pressure. Ser-Ap-Es incorporates three different drugs, each of which has a lowering effect on the blood pressure. Reserpine acts on the nervous system to block nerves causing constriction of blood vessels, hydrochlorothiazide causes loss of salt and water and also dilates the blood vessels, and hydralazine dilates the blood vessels. The actions of the drugs together are additive. Although this combination allows the use of smaller doses of each drug, thereby reducing the possibility of adverse side effects which occur with higher doses, it does not allow an individual drug regimen to be established by adjusting the dose of each ingredient, nor does it allow the doctor to identify which ingredient is causing any side effects that occur.

Adult dosage It is seldom that a multiple of the dose of all three components of Ser-Ap-Es in fact approximates the best dose of each drug for controlling blood pressure and minimizing side effects in a particular patient. The usual dosage is one or two tablets twice a day but this must be carefully determined for each individual patient.

Adverse effects Ser-Ap-Es can cause side effects related to any of its three components. Reserpine can cause depression, nasal stuffiness, stomach upset, and a drop in blood pressure on changing posture (for example, standing up too quickly). The side effects of hydrochlorothiazide are not usually prominent due to the relatively low dose; and the side effects of hydralazine are usually suppressed by the action of the reserpine component, although allergic rashes to either hydralazine or reserpine may occur.

Precautions Ser-Ap-Es should be used with caution by patients with gout or diabetes, depression or peptic ulcers. It should be avoided if possible by pregnant or potentially pregnant women. Women taking this drug for long periods should have regular breast examinations; this is because of a possible link between long-term use of reserpine and breast cancer, though this finding is controversial.

Drug interactions Drugs for weight loss, asthma, colds, depression, and heart conditions may interact with Ser-Ap-Es to increase the blood pressure and they should be taken together only under the supervision of the physician who prescribed the Ser-Ap-Es. Alcohol and other sedative drugs may also have enhanced effects when taken with Ser-Ap-Es. The thiazide diuretic may increase loss of potassium, and this is additive to the effects of steroids such as prednisone; excessive loss of potassium can also increase sensitivity to the toxic effects of digoxin.

See *High blood pressure,* page 58; *Diuretics,* page 63.

Serax

Generic name

oxazepam

Action and uses A minor tranquilizer used in the treatment of mild to severe anxiety and sometimes to relieve the symptoms of alcohol withdrawal. Serax is chemically similar to the tranquilizers Valium, Librium, and Tranxene, but it may, in some cases, be preferable to them because it does not share their tendency to accumulate in the body.

Adult dosage The usual dose of Serax ranges from 10–15 mg two to four times per day, to 15–30 mg three or four times per day. For those who experience anxiety only intermittently, one daily dose may be sufficient.

Adverse effects On the whole, Serax is a fairly safe tranquilizer. Its side effects may include sleepiness, lethargy, dizziness, fatigue, depression, irritability, headache, or nausea. These effects can sometimes be eliminated by lowering the dose. Sometimes there are other side effects, such as allergic skin reactions, but these are unusual.

Precautions Because of the possible connection between similar drugs and birth defects, the package insert for Serax warns against its use by pregnant or potentially pregnant women. It may interfere with driving or operating machinery.

Drug dependence Psychological and/or physical dependence are possible with extended use of this drug.

Drug interactions The sedative effects of Serax can be increased by alcohol, sleeping pills, other tranquilizers, antidepressants, and antihistamines.

See *Minor tranquilizers,* page 45.

Sinequan

Generic name

doxepin

Action and uses A commonly prescribed antidepressant drug. Like Elavil and Tofranil, it belongs to a group of closely related drugs called *tricyclic antidepressants* and is used to treat certain types of moderately severe and long-standing depression. The tricyclic antidepressants are not true tranquilizers, although they can cause some sedation. The antidepressant effect of Sinequan may take days or weeks to appear, although temporary sedative and other side effects occur immediately.

Adult dosage The effective dose of Sinequan must be adjusted for each individual patient, and the process of establishing the best dose may take one or two months. Initially the dose is usually 25–75 mg per day and may be increased to 150 mg per day. (The dose may be lower for elderly patients.) Because the drug is long-acting and may cause some sedation, it is usually taken just once a day, at bedtime.

Adverse effects Initially, Sinequan may cause dry mouth, blurred vision, drowsiness, constipation, and difficulty in urinating. These effects are particularly marked in older people, but they tend to disappear in 3–4 weeks. Other significant side effects may include effects on the heart rhythm, and sometimes confusion or dizziness.

Precautions Sinequan should be taken with caution by people with glaucoma, prostate gland problems, liver or heart disease, epilepsy, or hyperthyroid conditions. It should not be taken by pregnant or potentially pregnant women or nursing mothers. The drowsiness may interfere with driving or operating machinery.

Drug interactions Sinequan can cause oversedation when taken in combination with alcohol, sleeping pills, tranquilizers, antihistamines, and drugs containing narcotics. It can add to the side effects of antispasmodic drugs and decrease the effects of drugs to lower blood pressure such as Ismelin. It can dangerously interfere with drugs to regulate heart rhythm, thyroid drugs, and drugs of the MAO inhibitor family (such as Marplan, Parnate and Nardil). Taken with drugs of the latter type or with the sedative Placidyl, Sinequan can cause delirium.

See *Antidepressants and lithium,* page 52.

Slow-K

Generic name

potassium chloride (available by generic name)

Action and uses A special preparation of potassium chloride (KCl) used to replace potassium in cases of potassium loss. Slow-K is usually prescribed for patients who eliminate too much potassium because they are taking a diuretic ("water pill") for high blood pressure or some other reason. The active chemical ingredient, potassium chloride, is contained in a wax matrix to keep it from being released into the system too quickly. This is believed to prevent ulceration of the stomach and intestines, which can occur if potassium is released too quickly. Whether this actually works has been questioned. There is still a risk of ulceration, and this, added to the cost of Slow-K and the many pills required each day make it doubtful that this form of potassium is better than liquid KCl or powder preparations.

Adult dosage The dose varies from person to person and must be determined by the physician. The usual dose is 5 tablets (40 milliequivalents) to 10 tablets a day; the relatively high number of tablets that must be taken is a disadvantage of taking this preparation.

Adverse effects Slow-K can produce severe ulceration of the stomach and intestines if there is any obstruction to its movement through the system. Because it is specially designed to be released slowly, however, this is not a common problem. It may also cause nausea, vomiting, intestinal cramps, and diarrhea.

Precautions This drug should not be used by people with severe kidney disease, severe diabetes, and water deprivation, except under careful medical supervision.

Drug interactions Slow-K should not be used in conjunction with drugs which retain potassium, such as spironolactone (Aldactone, Aldactazide) or triamterene (Dyazide, Dyrenium).

See *High blood pressure,* page 58; *Diuretics,* page 63; *Vitamins and minerals,* page 134.

Sorbitrate

Generic name

> isosorbide dinitrate
> (available by generic name)

Action and uses A drug which is used to relieve the pain of angina pectoris, a heart condition characterized by pain (usually brought on by exercise, exertion, or emotion) in the chest or arm. The pain is caused by an inadequate supply of oxygen to the heart; the heart receives oxygen from the blood carried to it by the *coronary arteries.* Sorbitrate acts in two ways: to open up the coronary arteries, which are often partially obstructed, and to dilate peripheral blood vessels, thereby reducing the amount of work the heart must do.

Sorbitrate is also used sometimes to treat conditions where blood circulation is poor, such as Raynaud's disease, and in certain other heart failure conditions.

Adult dosage For acute attacks the usual dosage is 2.5 to 10 mg; the tablets are placed under the tongue and allowed to dissolve. The tablets each contain either 2.5 mg or 5 mg. For regular use tablets containing 5 mg, 10 mg, or 20 mg are *swallowed* to reduce the frequency of angina attacks. For this purpose the usual dosage is 5–30 mg taken four times per day by swallowing. Long-acting tablets and long-acting capsules called Tembrids, containing 40 mg isosorbide dinitrate, are also available. These should be taken every 6 to 12 hours.

Adverse effects Flushing is very common and is due to increased blood flow to the skin. Throbbing headache often occurs and is also associated with changes in blood flow. A feeling of faintness or dizziness can occur (particularly in hot weather), more commonly in people with high blood pressure.

296

Precautions	If more than two or three tablets do not relieve the pain, the doctor should be notified at once.
Drug interactions	Excessive alcohol intake tends to dilate blood vessels and increase the action of isosorbide, as do certain antihypertensive drugs, e.g. Apresoline.
See	*Poor circulation,* page 68; *Angina pectoris,* page 71.

Stelazine

| Generic name | trifluoperazine |

Action and uses	One of a large family of drugs known as *phenothiazines.* Stelazine is a major tranquilizer, or "antipsychotic" drug, used primarily in the treatment of serious psychological disorders. Though not capable of curing the underlying illness, Stelazine and the other drugs in this group do relieve the severe thought disorders (such as disorientation, delusions, and hallucinations) that characterize schizophrenia and manic-depressive psychoses, severe alcohol withdrawal, some cases of senility, some neurological diseases, and the effects of certain drugs such as LSD and amphetamines.
Adult dosage	For the treatment of thought disorders the initial dose may range from 2 mg to 15 mg per day, but may eventually go as high as 50 mg or more per day in some cases. The dose is likely to vary greatly according to the needs of each patient, because sensitivity to the drug varies widely from person to person. Generally speaking, however, the dose tends to be lower for older people and, whatever the patient's age, it may usually be taken just once a day and occasionally omitted on weekends.
Adverse effects	Stelazine may produce a number of significant side effects and can occasionally cause some serious drug reactions. Its use, therefore, must be carefully supervised. Unlike the other phenothiazine drugs such as Thorazine, Stelazine causes only mild sedation and seldom causes a significant fall in the blood pressure. It has a greater tendency, however, to produce tremors and restlessness—called "Parkinsonian" side effects due to their similarity to the symptoms of Parkinson's disease. These effects can usually be reduced by taking an anti-Parkinsonian drug such as Cogentin. Stelazine can cause jaundice, skin rash, or a fall in the white blood cell count (which increases the patient's vulnerability to infection) and

if so the drug must be discontinued. These side effects and adverse reactions are not common. A serious side effect, called "tardive dyskinesia" which is characterized by uncontrollable movements of the tongue and lips, occasionally occurs after the drug is discontinued.

Precautions Prolonged use of Stelazine requires regular medical evaluation at intervals.

Drug interactions Oversedation is possible when Stelazine is taken in combination with alcohol, other sedatives and tranquilizers, sleeping pills, antidepressants, antihistamines, and drugs containing narcotics. Stelazine can counteract the blood pressure-lowering effect of the antihypertensive drugs Ismelin and Aldomet.

See *Major tranquilizers,* page 49.

Sudafed

Generic name

> pseudoephedrine (available by generic name)

Action and uses Sudafed is a very popular, commonly prescribed decongestant used in the treatment of various allergic conditions such as allergic sinusitis or blocked Eustachian tubes (stuffy ears), as well as for the relief of similar symptoms associated with a cold. It is occasionally used in the treatment of asthmatic symptoms. Prolonged or continued use may result in decreased effectiveness.

Adult dosage 30–60 mg orally three or four times per day.

Adverse effects Occasionally some stimulation, insomnia, or jitteriness may be noted, and drowsiness or headache may also occur.

Precautions People who are taking medication for high blood pressure or heart trouble should take Sudafed only after consultation with a physician. Some people may experience pounding of the heart (palpitations).

Drug interactions Sudafed can interact with drugs used to treat high blood pressure and counteract their effects. It is also similar, and therefore additive, to ingredients in nasal sprays and in certain drugs given for asthma; you should check with your physician before using Sudafed in combination with such products.

See *Coughs and colds,* page 117.

Sulfamethoxazole (generic name). See GANTANOL.

Sulfisoxazole (generic name). See GANTRISIN.

Sultrin Triple Sulfa Cream & Suppositories

Generic ingredients

> sulfa antibacterials : sulfatriazole,
> sulfacetamide,
> sulfabenzamide

Action and uses Sultrin triple sulfa preparations are used to treat vaginal infections not due to yeast or to the protozoan *Trichomonas*. Although the effectiveness of these sulfa vaginal creams has been generally debated, it has been conceded that they are probably effective for certain types of infection. Because of the diversity of vaginal infections, the effectiveness of such preparations (see also AVC CREAM) has been difficult to prove.

Adult dosage One application of cream or one suppository once or twice daily for seven to ten days, or through one menstrual cycle, as directed.

Adverse effects Local sensitivity or burning may occur, and sensitivity to the sulfonamide may occur locally or throughout the body. If so, the drug should be discontinued.

Precautions This preparation should not be used by women who are allergic to sulfonamide drugs. Safety in pregnancy and during nursing has not been established.

Drug interactions Drug interactions are unlikely to occur with the local preparation.

See *Skin and local disorders,* page 125.

Sumycin (brand name for tetracycline). See
TETRACYCLINE.

Synalar Cream and Ointment

Generic name

> fluocinolone

Action and uses A commonly prescribed preparation of a synthetic corticosteroid (cortisone-like drug) for topical (local) application to the skin. It is used primarily for its anti-inflammatory effects in the treatment of many types of skin disorder, e.g.,psoriasis, certain types of neurodermatitis (inflammation of the skin associated with emotional factors) and a variety of other conditions where there is no infection. In many cases, the effects are dramatic. Because it retards formation of scar tissue, it can also prevent scarring.

Adult dosage The preparation is applied sparingly two or three times daily. It is available in ointments, lotions, and creams in several strengths, the choice depending upon where it is to be used.

Adverse effects If Synalar preparations are not used for long periods or on infected areas, there are virtually no important adverse effects; however, if they are used for long intervals on the face, they can cause eruptions and redness. If Synalar preparations are used for long periods on a large area of the body, the corticosteroid can be absorbed into the body through the skin. This can cause weight gain, ulcers or stomach upset, decreased resistance to infection and stress, and can be quite dangerous. If Synalar is used on an infected area of skin it can help the infection spread, and it can be very hazardous if used for any skin sores caused by a virus, such as those of herpes simplex ("cold sores"), shingles, or chickenpox.

Precautions Do not use for long periods of time or on large areas of the body except under continued medical supervision. If a skin eruption worsens with continued use, the physician should be notified and use of the preparation discontinued.

Drug interactions No significant interactions will occur although other topical preparations placed on the same skin area as Synalar may interfere with its effects.

See *Steroids, or cortisone-like drugs,* page 102; *Skin and local disorders,* page 125.

Synalgos-DC

Generic ingredients

```
narcotic pain reliever : dihydrocodeine
sedative : promethazine
pain relievers : aspirin, phenacetin
mild stimulant : caffeine
```

Action and uses A combination product used to relieve pain. This particular combination contains both narcotic and non-narcotic pain relievers as well as a major tranquilizer which was added as a sedative. A similar product, Synalgos, is identical except for the absence of the narcotic. Whether all of these components act together to give greater relief of pain and anxiety than the less costly codeine or aspirin with codeine is not known. The problematic side effects of some ingredients tends to make such a mixture less desirable than simpler drugs.

Adult dosage One or two capsules every four to six hours as needed for pain.

Adverse effects Undesired effects can result from several of the components. The dihydrocodeine can cause constipation, and both it and the aspirin can cause stomach upset. The promethazine, though present in small amounts, can cause sedation with repeated doses, as can the narcotic. Promethazine can also rarely cause allergies, effects on the white blood cell count, and jaundice, as can other phenothiazines (major tranquilizers). Allergies can also occur to either the aspirin, phenacetin, or codeine. Prolonged use of this drug can also lead to kidney damage caused by the phenacetin component, and to habituation caused by the dihydrocodeine.

Precautions If sedation occurs, driving or operating heavy machinery may be hazardous. This drug should be avoided by pregnant or potentially pregnant women and nursing mothers, and by those sensitive to aspirin, codeine, or phenothiazines.

Drug dependence Synalgos-DC may cause psychological and/or physical dependence; prolonged use should therefore be avoided to prevent habituation.

Drug interactions The sedative effects of the dihydrocodeine and promethazine can add to the effects of other tranquilizers, sedatives, alcohol, or sleeping pills. Aspirin adds to the effects of oral anticoagulants, increasing the risk of bleeding, and to the effects of cortisone-like drugs, increasing the risk of peptic ulcer.

See *Narcotic pain relievers,* page 41.

Synthroid

Generic name

> levothyroxine (available by generic name)

Action and uses A synthetic form of thyroid hormone. Thyroid hormones help to regulate many of the body's functions, especially the metabolism, including the rate at which cells use oxygen. Certain thyroid conditions, for example myxedema (hypothyroidism) and simple goiter, may be caused by a deficiency of thyroid hormone, and synthetic hormones such as Synthroid are used as "replacement therapy." In most cases today pure hormones such as Synthroid are used in preference to the animal gland extracts which were widely used before purified synthetic hormones became available. Synthroid, like other thyroid preparations, has no place in weight control therapy.

Adult dosage The dose must be adjusted according to the individual patient's requirements. Synthroid is produced in six different strengths. Synthroid tablets are ten times stronger than other thyroid preparations and cannot be simply substituted for them. Laboratory tests are usually necessary to determine the correct dosage.

Adverse effects If too high a dose of Synthroid is given, symptoms of overdose will occur. These include nervousness, sweating, irregular and rapid heartbeats, chest pains (angina), and, in women, irregular menstruation.

Precautions The required amount of Synthroid may vary over time, and therefore regular checks of thyroid function may be needed. Careful regulation of the dose is also important if high blood pressure or heart disease is also present.

Drug interactions When taken with thyroid drugs, certain tricyclic antidepressant drugs (e.g.,Elavil) and decongestants or drugs for asthma can increase the likelihood of palpitations, rapid heart rate, and elevation of the blood pressure.

See *Thyroid disorders,* page 89.

Tagamet

Generic name

> cimetidine

Action and uses A new and widely used drug for the treatment of duodenal ulcer and diseases where there is severe excessive secretion of stomach acid. Stomach acid (hydrochloric acid, or HCl) is secreted at all times but is produced in greater quantities in response to food and other factors, e.g.,caffeine. It is beleived that stomach acid prevents an ulcer from healing once it develops. Tagamet blocks the secretion of acid by acting on special "histamine-2 receptors" (not the receptors related to common allergies) in special cells in the lining of the stomach. This contrasts with the action of antacids (which have long been the mainstay of ulcer therapy), that *neutralize* the acid in the stomach after it is secreted. At the present time, Tagamet is used only for fairly short periods (two months or less) during the acute illness, although its potential for use over longer time periods by people who have recurrent severe ulcer problems is being studied. Tagamet and antacids accomplish the same goal (less acid in the stomach) by different means and the overall risks and benefits of the two therapies are still under analysis (in fact, antacids are still used along *with* Tagamet).

Adult dosage Usually 300 mg orally four times daily with meals and at bedtime.

Adverse effects Since Tagamet is a new drug, the frequency with which side effects occur is still being clarified. Diarrhea, muscle pain, dizziness, and rashes may occur, and (much less frequently) effects on white blood cells and liver function have been observed, and also breast enlargement in men. Older people may be at greater risk of developing confusion when taking the drug.

Precautions Tagamet should not be taken by pregnant or potentially pregnant women or nursing mothers and should not be taken for longer periods than recommended unless discussed fully with the prescribing physician.

Drug interactions Tagamet may interact with the anticoagulant drug Coumadin to increase the risk of bleeding.

See *Nausea, stomach upset, and ulcers,* page 75.

Talwin

Generic name

pentazocine

Action and uses A pain reliever closely related in some respects to the narcotic analgesics, although it is not yet subject to the same restrictions as narcotics. Like codeine, Talwin is used for relief of moderate pain, but it is more expensive than codeine and appears to offer few advantages. Its potential side effects (see below) and its cost tend to limit its usefulness, although it does offer an alternative strong oral analgesic when such a drug is needed, as it is sometimes in cases of terminal cancer.

Adult dosage Talwin may be given by intramuscular injection or taken orally in doses of 15–60 mg every three to six hours as needed for pain.

Adverse effects Talwin can depress breathing, and, like codeine, can cause constipation, nausea, drowsiness, and dizziness. Additionally, unlike most of the narcotic drugs, Talwin can increase blood pressure and strain on the heart and also can produce unpleasant sensations of anxiety and/or strange thoughts and hallucinations. Allergic skin rashes are another possible side effect.

Precautions Talwin should be avoided by patients with severe respiratory disorders, a history of mental disorders or epilepsy, and by pregnant or potentially pregnant women and nursing mothers.

Drug dependence Talwin can cause psychological and/or physical dependence.

Drug interactions Talwin may increase the sedative effect of tranquilizers, sleeping pills, antidepressants, sedatives, and alcohol.

See *Non-narcotic pain relievers,* page 42.

Tandearil

Generic name

oxyphenbutazone

Action and uses A drug used to reduce inflammation, especially in the joints. Tandearil relieves the painful symptoms of inflammation but does not cure the disease which causes the inflammation. It is not known how it works. It is not a steroid hormone and is not related to steroids, although its anti-inflammatory actions are similar. Because of very serious side effects it is used only when milder drugs, such as aspirin, do not relieve the symptoms of inflammation. It is useful for the treatment of isolated severe pains of inflamed tendons and joints, and occasionally for acute gout and for acute flare-ups of rheumatoid arthritis.

Adult dosage The optimum dose of Tandearil varies from person to person and must be determined by the physician for each individual case. It is available in 100 mg tablets, and the daily dose ranges from 300–600 mg, usually taken in divided doses with meals or milk.

Adverse effects While Tandearil is an effective and useful drug, it is also a dangerous and poisonous one. Many severe reactions occur, particularly if it is used for longer than seven days, especially in people over the age of 60. It may poison the bone marrow and prevent the body from producing red blood cells, thereby causing anemia, and white blood cells, causing loss of resistance to infection. If such a reaction occurs the effects may be irreversible if the drug is not stopped immediately. Hives, skin rashes, itching and sores in and around the mouth can be signs of serious reactions to the drug and should be reported to the physician immediately. Tandearil also may cause stomach upsets, nausea, vomiting, and indigestion, though this may be avoided by taking it with meals. It can also cause liver damage and fluid retention.

Precautions Tandearil should not be used by children under the age of 14, or by pregnant or potentially pregnant women or nursing mothers. It should never be used for more than seven days by any person over the age of 60 unless specifically ordered by, and discussed with, a physician, and it should be followed up with regular blood counts. It should be used cautiously by people who have stomach or intestinal trouble or ulcers.

Drug interactions Tandearil interacts with many drugs, including antidiabetic drugs, other anti-inflammatory drugs (e.g., Motrin), sulfa drugs, Dilantin and Coumadin, increasing the risk of toxicity of each.

See *Pain with inflammation,* page 43.

Tedral

Generic ingredients

> bronchodilators : theophylline; ephedrine
> sedative : phenobarbital

Action and uses A combination of three drugs used to treat asthma. Theophylline and ephedrine both act on the muscles of the bronchi (the airways in the lungs) to relax and dilate them (open them up). Phenobarbital is included on the theoretical basis that it provides a mild sedative for anxious asthmatic patients and counteracts any stimulant effect of the ephedrine. However, neither effect is proven and, at the small dose of phenobarbital used, neither is very likely. Most often, theophylline alone in proper doses is equally effective, less costly, and has fewer side effects. Further, this fixed combination does not allow the dose of each ingredient to be adjusted individually.

Adult dosage One or two tablets every four hours (to treat attacks or to prevent them).

Adverse effects Adverse effects from the ephedrine component can include nervousness, high blood pressure, fast heart rate, and palpitations. The theophylline can cause nausea, headaches or muscle cramps, and also palpitations. The phenobarbital can cause allergic reactions.

Precautions Tedral should be used with caution by people who have heart disease or high blood pressure. It can be additive to certain over-the-counter drugs for asthma; therefore the prescribing physician should be made aware of *all* drugs being used, including aerosols or inhalers.

Drug interactions The ephedrine can be additive to drugs for coughs and colds and can therefore increase their side effects, but it can counteract antihypertensive drugs.

The theophylline and phenobarbital can interact with anticoagulant drugs (e.g.,Coumadin) to decrease their effect.

See *Asthma and lung disease,* page 109.

Teldrin

Generic name

chlorpheniramine (available by generic name)

Action and uses A commonly prescribed antihistamine which is frequently used to treat allergic conditions, especially allergic rhinitis, sinusitis, or conjunctivitis (redness of the eye). In common with most other antihistamines it blocks the effects of histamine (a substance which is released by the body in response to various noxious stimuli and which causes many of the symptoms of inflammation and allergic reactions); the drug can therefore relieve itching of the skin due to allergies, hives, or rashes. It also can sometimes have a sedating effect, although it is not customarily used for this. It is not useful for treatment of asthma. It is usually much less expensive in generic form, as chlorpheniramine.

Adult dosage Teldrin is available in long-acting 12 mg capsules. The usual oral dose is one 12 mg capsule once or twice daily as needed for treatment of allergic conditions.

Adverse effects Teldrin may also cause significant sedation in some people, although it may do so less frequently than some other antihistamines. Other side effects are relatively rare, but can include dry mouth, blurred vision, or difficulty in urinating, especially in older people or those with glaucoma or prostate trouble.

Drug interactions Teldrin is additive to other sedative or tanquilizing drugs and to alcohol. It is also additive to other antispasmodic drugs used to treat ulcers or stomach problems (e.g., Pro-Banthine and Librax) causing excessive dry mouth, constipation, and difficulty in urinating.

Precautions	If sedation occurs, it may make driving or operating machinery dangerous. This drug should be used with caution by those with glaucoma or prostate trouble. It should also be avoided by pregnant or potentially pregnant women and nursing mothers.
See	*Antihistamines,* page 121.

Tenuate

Generic name	diethylpropion (available by generic name)

Action and uses	An appetite suppressant used as an aid in weight reduction. Its effect in decreasing the appetite tends to diminish after 7–14 days. Its true effectiveness in causing weight loss is questionable. Like amphetamine sulfate, to which it is related, it also stimulates the nervous system, producing an increase in energy and mental alertness and a lift in mood. Though Tenuate is less effective in suppressing appetite than amphetamine sulfate, it is probably preferable because it may have less tendency to cause dependence.
Adult dosage	Usually 25 mg before meals, three times daily.
Adverse effects	Like amphetamine sulfate, Tenuate can cause dry mouth, nervousness, headache, anxiety, nausea, vomiting, rapid and irregular heartbeat, and elevation of the blood pressure. (In most patients, however, the side effects of Tenuate on the nervous system and cardiovascular system are less marked than those of amphetamine sulfate.) Withdrawal symptoms of fatigue and depression are likely to occur when the drug is stopped, particularly if it has been taken in doses exceeding those prescribed.
Precautions	Tenuate should be used only for short periods and under careful supervision. It should not be used by anyone with any type of heart disease, irregular heart rhythm, or high blood pressure.
Drug dependence	Like amphetamine sulfate, Tenuate can cause severe psychological and/or physical dependence, and tolerance to its effects develops quickly.
Drug interactions	Tenuate can counteract the effect of drugs for high blood pressure, and of some drugs used to regulate heart rhythms. Its effects can be additive to those of decongestants, nasal

sprays, and drugs for asthma, and if used with them can increase the likelihood of side effects.

See *Weight loss,* page 106.

Tetracycline

Trade names

> Achromycin-V, Retet, Robitet, Sumycin,
> Panmycin, Tetrex

Action and uses One of the most commonly used oral antibiotics. In the generic form it was the fourth most frequently prescribed drug in 1976. There are a number of tetracycline drugs available, and most are comparable in their actions and side effects, with the exceptions of Minocin and Vibramycin. Tetracycline is known as a "broad-spectrum" antibiotic because it can be used in a wide variety of different infections, although it is the first-choice drug in very few common infections. It acts by stopping the production of proteins in sensitive bacterial cells, but has little effect on human cells. Tetracycline is currently very commonly used in low doses to inhibit the growth of the bacteria on the face which are believed to contribute to acne. It is also frequently used by those with chronic bronchitis or other lung disease. Less frequently it is used to treat urinary tract infections or venereal disease when the patient is allergic to penicillin. It has no effect on viral illnesses, including colds or fungal infections.

Adult dosage The usual oral dose is 250 or 500 mg every six hours for a prescribed number of days as specified by the physician. It is very important to take this on an empty stomach. The dose may vary in some conditions, e.g.,in acne, where it may be lower.

Adverse effects Tetracycline commonly can cause various gastrointestinal symptoms including nausea and vomiting, burning stomach or belching, cramps, and diarrhea. The latter symptom is often due to the fact that tetracycline inhibits some bacteria in the lower intestine and elsewhere and thus allows overgrowth of other bacteria (normally held in check) and minor fungi. This can also result in vaginal infections, anorectal itching, and a sore mouth (thrush). These symptoms tend to disappear when the drug is discontinued. Less commonly, tetracycline can cause rashes or other allergic reactions and sensitivity of the skin to sunlight (photosensitivity), which can also cause rashes. In addition, it tends to worsen certain types of kidney disease and in rare instances may cause liver damage or blood-cell abnormalities.

Precautions Tetracycline should not be taken by pregnant or potentially pregnant women or nursing mothers and should be used with caution when significant liver or kidney disease is present. This antibiotic, like all others, should be taken for the full course prescribed, and every dose should be taken. Failure to do this can result in inadequate treatment of the infection, which may lead to recurrence of the infection or the development of resistant strains of bacteria.

Drug interactions The most common drug interaction occurs with antacids or milk products; tetracycline binds to these and is prevented from being absorbed into the body. Tetracycline can potentially increase the effect of the anticoagulant Coumadin and increase the hazard of bleeding.

See *Infections,* page 111.

Theophylline (generic name). See ELIXOPHYLLIN.

Thorazine

Generic name

chlorpromazine (available by generic name)

Action and uses The prototype of a large family of major tranquilizers, or "anti-psychotic" drugs, primarily used in the treatment of serious psychological disorders. Though not capable of curing the underlying illness, Thorazine and the other drugs in this group do relieve the severe thought disorders (such as disorientation, delusions, and hallucinations) that characterize schizophrenia and manic-depressive psychoses, severe alcohol withdrawal, some cases of senility, some neurological diseases, and the effects of certain drugs such as LSD and amphetamine. First introduced as a "tranquilizer" in the early 1950s, Thorazine revolutionized the treatment of mental patients by making it possible for them to receive therapy in the community rather than being confined to locked hospital wards.

Thorazine also has sedative effects, but is usually used for this purpose only when the patient is also suffering from a thought disorder. Thorazine can also be used to decrease nausea and vomiting, and to suppress constant hiccoughs (when they cannot be stopped in other ways).

Adult dosage   For the treatment of thought disorders, the initial dose of Thorazine may be 50–200 mg per day, eventually rising to 750–1000 mg per day in some cases. The dose is carefully adjusted for each patient because sensitivity to the drug varies widely from person to person. Generally speaking, however, the dose tends to be lower for older people, and, whatever the patient's age, it may usually be taken just once a day (often at bedtime, to take advantage of its sedative effect) when used over a long period of time.

Adverse effects   Thorazine may produce a number of significant side effects, and can occasionally cause serious drug reactions. Its use, therefore, must be carefully supervised. When first taken, Thorazine is likely to produce heavy sedation, a sensation of mental dullness, and, in some cases, blurred vision, dry mouth, and constipation. These effects usually diminish if the drug is continued for two to three weeks or more. Thorazine also lowers the blood pressure, an effect which may manifest itself in a sensation of dizziness when a person stands up suddenly. In some people, Thorazine causes restlessness, a fixed facial expression, and trembling in the hands, arms or legs. These side effects resemble the symptoms of Parkinson's disease and usually they can be controlled with an anti-Parkinsonian drug like Cogentin. A few people who have taken Thorazine for a long time experience an involuntary movement of the tongue and lips. Occasionally, Thorazine can cause skin rash, jaundice, or a fall in the white blood cell count (which increases the patient's vulnerability to infection). If these latter symptoms occur, the drug must be discontinued.

Precautions   Prolonged use of Thorazine requires regular medical evaluation at intervals. Its effects may make driving or operating machinery dangerous.

Drug interactions   Oversedation is possible when Thorazine is taken in combination with alcohol, other sedatives and tranquilizers, sleeping pills, antidepressants, antihistamines, and drugs containing narcotics. If taken with the antihypertensive drugs Ismelin and Aldomet, it can counteract their blood-pressure-lowering effect. It can also cause constipation or bladder dysfunction in some people when combined with antispasmodic drugs, anti-Parkinsonian drugs such as Cogentin, and tricyclic antidepressants such as Elavil.

See   *Major tranquilizers,* page 49.

Thyroglobulin (generic name). See PROLOID.

Thyroid

Trade names

Thyrolar, Thyrocrine

Action and uses　An extract from the thyroid glands of animals containing the natural thyroid hormones, sometimes called T-3 and T-4. Thyroid hormones regulate many body functions, especially the metabolic rate (including the rate at which the cells of the body use oxygen). Thyroid hormones are given to make up for a deficiency in thyroid conditions such as myxedema (hypothyroidism) and simple goiter. In recent years animal thyroid extracts have been largely superseded by the newer synthetic hormones (e.g., Synthroid). Like other thyroid drugs, Thyroid has no place in weight-control programs.

Adult dosage　There is no standard dose for thyroid. The dose must be adjusted for each patient individually and depends on the results of tests of thyroid function and the patient's response to the drug. The tablets come in eight different strengths from 15 mg to 300 mg.

Adverse effects　If too high a dose of thyroid is given, symptoms of overdose will occur. These include nervousness, sweating, irregular and rapid heartbeat, chest pains (angina) and, in women, irregular menstruation.

Precautions　The required dose of thyroid may vary over time, and therefore regular checks of thyroid function may be needed. Careful regulation of the dose is important if high blood pressure or heart disease is also present.

Drug interactions　When taken with thyroid drugs, certain tricyclic antidepressant drugs (e.g.,Elavil) and decongestants or drugs for asthma can increase the likelihood of palpitations, rapid heart rate and elevation of the blood pressure.

See　*Thyroid disorders,* page 89.

Thyroxine (generic name). See SYNTHROID.

Tigan

Generic name

benzamide hydrochloride

Action and uses	A drug used for the control of nausea and vomiting. Tigan is often prescribed for the treatment of motion sickness and nausea and vomiting in other disorders. It should be used only when the cause of nausea is known. The exact way in which Tigan helps to control these symptoms is not known, but it is thought to act on the centers in the brain which stimulate vomiting.
Adult dosage	Usually 250 mg three or four times per day, as needed. Tigan is also available as suppositories. The usual dose of these is one 200 mg suppository three or four times per day.
Adverse effects	Side effects are relatively infrequent. Occasionally, however, drowsiness, skin rash, tremors of the hands, dizziness and headache may occur.
Drug interactions	Tigan may be additive in its sedative effects to major or minor tranquilizers, sleeping pills, or antihistamines.
See	*Nausea, stomach upset and ulcers,* page 75.

Tofranil

Generic name

imipramine (available by generic name)

Action and uses	A commonly prescribed antidepressant drug. Like Elavil and Sinequan, Tofranil belongs to a group of closely related drugs called *tricyclic antidepressants* and is used to treat certain types of moderately severe and long-standing depression. The tricyclic antidepressants are not true tranquilizers, although they can cause some sedation. Though effective, the antidepressant effect of Tofranil may take days or weeks to appear, and a truly depressed person should be aware of this, as well as the initial side effects. Tofranil is sometimes used to treat childhood bedwetting.
Adult dosage	The effective dose of Tofranil varies for each individual patient and one or two months of adjustment may be necessary before the optimum dose is established. Initially the dose is 50–100 mg per day and may be increased to 150 or 200 mg per day. (The dose may be lower for elderly patients.) Because the drug is long-acting and may cause some sedation, it is usually taken just once a day, at bedtime.
Adverse effects	Initially, Tofranil may cause dry mouth, blurred vision, drowsiness, constipation, and difficulty in urinating. These effects are especially a problem in older people, but they tend

to disappear in three or four weeks. Other significant side effects may include effects on the heart rhythm and sometimes confusion or dizziness.

Precautions Tofranil should be taken with caution by people with glaucoma, prostate gland problems, liver or heart disease, epilepsy, or hyperthyroid conditions. It should not be taken by pregnant or potentially pregnant women or nursing mothers. The drowsiness may interfere with driving or operating machinery.

Drug interactions Tofranil can cause oversedation when taken in combination with alcohol, sleeping pills, tranquilizers, antihistamines, and drugs containing narcotics. It can add to the side effects of drugs such as Ismelin to lower blood pressure. It can dangerously interfere with drugs to regulate heart rhythm, thyroid drugs, and drugs of the MAO inhibitor family (e.g.,Marplan, Parnate and Nardil). Taken with drugs of the latter type, or with the sedative Placidyl, Tofranil can cause delirium.

See *Antidepressants and Lithium,* page 52.

Tolbutamide (generic name). See ORINASE.

Tolectin

Generic name

tolmetin

Action and uses One of several recently introduced drugs, called "non-steroidal anti-inflammatory drugs," used to treat the symptoms of various types of arthritis. It has some ability to relieve pain and also acts to decrease inflammation. Tolectin, like the similar new drugs Indocin, Motrin, Nalfon, Naprosyn, and Clinoril, is often used as an alternative to aspirin for rheumatoid and other types of arthritis. In some cases, its effect is seen in a few days, but, in others, it may take longer to act.

Adult dosage Usually, two 200 mg tablets three times a day with adjustment of dosage as needed.

Side effects Like the other non-steroidal anti-inflammatory drugs, which Tolectin resembles chemically, gastrointestinal side effects may occur in as many as 15% of those taking it and 2% may develop peptic ulcers, especially if there is a history of ulcers. Nervousness, dizziness, rashes, ringing in the ears, and fluid retention may also occur in as many as 1% of people taking the drug.

Precautions Tolectin should be avoided by pregnant or potentially pregnant women and nursing mothers. It should be used with caution by people with a history of allergy to aspirin or other non-steroidal anti-inflammatory drugs, heart failure, history of peptic ulcer, and history of kidney failure, and also by people who are taking anticoagulants, anti-epileptic drugs, and oral drugs for diabetes. If bleeding, rash, or unusual changes occur, the prescribing physician should be notified at once.

Drug interactions Tolectin may interact with the oral anticoagulant Coumadin to increase the risk of bleeding, and with Dilantin and oral drugs for diabetes to increase their toxic effects. Aspirin and phenobarbital may reduce the effectiveness of Tolectin.

See *Pain with inflammation,* page 43.

Tolinase

Generic name

tolazamide

Action and uses A drug which lowers the levels of sugar (glucose) in the blood, used to treat diabetes. Because Tolinase can be taken orally (unlike insulin) it is termed an "oral hypoglycemic" drug (hypoglycemic means "blood-sugar-lowering"). It is similar to other oral antidiabetic drugs such as Orinase and Diabinese, but not to DBI. Tolinase works by stimulating the pancreas to produce insulin and by helping the cells to use glucose. It is of value only for diabetics who are able to make insulin. Such patients usually have the mild type of diabetes which often becomes evident toward middle age (and is therefore known as maturity-onset diabetes). Oral hypoglycemic drugs should be taken only if dietary measures alone have failed to control the condition. Resistance to the effects of Tolinase often develops after a few months or years. It is recommended that withdrawal of oral antidiabetic drugs be tried every six months to one year, since their continued use may not be needed. The long-term benefits versus risks of this and related drugs are now widely debated.

Adult dosage Dosage is adjusted to suit the needs of each patient. Initially it is 100–250 mg daily, taken with breakfast; adjustment is made according to response.

Adverse effects The most common and hazardous adverse effect is excessive *lowering* of the blood sugar, which can cause symptoms of dizziness, weakness, cold sweats, and mental dullness. Older people and those taking certain other drugs (see drug interactions below) or with liver or kidney disease, are more prone to this. In proper dosage, other side effects are unusual, but rashes, blood or liver abnormalities, and water retention can occur.

Precautions This drug should be avoided by pregnant or potentially pregnant women and nursing mothers and also by those with significant kidney or liver disease. Those allergic to sulfa drugs may develop an allergy to this drug.

Drug interactions Thiazide diuretics (as hydrochlorothiazide, Diuril, Hygroton) can aggravate diabetes and may increase the dose requirement of the oral antidiabetic drug. A number of drugs can increase the risk of low blood sugar if taken at the same time as Tolinase. These include insulin, sulfa drugs, anti-inflammatory drugs such as aspirin, Butazolidin, and Tandearil, and the anticonvulsant Dilantin. Inderal (propranolol) can also cause dangerous interactions and disguise the symptoms of hypoglycemia. Alcohol can cause a flushing reaction when taken with this drug.

See *Diabetes,* page 90.

Tranxene

Generic name

clorazepate

Action and uses A minor tranquilizer chemically related to Valium and Librium. Primarily used to relieve anxiety and nervous tension, Tranxene is also sometimes used to induce sleep and to treat the symptoms of alcohol withdrawal.

Adult dosage Usually 3.75 mg to 7.5 mg one to three times per day. Because it is eliminated from the body rather slowly, it can also be taken once a day, at bedtime, in order to take advantage of its sleep-inducing effects. Accordingly, it is available in a once-daily dosage form, Tranxene-SD, which contains 22.5 mg (in other words, three 7.5 mg doses).

Adverse effects Drowsiness, dizziness, and blurred vision are possible side effects of Tranxene, but these effects are usually dose-related, and can be reduced by lowering the dose. Though other side effects are possible, they are relatively unusual.

Precautions Because of the possible connection between similar drugs and birth defects, Tranxene should not be taken by pregnant or potentially pregnant women.

Drug dependence Because of its sedative effects, Tranxene may interfere with driving or operating machinery. Prolonged use of Tranxene may cause habituation and withdrawal symptoms when discontinued.

Drug interactions The sedative effects of Tranxene can be increased by alcohol, antihistamines, sleeping pills, and other sedatives, tranquilizers, and antidepressants.

See *Minor tranquilizers,* page 45.

Triamcinolone (generic name). See ARISTOCORT, KENALOG.

Triavil

Generic ingredients

antidepressant : amitriptyline
major tranquilizer : perphenazine

Action and uses A combination drug promoted and used to treat moderate to severe anxiety with depression. Triavil contains two potent drugs: amitriptyline, a tricyclic antidepressant used in the treatment of moderate to severe depression; and perphenazine, an antipsychotic drug, or major tranquilizer, used in the treatment of psychoses (thought disorders). There is some debate among medical authorities as to the wisdom or efficacy of using these two drugs in a fixed-combination form.

In the first place, when used alone, both drugs require careful adjustment of dose to suit each individual patient; in a combination, it is not possible to alter the relative proportions of each ingredient, and as a result dose adjustment cannot be made with any subtlety. Second, the adverse effects of the two drugs (described below) are very similar and can be additive. Third, although Triavil is promoted for the treatment of anxiety with depression, neither of its two components is a true anti-anxiety drug. One possible justification for the use of this combination drug is that the antidepressant amitriptyline will on occasion produce a thought disorder which can be suppressed by perphenazine; however, whether this is true has not been carefully established in clinical testing. In the final analysis, it is questionable whether, in view of their additive side effects, the use of these two potent drugs is justified in any situation other than a truly serious mental disorder, and then it is possible that only one is really needed.

Adult dosage Triavil is available in four tablet sizes; it is recommended that they should be taken three or four times per day, but since both ingredients are long-acting, they can be taken once daily, usually in the evening to make use of the sedative effect.

Adverse effects Triavil has the combined side effects of its two components, which are significant and additive. Amitriptyline and perphenazine can both cause dry mouth, blurred vision, urine retention, constipation, and rapid or irregular heartbeat. Perphenazine can also cause "Parkinsonian symptoms" (symptoms resembling those of Parkinson's disease—a rigid facial expression, stiff gait, and trembling in the hands, arms, and feet), as well as dizziness, jaundice, blood disorders, and severe skin rashes.

Precautions Triavil should not be used by pregnant or potentially pregnant women or nursing mothers. Triavil should be used with caution by patients with glaucoma, prostate gland trouble, heart disease, epilepsy, impaired liver function, or hyperthyroidism.

Drug interactions Oversedation is possible when Triavil is combined with alcohol, other tranquilizers and antidepressants, sleeping pills, sedatives, and drugs containing narcotics. The amitriptyline in Triavil can interfere with drugs to lower blood pressure, thyroid drugs, and drugs of the MAO inhibitor family (e.g. Marplan, Parnate, and Nardil). The perphenazine in Triavil can also dangerously interfere with drugs to lower blood pressure. Both drugs can be additive to antispasmodic drugs and anti-Parkinsonian drugs such as Cogentin to cause constipation.

See *Major tranquilizers,* page 49; *Antidepressants and Lithium,* page 52.

Trihexyphenidyl (generic name). See ARTANE.

Tri-Vi-Flor

Generic ingredients

vitamins : A,D,C
minerals : fluoride

317

Action and uses	A fixed-combination vitamin and mineral supplement used for infants. The vitamins are intended to supplement the regular food of infants. The fluoride is intended to help prevent dental cavities, for use in areas where there is no fluoride in the water supply.
Dosage	Usually one dropperful (1 ml) per day or one chewable tablet per day.
Adverse effects	Both vitamin A and vitamin D can cause serious adverse effects if taken in excess. Vitamin A can cause liver and skin abnormalities, and vitamin D, bone abnormalities.
Precautions	Tri-Vi-Flor should not be used if the local water supply already contains fluoride. Only the dose recommended should be used, preferably with a doctor's advice.
Drug interactions	No significant interactions occur at the recommended dose.
See	*Vitamins and minerals,* page 134.

Tuss-Ornade

Generic ingredients

> cough suppressant and anticholinergic : caramiphen
> antihistamine : chlorpheniramine
> decongestant : phenylpropanolamine
> anticholinergic : isopropamide iodide

Action and uses	This mixture of ingredients is available as a long-acting, time-released Spansule or as a liquid; it is identical to Ornade, except for the addition of ingredients which can reduce coughing and have a drying (anticholinergic) action. Because of the presence of the cough-suppressant ingredient (although it is less effective in reducing coughing than codeine), Tuss-Ornade should be primarily reserved for occasions when it is desirable and necessary to suppress coughing. The other ingredients are aimed at relieving the symptoms of nasal stuffiness and a runny nose.
Adult dosage	Spansule: one capsule every twelve hours, as needed for symptoms. Liquid: one or two teaspoons three or four times per day.
Adverse effects	The antihistamine component and caramiphen may cause drowsiness, and the anticholinergic ingredients may cause an excessively dry nose and mouth. There may be palpitations or dizziness. People with heart disease, high blood pressure, diabetes, or prostate trouble may be more susceptible to these effects.

Precautions This drug should be avoided by pregnant or potentially pregnant women and nursing mothers. This drug should not be taken by a person allergic to iodine. Because the preparation may decrease alertness, driving or operating machinery may be hazardous. Those with heart trouble or high blood pressure should check with their doctor since this drug can increase blood pressure.

Drug interactions The sedative effects of the antihistamine and cough-suppressant ingredients can add to the effects of alcohol and tranquilizing drugs. The effects of the two anticholinergic components (dry mouth or bladder problems) can be additive to those of antispasmodic drugs (e.g.,Pro-Banthine, Librax) and tricyclic antidepressant drugs (e.g.,Elavil). The iodide present can interfere with tests of thyroid function.

See *Coughs and colds,* page 117.

Tylenol

Generic name

acetaminophen (available by generic name)

Tylenol with Codeine

Generic ingredients

narcotic : codeine
pain reliever : acetaminophen

Action and uses A popular mild analgesic drug available with or without the addition of codeine, a narcotic analgesic. With codeine it is used to treat more severe pain than can be relieved by simple analgesics such as aspirin or acetaminophen alone.

Adult dosage One or two tablets, every four to six hours as needed for pain.

Adverse effects The major side effects that can occur are due to the codeine, which can cause constipation, occasional nausea and vomiting, and occasional dizziness. Large doses of acetaminophen can cause serious liver damage.

Precautions Because habitual use involves the risk of dependence (habituation), the forms containing codeine should be used only when non-narcotic analgesics are not effective.

Drug dependence Prolonged use of codeine may cause dependence.

Drug interactions The effects of the codeine can be additive to those of other narcotic drugs and other sedative drugs such as tranquilizers or alcohol.

See *Narcotic pain relievers,* page 41.

Valisone Cream, Ointment, Lotion & Spray

Generic name

betamethasone

Action and uses A commonly used preparation of a synthetic corticosteroid (cortisone-like drug) for local (topical) application to the skin. It is used primarily for its anti-inflammatory effects in the treatment of many types of skin disorders such as psoriasis, certain types of neurodermatitis (inflammation of the skin associated with emotional factors), and a variety of other conditions where there is no infection. In many cases, the effects are dramatic. Because it retards formation of scar tissue, it can also prevent scarring.

Adult dosage The preparation is applied sparingly two or three times daily. It is available in ointments, lotions, creams, and as a spray, in several strengths, depending upon where it is to be used.

Adverse effects If Valisone preparations are not used for long periods or on infected areas, there are virtually no important adverse effects; however, if they are used for long intervals on the face, they can cause eruptions and redness. If Valisone preparations are used for long periods on a large area of the body, the corticosteroid can be absorbed into the body through the skin. This can cause weight gain, ulcers or stomach upset, decreased resistance to infection and stress, and can be quite dangerous. If used on an infected area of the skin it can help the infection spread, and it can be very hazardous if used for any viral skin lesions such as those of herpes simplex ("cold sores"), shingles, or chickenpox.

Precautions Do not use for long periods or on large areas of the body except under continued medical supervision. If a skin eruption worsens with continued use, the physician should be notified and the preparation discontinued.

Drug interactions No significant interactions will occur, although other topical preparations placed on the same skin area as Valisone may interfere with its effects.

See *Steroids, or cortisone-like drugs,* page 102; *Skin and local disorders,* page 125.

Valium

Generic name	diazepam

Action and uses

A minor tranquilizer widely used to treat anxiety and nervousness. The primary effect of Valium is to produce calm and decrease the feeling of anxiety. Valium is one of a group of related drugs which includes Librium, Serax, Dalmane, and Tranxene; they are the most frequently prescribed drugs in the United States. Valium is usually prescribed to relieve the symptoms of a condition in the same way that narcotics are used to relieve pain. In general it has no effect on the *cause* of the symptoms. Valium is also often used in the treatment of withdrawal from certain drugs, especially alcohol. It can also be used as a sleeping medication in a similar way to the related drug, Dalmane. It is not known exactly how these drugs work.

Adult dosage

The usual dose of Valium ranges from 10 mg per day to 2–10 mg, two to four times per day, depending on individual requirements. Some people are strongly sedated by 2 mg or 5 mg, while others are not especially affected by these amounts.

Adverse effects

The most common side effect of Valium is sedation and depression, and sometimes dizziness, but this can usually be relieved by lowering the dosage. In some cases the sedation may interfere with working, driving, or operating machinery. Other side effects are relatively uncommon. A few individuals may suffer from increased anxiety when taking Valium, but this is rare. When Valium is taken in combination with alcohol the two drugs act together and marked sedation may occur.

Drug dependence

Valium is not addictive in the same way as narcotics but, like other sedatives, it can be habit-forming to a certain extent if taken for a long period of time. If it is then stopped suddenly some withdrawal symptoms may occur, especially after large doses. These can include anxiety, insomnia and nightmares.

Precautions

There is a possibility that minor tranquilizers may cause birth defects and the manufacturers therefore warn against the use of Valium by pregnant or potentially pregnant women.

Drug interactions

Valium can enhance the sedative effect of alcohol, antihistamines, sleeping pills, and narcotics, sometimes to a dan-

gerous extent. Unlike many sedatives, Valium does not interfere with the actions of the anticoagulant Coumadin.

See   *Minor tranquilizers,* page 45.

Vasodilan

Generic name

isoxsuprine (available by generic name)

Action and uses   This drug is promoted and used for disorders causing decreased circulation to the brain, feet, or hands. However, although it relaxes normal blood vessels (and therefore increases the flow of blood) in the muscles of the extremities,
there is no clear evidence that it can increase blood flow in
abnormal states, such as when there is fatty obstruction of
the blood vessels (*arteriosclerosis*), or when a person experiences coldness of the extremities or pain with exercise (*intermittent claudication*). It is also used in conditions where there
is temporary spasm of the arteries, such as Raynaud's phenomenon, but in such cases its effectiveness is again
questionable.

Adult dosage   10–20 mg three or four times a day.

Adverse effects   Vasodilan is well tolerated, but may cause dizziness, especially with rapid changes in position (for example, when the
patient stands up suddenly), and rapid heart rate. Allergic
rashes may also occur.

Precautions   This drug should not be used directly after minor or major
surgery or childbirth. It should be avoided by pregnant and
potentially pregnant women.

Drug interactions   Vasodilan may add to effects of other more effective blood-
vessel relaxing drugs, such as nitroglycerin or Apresoline, to
lower blood pressure.

See   *Poor circulation,* page 68.

V-Cillin K

Generic name

phenoxymethyl penicillin (available by generic name)

Action and uses   A semi-synthetic penicillin antibiotic which is almost identical to penicillin G in its action and adverse effects except
that due to a small difference in its chemical structure, it is

more effective when taken orally. This is because it is not easily destroyed by stomach acid. V-Cillin K acts to prevent formation of the cell walls of bacteria; this prevents their growth and multiplication. There is no effect on human cells, which have a different structure. It is most effective against the group of bacteria which commonly cause sore throats (*Streptocócci*—hence the term "strep throat"), pneumonia, and certain abscesses, although some bacteria in abscesses (*Staphylococci,* or "staph") can become resistant to penicillin, especially in hospitals. V-Cillin K, like the other penicillins, is not so effective for the treatment of serious infections by the group of bacteria called "gram-negative bacilli," which cause infections in the urinary tract, bowel, and elsewhere. It has no effect on viral or fungal infections.

Adult dosage The usual oral dose is 250–500 mg (equivalent to 0.4–0.8 million units) every six hours on an empty stomach, but this is adjusted for each patient according to the infection.

Adverse effects The most common adverse effect is gastrointestinal upset, cramps, or diarrhea. A more serious complication, which may occur when V-Cillin K is either given by injection or taken orally, is the occurrence of allergic reactions, which can include skin rashes, or hives, swelling of the face or throat, difficulty in breathing, or joint pains and fever (which may occur some time after the drug is taken).

Precautions V-Cillin K should not be taken when there is known allergy to any of the penicillin drugs. Once a course of V-Cillin K is begun, it should be taken for the full course prescribed (usually five to ten days), and every dose should be taken, even though symptoms may disappear. This is very important since the infection may otherwise recur and even develop resistance to the antibiotic.

Drug interactions In some cases, the effect of V-Cillin K may be decreased if erythromycin or chloramphenicol is also taken.

See *Infections,* page 111.

Vibramycin

Generic name

doxycycline (available by generic name)

Action and uses A slightly different and more costly form of one of the most commonly used oral antibiotics, tetracycline. There are a number of tetracycline drugs available, and most are comparable in their actions and side effects; Vibramycin, however, forms an exception, as does Minocin. Doxycycline is known as a "broad-spectrum" antibiotic because it can be used in a wide variety of different infections, although it is the first choice drug in very few common infections. Like other antibiotics, it acts by stopping the production of proteins in sensitive bacterial cells and has little effect on human cells. Doxycycline sometimes is used for chronic brochitis or other lung disease, for other minor infections, and occasionally for acne. Because of its cost, it is generally reserved for use as an alternative to tetracycline when kidney disease is present, since unlike other tetracyclines it does not harm the diseased kidney.

Adult dosage *The dose and schedule for doxycycline are not the same as for other tetracyclines.* The usual oral dose is 100–200 mg the first day, then 50–100 mg once or twice a day for a prescribed number of days as specified by the physician. It is very important to take the drug on an empty stomach. The dose may vary in some cases such as acne, where it may be lower.

Adverse effects Doxycycline can cause various gastrointestinal symptoms, including nausea and vomiting, burning stomach or belching, cramps, and diarrhea. The latter symptom, which is due to the fact that tetracycline inhibits some bacteria in the lower intestine and elsewhere and allows overgrowth of other bacteria and minor fungi, may occur less frequently with doxycycline than with other tetracyclines. These symptoms tend to disappear when the drug is discontinued. Less commonly, doxycycline can cause rashes or other allergic reactions and sensitivity of the skin to sunlight (photosensitivity), which may also cause rashes. In rare instances it can also cause liver damage or blood-cell abnormalities.

Precautions Doxycycline should not be taken by pregnant or potentially pregnant women or nursing mothers and should be used with caution when significant liver disease is present. This antibiotic, like all others, should be taken for the full time period directed, and every dose should be taken. Failure to do this can result in inadequate treatment of the infection, leading to recurrence or to the development of resistant infections.

Drug interactions The most common drug interaction occurs with antacids or milk products, since the doxycycline can bind to these and fail to be absorbed into the body. Doxycycline can potentially increase the effect of the anticoagulant Coumadin to increase the hazard of bleeding.

See   *Infections,* page 111.

Vioform-Hydrocortisone

Generic ingredients

> antibacterial/antifungal : iodochlorhydroxyquin
> corticosteroid : hydrocortisone

Action and uses   A topical preparation used to treat a wide variety of skin conditions associated with local infection of the skin, including various types of eczema, and fungal infections of the foot (athlete's foot) and other areas. The preparation is available without the corticosteroid ingredient as Vioform. There is some controversy whether the addition of the hydrocortisone, which decreases inflammation and scarring, is useful or not, since it may also help to spread the infection. It is available as a cream, lotion, or ointment, the choice depending on where it is to be used. Ointments are customarily used on dry areas, lotions on moist areas.

Adult dosage   The preparation of 3% iodochlorhydroxyquin and 1% hydrocortisone is applied sparingly to the affected area, three or four times daily.

Adverse effects   Allergies can occur to the ointment, and these may be hard to detect, except when there is increased itching and failure of an area to heal. Both ingredients may be absorbed into the body if used on large areas for long periods. If so, the iodine-containing product can cause interference with tests of thyroid function; the hydrocortisone can also cause weight gain, stomach upset, or ulcer, and decreased resistance to infection or illness. Very long-term use can also cause local breakdown of the skin (similar to stretch marks).

Precautions   Do not use for long periods of time or on large areas of the body except under continued medical supervision. If a skin eruption worsens with continued use, the physician should be notified and use of the preparation discontinued.

Drug interactions   The iodine-containing compound can interfere with tests of thyroid function.

See   *Steroids, or cortisone-like drugs,* page 102; *Skin and local disorders,* page 125.

Vistaril

Generic name

hydroxyzine

Action and uses An antihistamine which is promoted primarily for its anti-anxiety and sedating actions. It has a chemical structure similar to other antihistamines which are used for motion sickness (e.g.,Marezine), and it is essentially identical to the drug Atarax. Vistaril is also used on occasion for its antihistamine effects and in the treatment of conditions which cause itching of the skin.

Adult dosage Because sensitivity to its effects varies, the dose ranges from 25 to 100 mg two or three times a day.

Adverse effects Excessive sedation or decreased mental alertness may create a significant problem. Other side effects are relatively unusual.

Precautions Vistaril may interfere with driving or operating machinery. It should not be used by pregnant or potentially pregnant women or nursing mothers.

Drug interactions Vistaril is additive to other drugs causing sedation, such as sleeping pills, tranquilizers, alcohol, and narcotics such as morphine; these combinations should be avoided unless a greater degree of sedation is desired.

See *Antihistamines,* page 121; *Minor tranquilizers,* page 45.

Zyloprim

Generic name

allopurinol

Action and uses A drug used in the treatment of gout. Zyloprim is a chemical which helps to lower the level of uric acid in the blood. If uric acid levels rise too high, crystals of uric acid salts collect in joints and other places, especially the big toes and ears, causing sharp attacks of pain and forming deposits called *tophi.* It can gradually destroy the joints and may also form crystals in the kidneys to cause stones. This general condition is known as gout. Zyloprim prevents uric acid from forming and thus prevents the deposition of the crystals in the joints and in the kidneys. It is also used to reduce uric acid levels in other diseases such as leukemia, certain other types of cancer, and kidney disease.

Adult dosage The average dose is 200 to 300 mg per day, in a single dose, with adjustment made according to the levels of uric acid in the blood.

Adverse effects Some people develop sensitivity to Zyloprim and may suffer from skin rash, itching, or hives. Severe allergic reactions can develop. Drowsiness can also occur and liver abnormalities may develop. When the drug is first started, acute attacks of gout may be produced, so another antigout drug, colchicine, is usually added for several days to prevent this.

Precautions Zyloprim should not be used during pregnancy or by nursing mothers. The dose must be adjusted when taken with certain other drugs used for tumors or to suppress immunity.

Drug interactions Zyloprim can increase the effect of the anticoagulants Coumadin and dicumarol and some other drugs. The dose of Zyloprim may need to be reduced when the drugs mercaptopurine and Imuran are also used.

See *Gout,* page 132.

TABLE 1 • A Summary of Drugs by Use, Category, Generic and Trade Names

Health Problem or Drug Type	Specific Drug Group	Generic Name	Trade Name(s)
ALLERGIES AND COLD SYMPTOMS	antihistamines	brompheniramine[1]	Drixoral[2]
			Dimetane Expectorant[2]
			Dimetane Expectorant DC[2]
			Dimetane Tablets[2]
			Dimetapp[2]
		chlorpheniramine[1]	Chlor-Trimeton Tablets
			Naldecon[2]
			Novahistine-DH[2]
			Ornade[2]
			Polaramine
			Teldrin
			Tuss-Ornade[2]
		cyproheptadine	Periactin
		diphenhydramine[1]	Ambenyl Expectorant[2]
			Benadryl
			Benadryl Elixir
			Benylin Cough Syrup
		phenyltoloxamine	Tussionex[2]
		triprolidine	Actifed[2]
			Actifed-C Expectorant[2]
	decongestants	d-Isoephedrine	Drixoral[2]
		phenylephrine[1]	Phenergan Expectorant / Codeine[2]
			Phenergan VC Expectorant[2]
			Phenergan VC Expectorant / Codeine[2]
		phenylpropanolamine	Ornade[2]
			Novahistine-DH[2]
			Tuss-Ornade[2]
		phenylpropanolamine plus phenylephrine	Dimetane Expectorant[2]
			Dimetane Expectorant-DC[2]
			Dimetapp[2]
			Naldecon[2]
		pseudoephedrine[1]	Actifed[2]
			Actifed C Expectorant[2]
			Drixoral[2]
			Sudafed
	narcotic cough suppressants	codeine	Actifed C Expectorant[2]
			Ambenyl Expectorant[2]
			Dimetane Expectorant-DC[2]
			Novahistine DH[2]
			Phenergan Expectorant / Codeine[2]
			Phenergan VC Expectorant / Codeine[2]
		hydrocodone	Tussionex[2]
	phenothiazines[3]	promethazine	Phenergan Expectorant[2]
			Phenergan Expectorant / Codeine[2]
			Phenergan VC Expectorant[2]

329

Table 1—*continued*

Health Problem or Drug Type	Specific Drug Group	Generic Name	Trade Name(s)
ANALGESICS AND ANTI-INFLAMMATORIES	mild analgesics	acetaminophen[1] (APAP, paracetamol)	Darvocet N-100[2] Parafon Forte[2] Phenaphen/Codeine[2] Tylenol/Codeine[2]
		acetylsalicylic acid[1] (ASA, aspirin)	Aspirin Darvon Compound-65[2] Empirin Compound/Codeine[2] Equagesic[2] Fiorinal[2] Fiorinal/Codeine[2] Norgesic[2] Norgesic Forte[2] Synalgos-DC[2]
	narcotic analgesics	codeine[1]	Empirin/Codeine[2] Fiorinal/Codeine[2] Phenaphen/Codeine[2] Synalgos-DC[2] Tylenol/Codeine[2]
		oxycodone	Percodan[2]
		pentazocine	Talwin
		propoxyphene[1]	Darvon Darvon Compound-65[2] Darvocet-N-100[2]
	non-steroids/ anti-inflammatory	fenoprofen	Nalfon
		ibuprofen	Motrin
		indomethacin	Indocin
		naproxen	Naprosyn
		oxyphenbutazone	Tandearil
		phenylbutazone[1]	Butazolidin Alka[2]
		tolmetin	Tolectin
ANTI-ASTHMA DRUGS (Bronchial Dilators)	beta adrenergic stimulators	pseudoephedrine[1]	Marax[2] Sudafed
		terbutaline	Brethine
	methylxanthines	aminophyllin[1] oxtriphyllin	Choledyl
		theophylline[1]	Elixophyllin Marax[2] Quibron
ANTIBIOTICS AND ANTI-INFECTIVES	cephalosporins	cephalexin[1]	Keflex

Table 1—*continued*

Health Problem or Drug Type	Specific Drug Group	Generic Name	Trade Name(s)
	erythromycins	erythromycin estolate	Ilosone
		erythromycin ethyl-succinate[1]	E.E.S.
		erythromycin stearate	Erythrocin
		erythromycin base[1]	E-mycin
	miscellaneous	clotrimazole (topical)	Lotrimin[4]
		gamma benzene hexachloride (shampoo)	Kwell
		metronidazole	Flagyl
		miconazole (topical)	Monistat[4]
		nitrofurantoin[1]	Macrodantin
		nystatin (topical)	Mycostatin[4], Mycolog[2]
		polymyxin B-Bacitrac-in-neomycin (topical)	Neosporin
		polymyxin-gramicidin-neomycin	Cortisporin OTIC
	penicillins	amoxicillin[1]	Amoxil / Larotid
		ampicillin[1]	Amcill
		penicillin[1]	Omnipen
		penicillin G[1]	Pentids
		penicillin V[1]	Pen-Vee K / V-Cillin K
	sulfonamides ("sulfa" drugs)	sulfamethoxazole[1]	Gantanol
		sulfamethoxazole-trimethoprim	Bactrim[2] / Septra[2] / Septra DS[2]
		sulfanilamide (topical)	AVC[4]
		sulfathiazole, ("triple sulfa," topical)	Sultrin[4] / Triple Sulfa Cream
		sulfisoxazole[1]	Azo Gantrisin[2] / Gantrisin
	tetracyclines	doxycycline	Vibramycin
		minocycline	Minocin
		tetracycline[1]	Achromycin V / Sumycin
ANTICONVULSANTS		phenobarbital[1]	
		phenytoin[1]	Dilantin

Table 1—*continued*

Health Problem or Drug Type	Specific Drug Group	Generic Name	Trade Name(s)
ANTIDEPRESSANTS	tricyclic anti-depressants	amitriptyline[1]	Elavil Triavil[2]
		doxepin	Sinequan
		imipramine[1]	Tofranil
ANTI-INFECTIVES (See "Antiobiotics")			
ANTI-INFLAMMATORIES (See "Analgesics")			
BRONCHIAL DILATORS (See "Anti-Asthmatics")			
COLD SYMPTOMS (See "Allergies")			
GASTRO-INTESTINAL DISORDERS	anti-diarrheal drugs	diphenoxylate	Lomotil[2]
	anti-nausea drugs:		
	antihistamines[1]	doxylamine	Bendectin[2]
		meclizine[5]	Antivert
	phenothiazines	prochlorperazine	Combid[2] Compazine
		trimethobenzamide	Tigan
GLAUCOMA		pilocarpine[1]	Isoptocarpine
GOUT		allopurinol	Zyloprim
HEART AND VASCULAR DISORDERS	antiarrythmics	procainamide[1] quinidine[1]	Pronestyl
	anticoagulants ("blood thinners")	acetylsalicylic acid[1]	Aspirin
		warfarin[1]	Coumadin
	"cardiotonic" drugs	digoxin[1]	Lanoxin
	coronary-peripheral vasodilators	dipyridamole	Persantine
		isosorbide dinitrate[1]	Isordil Sorbitrate
		nitroglycerin[1]	Nitro-Bid Nitrostat
	non-specific blood vessel dilators	cyclandelate	Cyclospasmol
		dihydroergotoxine	Hydergine
		isoxsuprine	Vasodilan
		papaverine	Pavabid

Table 1—*continued*

Health Problem or Drug Type	Specific Drug Group	Generic Name	Trade Name(s)
HIGH BLOOD PRESSURE	potassium-retaining diuretics	spironolactone[1]	Aldactone Aldactazide[2]
		triamterene[1]	Dyazide[2]
	"potent" diuretics	furosemide[1]	Lasix
	sympathetic-blocking drugs	clonidine	Catapres[2]
		methyldopa[1]	Aldomet Aldoril[2]
		prazosin	Minipress
		propranolol[1]	Inderal
		reserpine[1]	Diupres[2] Hydropres[2] Regroton[2] Salutensin[2] Ser-Ap-Es[2]
	thiazide diuretics	chlorothiazide[1]	Diupres Diuril
		chlorthalidone[1]	Hygroton Regroton[2]
		hydrochlorothiazide[1]	Aldactazide[2] Aldoril[2] Dyazide[2] Esidrix HydroDIURIL Hydropres[2] Ser-Ap-Es[2]
		hydroflumethiazide	Salutensin
		methyclothiazide	Enduron
	vasodilators	hydralazine[1]	Apresoline Ser-Ap-Es[2]
HORMONES	cortisone-like drugs	betamethasone	Valisone (topical)
		flurandrenolide	Cordran (topical)
		fluocinolone	Synalar (topical)
		fluocinonide	Lidex (topical)
		hydrocortisone[6]	Anusol HC Vioform (topical)
		methylprednisolone	Medrol
		prednisone[1]	
		triamcinolone[6]	Aristocort (topical) Kenalog (topical) Mycolog[2]

Table 1—*continued*

Health Problem or Drug Type	Specific Drug Group	Generic Name	Trade Name(s)
	estrogens	conjugated estrogens[1]	Premarin
	insulin	insulin[1]	Insulin-NPH
	progesterone	medroxyprogesterone	Provera
	thyroid	levothyroxine[1]	Synthroid
		thyroglobulin	Proloid
METABOLIC DISORDERS	lipid (fat)-lowering agents	clofibrate	Atromid-S
	oral antidiabetic drugs (sulfonureas)	chlorpropamide[1]	Diabinese
		tolazamide	Tolinase
		tolbutamide[1]	Orinase
	potassium replacements	potassium bicarbonate, citrate and chloride[2]	K-lyte
		potassium chloride[1]	Slow-K
MUSCLE RELAXANTS		chlorzoxazone	Parafon Forte[2]
		diazepam	Valium
		meprobamnate[1]	Equanil[2]
			Equagesic[2]
		orphenadrine	Norgesic[2]
			Norgesic Forte[2]
ORAL CONTRACEPTIVES	combination Estrogen-Progestogen	ethinyl estradiol-(containing) as estrogen	Demulen-21[2]
			Lo/Ovral[2]
			Norlestrin-21[2]
			Ovral[2]
			Ovral-28[2]
		ethynodiol as progestogen	Demulen-21[2]
			Ovulen-21[2]
		mestranol as estrogen	Norinyl 1/50-21[2]
			Ortho Novum 1/50-21[2]
			Ortho Novum 1/50-28[2]
			Ortho Novum 1/80-21[2]
			Ovulen-21[2]
		norethindrone as progestogen	Norinyl 1/50-21[2]
			Norlestrin-21[2]
			Ortho-Novum 1/50-21[2]
			Ortho-Novum 1/50-28[2]
			Ortho-Novum 1/80-21[2]
		norgestrel as progestogen	Lo-Ovral[2]
			Ovral[2]
			Ovral-28[2]
	progestogen only	*None currently listed in top 200 drugs*	

Table 1—*continued*

Health Problem or Drug Type	Specific Drug Group	Generic Name	Trade Name(s)
TRANQUILIZERS (MAJOR)	butyrophenones	haloperidol	Haldol
	phenothiazines	chlorpromazine[1]	Thorazine
		perphenazine	Triavil[2]
		thioridazine	Mellaril
		trifluoperazine	Stelazine
TRANQUILIZERS (MINOR), SEDATIVES, AND SLEEPING PILLS	antihistamines	hydroxyzine[1]	Atarax Vistaril
	benzodiazepines	chlordiazepoxide[1]	Librium, Librax[2]
		clorazepate	Tranxene
		diazepam	Valium
		flurazepam	Dalmane
		lorazepam	Ativan
		oxazepam	Serax
	carbamic acid ester	meprobamate[1]	Equanil
	short-acting barbituates	butabarbital[1]	Butisol
URINARY ANTISEPTIC-DYE		phenazopyridine[1]	Azo Gantrisin[2] Pyridium
VASCULAR PROBLEMS (See "Heart Disorders")			
VITAMINS		multivitamins	Poly-Vi-Flor Chewable[2] Tri-Vi-Flor Drops[2]
WEIGHT LOSS	anorectic drugs	diethylpropion[1]	Tenuate
		phentermine[1]	Fastin
		phentermine resin	Ionamin

NOTE: All salts have been deleted except where they are significant.

[1] Also available by generic name

[2] Combination product

[3] Also has antihistamine action

[4] Vaginal cream

[5] Also has anti-motion sickness effect

[6] Available in tablets, injection, creams by generic name

TABLE 2 • Major Hazardous Drug Interactions

Type of Drug	Interacts with	Possible effect(s)
1. TRANQUILIZERS and SLEEPING PILLS* (Atarax, Ativan, Butisol, Dalmane, Librax, Librium, Meprobamate, Serax, Tranxene, Valium, Vistaril)	ALCOHOL, ANTIHISTAMINES*, and NARCOTIC PAIN RELIEVERS (See 2 and 3 below.)	Excess sleepiness and dizziness
2. ANTIHISTAMINES and COLD AND ALLERGY DRUGS* (Actifed, Benadryl, Chlor-Trimeton, Dimetapp, Drixoral, Ornade, and others)	ALCOHOL	Dizziness (sometimes severe), excess sleepiness, and unsteadiness
3. NARCOTIC-CONTAINING Drugs* (Codeine, Darvon, Percodan, and codeine-cough medicines)	ALCOHOL	Dizziness (sometimes severe), excess sleepiness, and unsteadiness
4. DRUGS FOR HIGH BLOOD PRESSURE, especially sympathetic-blocking drugs*	Over-the-counter NASAL SPRAYS and all DECONGESTANTS, such as Sudafed, Actifed, and Ornade	Decreased effect of antihypertensive drug, resulting in *increased* blood pressure
5. BLOOD-THINNING Drugs (Coumadin)	ASPIRIN and NON-STEROIDAL ANTI-INFLAMMATORY drugs* used for arthritis	Increased risk of bleeding

*See Table 1.

Index

This Index is compiled of all references to medical disorders and the medications related to them. References to medical disorders can be found under general or specific symptoms (e.g., "gastrointestinal disorders" or "constipation").

References to medications in general are compiled under the names of drug categories (e.g., "antihistamines;" "hormonal drugs;" "tranquilizers"). References to specific drugs are listed under the brand name of the drug (beginning with a capital) and/or under the generic name of the drug (beginning with a lower-case letter).

Numerals in italics indicate a major discussion of the topic cited.

341

345

Sultrin Triple Sulfa Cream and Suppositories (combination), 127, *299*
Sumycin (tetracycline), 307–308
Supen (ampicillin), 150–51
suppressants, cough, *119–20*
surgery, circulation problems and, *70*
Symmetrel (amantadine), 116, 132
sympathetic blocking drugs, 61
Synalar Cream and Ointment (fluocinolone), 125, *299–300*
Synalgos-DC (combination), *300–301*
Synthroid (levothyroxine), 90, 282, *301–302*, 311

T
T.A.C. (triamcinolone), 125
Tagamet (cimetidine), 78, *302–303*
Talwin (pentazocine), *303–304*
Tandearil (oxyphenbutazone), 133, 185, 257, *304–305*, 315
Tapazole (methimazole), 90
tardive dyskinesia, 50
Tedral (combination), 110, *305–306*
Tegretol (carbamazepine), 217
Teldrin (chlorpheniramine), *306–307*
Tempra (acetaminophen), *139*
Tenuate (diethylpropion), *307–308*
terbutaline, *166*
terpin hydrate, 120
Tes-Tape (glucose enzymatic test strip), 93
tetracycline, 25, 26, 114, 126, *140–141*, 205, *308–309*
Tetrex (tetracycline), *308–309*
thalidomide, 15–16, 25
theophylline, 75, 110, 111, 166, 172, *199*, 235, 236, 285, 286, 305, 306
thiazide-type diuretics, *63–64*
thioridazine, *239–40*
Thorazine (chlorpromazine), 17, 29, 51, 53, 77, 131, 146, 147, 155, 175, 176, 188, 209, 239, 297, *309–10*
thought, medications for problems with. *See* sleep disorders
thrombosis, anticoagulants and, *72*
Thyrocrine (thyroid), *311–12*
thyroglobulin, *282*
thyroid, *311–12*
thyroid disorders, drugs for, *89–90*
side effects, 90
treatment, 89–90
thyroid hormone, weight loss and, *108–109*
Thyrolar (thyroid), *311–12*
thyroxin, 89, 90
Tigan (trimethobenzamide hydrochloride), 77, *311–12*
Tinactin (tolnaftate), 117, 126
tincture of belladonna, 76, 79
Titralac (calcium carbonate), 78

Tofranil (imipramine), 27, 53, 146, 147, 198, 220, 294, *312–13*
tolazamide, 95, *314–15*
tolbutamide, 95, *256–57*
Tolectin (tolmetin), 217, 243, 246, 247, *313–14*
Tolinase (tolazamide), 95, 185, 257, *314–15*
tolmetin, *313–14*
tolnaftate, 117, 126
Totacillin (ampicillin), *150–51*
tranquilizers, 45–49
major, *49–52*
anxiety and nausea problems, 50
dosages, 50
other side effects, 51–52
phenothiazines and thinking disorders, 49–50
side effects, 50–51
minor, 45–47
antihistamines, 45–46
barbiturates, 45
benzodiazepines, 45
dosages, 46
side effects, 46–47
Tranxene (clorazepate), 45, 159, 229, 293, *315–16*, 321
triamcinolone, 103, *154–55*, 223–24
triamcinolone acetonide, 244
triamterene, 197, 225
Triavil (combination), 51, 54, *316–17*
tricrynafen, 64
tricyclics, 53
trifluoperazine, *297–98*
trihexphenidyl, 131, *155–56*
Trilafon (perphenazine), 54, 209
trimethobenzamide, *311–12*
trimethoprim, 116, 162, 291
tripolidine hydrochloride, 141, 142
Tri-Vi-Flor (combination), 317–18
tropic hormones, 88
Tuinal (combination), 47
Tuss-Ornade (combination), *318–19*
Tylenol with Codeine (combination), 173, *319–20*

U
ulcers. *See* stomach upset
unipolar endogenous depression, 52
urine testing, diabetes and, *93*
U.S. Drug Enforcement Agency, 41

V
vaccines, *122–25*
active and passive immunity, 122–23
common, 123–24
for influenza, 124–25
vaginal medications, *126–27*
Vagitrol (combination), 127
Valisone Cream, Ointment, Lotion and Spray

(betamethasone), 125, *320*
Valium (diazepam), 16, 24, 26, 27, 42, 45, 46,
    49, 159, 180, 203, 210, 229, 240, 273,
    293, 315, *321–22*
Vanceril (beclomethasone), 105, 111
vascular disorders *See* heart and vascular dis-
    orders
Vasodilan (isoxsuprine), 58, 70, *322*
vasodilators, *61–62*
V-Cillin K (phenoxymethyl penicillin),
    322–23
Veracolate (combination), 83
Vibramycin (doxycycline), 140, 241, 308,
    323–25
Vioform-Hydrocortisone (combination), 126,
    325
Vistaril (hydroxyzine), 45, 77, 121, 158, *326*
vitamin A, 275, 317, 318
vitamin B complex, 275
vitamin C, 118, 275, 317, 318
vitamin D, 275, 317, 318
vitamin E, 275
vitamin K, 74
vitamins and minerals, *134–38*
    fat-soluble vitamins, 136

minerals, 136
multivitamins, 137–38
Recommended Daily Allowances, 137
supplements, uses of, 135–37
water-soluble vitamins, 136

W
warfarin, 54, *178–79*
water-soluble vitamins, *136*
"water pills." *See* diuretics
weight loss, medications for *106–109*
    anorexiants, *107*
    bulk fillers, 107
    diuretics, 108
    HCG, 109
    thyroid hormone, 108–109
Wigraine (combination), 129

X
Xylocaine (lidocaine), 54, 68, 127

Z
Zarontin (ethosuximide), 130
Zaroxolyn (metolazone), 64
Zyloprim (allopurinol), 133, *326–27*